PRIMARY CARE
of the Functionally Disabled
Assessment and Management

Additional Contributors

Michael E. Msall, M.D.
Assistant Professor
Pediatrics, Genetics, and Rehabilitation
State University of New York at Buffalo
Robert Warner Center and Children's Hospital of Buffalo
Chapter 7

Richard A. Carleton, M.D.
Physician-in-Chief
Department of Medicine
Memorial Hospital of Rhode Island
Pawtucket, Rhode Island
and
Professor
Brown University Program in Medicine
Chapter 8

Ronald J. Kulich, Ph.D.
Director, Outpatient Pain Management Program
Lahey Clinic Medical Center
Burlington, Massachusetts
and
Daniel W. Bienkowski, M.D.
Clinical Assistant Professor
University Hospital
Boston, Massachusetts
and
Attending Physician
New England Memorial Hospital
Chapter 12

PRIMARY CARE
of the Functionally Disabled
Assessment and Management

Carl V. Granger, M.D.
Professor, Rehabilitation Medicine
School of Medicine
State University of New York at Buffalo
Head, Department of Rehabilitation Medicine
Buffalo General Hospital, Buffalo, New York

Gary B. Seltzer, Ph.D.
Associate Professor
Boston University
School of Social Work
Boston, Massachusetts

Carol Farb Fishbein, M.S.W.

Seven Contributors

J. B. LIPPINCOTT COMPANY   Philadelphia
London • New York • São Paulo • Mexico City • St. Louis • Sydney

Acquisitions Editor: Lisa Biello
Sponsoring Editor: Sanford J. Robinson
Production Editor: Carol A. Florence
Indexer: Catherine Battaglia
Art Director: Tracy Baldwin
Interior and Cover Designer: Katherine Nichols
Design Coordinator: Anne O'Donnell
Production Manager: Kathleen P. Dunn
Production Coordinator: Caren Erlichman
Compositor: Bi-Comp, Inc.
Printer/Binder: R. R. Donnelley & Sons Company

6 5 4 3 2 1

Library of Congress Cataloging-in-Publication Data

Granger, Carl V.
  Primary Care of the Functionally Disabled

  Includes bibliographies and index.
  1. Medical history taking. 2. Medical protocols.
3. Function tests (Medicine) I. Seltzer, Gary B.
II. Fishbein, Carol. III. Title. [DNLM: 1. Primary
Health Care—methods. W 84.6 G758p]
RC65.G73 1987   616   86-18512
ISBN 0-397-50673-2

The authors and publisher have exerted every effort to ensure
that drug selection and dosage set forth in this text are in
accord with current recommendations and practice at the time
of publication. However, in view of ongoing research,
changes in government regulations, and the constant flow of
information relating to drug therapy and drug reactions, the
reader is urged to check the package insert for each drug for
any change in indications and dosage and for added warnings
and precautions. This is particularly important when the
recommended agent is a new or infrequently employed drug.

Preface

The long-term limitations in functional performance that are associated with physical and mental impairments due to chronic illness are major health-care problems in the United States today. Medical advances not only have reduced mortality from infectious diseases and other acute illnesses, but have enabled persons with chronic, disabling conditions to live longer. Chronically ill persons with limitations in functional performance are restricted in ability to engage in activities expected of their age group and culture. Initially, these include vocational pursuits and traveling about the community. As the functional limitations become more severe, functionally limited persons experience difficulties with maintaining the household and even personal care. The performance of these basic activities and maintenance of usual roles are important to self-esteem. Restrictions in performance of these activities and a diminished life role can have deleterious effects on the impaired person's sense of dignity and life satisfaction. Physicians, therefore, need to evaluate not only the patient's medical condition and degree of stability, but also the degree to which the patient is able to maintain his customary living arrangements, physical activities, interpersonal relationships, and autonomy.

PRIMARY CARE OF THE FUNCTIONALLY DISABLED: ASSESSMENT AND MANAGEMENT is written from the point of view of disablement. *Disablement* is a term that incorporates the impairment of organ functioning, the consequential restriction of activities, and the associated reduction in fulfillment of expected and desired social roles. The interplay between organic impairments and deficits in functional performance is often complex and overlapping. Although practitioners routinely inquire about deficits related to functioning of any particular organ system, they are less likely to do the inverse—evaluate functional performance once organic pathology is known. Yet, functional levels vary even when their pathological bases do not. Therefore, it is important to monitor functional ability for its own sake when managing patients with chronic illness. This manual highlights such an approach.

Rehabilitation medicine, a medical discipline that specializes in the treatment of patients with long-term conditions, has adopted the functional approach to medical care. A new frontier in medical education, the functional approach complements traditional clinical indicators of well-being by measuring a patient's health status as determined by how well he functions. Functional status is assessed first by questioning the patient regarding the ease of performance of a number of physical, social, and vocationally related activities that are normally performed by people in good health. Body systems that may be involved in the reported functional difficulties are then evaluated during the physical examination. Functionally oriented case management, rather than focusing solely on the diagnostic and curative aspects of a disease process, an approach that encourages sporadic interventions during acute exacerbations and little continuity, requires continual appraisal of the chronically ill patient's medical and functional status. Treatment is aimed at alleviating new medical problems, increasing independence, and improving satisfaction and quality of life.

This manual is designed to introduce students and practitioners of ambulatory care medicine to the functional approach. Readers are expected to be physicians in the primary care specialities such as family medicine, general internal medicine, and pediatrics, or to be nurses and other health practitioners. The manual emphasizes the interplay between rehabilitation medicine and ambulatory primary care practice. As the incidence and prevalence of chronic illness continue to rise, the amount of attention that primary care physicians must give to the long-term rehabilitation of these patients will grow in a corresponding fashion. Although patients with chronic health impairment might benefit from the services of a rehabilitation specialist, it is usually the primary care physician who is the first to evaluate a patient's need for rehabilitation services, and in some instances the primary care physician may be the *only* medical practitioner available to identify and manage the patient's chronic condition. Although primary care physicians provide outpatient services mainly, their rehabilitation training, if at all, is likely to have occurred in the inpatient setting. As a result, many primary care physicians may not perceive somewhat mild disabilities that might be improved or eliminated by early intervention and the use of adaptive or corrective aids.

The authors of this manual believe that physicians with a functional approach are likely to provide systematic and comprehensive care and to address the functional consequences of long-term illness frequently overlooked by an organ-focused, traditional approach. Specifically, primary care physicians practicing from a functional and rehabilitation perspective will be able to (1) prevent disability through early identification of functional loss, (2) develop a problem list on the patient that includes limitations in functional performance, (3) develop treatment plans that address organic and behavioral problems and enhance functional performance, (4) assure that the program of care addresses issues that are most likely to maximize the quality of life for the patient, (5) improve patient compliance by focusing on problems the patient feels are most limiting, (6) determine the effectiveness of treatment modes by measuring changes in functional performance over time, and (7) establish a standardized data base for use in research and treatment evaluations, and for improving communication with other health-care providers.

Chapters 1 and 2 introduce the primary care practitioner to the principles and methods of functional assessment. The second chapter presents the functional assessment screening questionnaire (FASQ), which can be used during a normal office visit to assess those tasks and body systems most frequently associated with early functional limitations. Chapter 3 provides the foundations for the functionally oriented physical examination. An abbreviated neuromuscular screening examination is presented, and the common pitfalls in muscle strength testing are discussed. Examples of neuromusculoskeletal disorders commonly seen in the outpatient setting are presented. Chapter 4 describes documenting functional assessment in the medical record by means of the SOAP note, an acronym for subjective data, objective data, analysis, and plan. Through presentation of case histories and a functional staging system, this chapter provides evidence of the applicability of the functional approach to comprehensive medical care. Chapter 5 provides an overview of physical interventions commonly used to treat neuromusculoskeletal problems. Therapeutic heat, cold, hydrotherapy, ultraviolet therapy, traction, therapeutic electric stimulation, exercise, massage, and biofeedback are described. Knowledge about these modalities should enable the primary care practitioner to make more appropriate and timely referrals to rehabilitation clinicians. Chapter 6 highlights the roles of the clinical treatment team members to whom the primary care physician may look for advice and assistance when managing the patient with long-term problems.

Chapters 7, 9, 10, and 11 present examples of severely disabling conditions that require long-term management by primary care physicians. Included are descriptions of developmental disabilities, Parkinson's disease, and multiple sclerosis. These conditions represent disorders affecting all age groups and continuing for long periods of time. They are characterized by varying types of onset and courses of illness. Chapter 8 presents considerations in the management of the patient with chronic cardiac or pulmonary problems. The METs system, which relates functional activity to specific levels of energy requirement, is discussed as a useful guideline for cardiac rehabilitation patients. Chapter 12 focuses on back pain, while Chapters 13 and 14 discuss management of the patient with sensory impairments. Since most physicians-in-training have little opportunity to interact with blind or deaf patients in the outpatient setting, these chapters are included to acquaint physicians with the many community resources and aids that are available to increase functional performance substantially.

Chapter 15 explores the problems of organic mental disorders and dementia, and Chapter 16 presents mental retardation. These chapters provide insights into the psychosocial adaptions to chronic illness and emphasize the fact that functional performance can be compromised not only by physical impairments, but by mental and psychological disturbances as well.

Perhaps this book's most important message with respect to the provision of primary care is that there are numerous benefits to be derived by employing a functional approach to the care of the patient with disabilities. These benefits are realized by providing comprehensive care more efficiently in order to enhance satisfaction and quality of life for the patient and the family.

Carl V. Granger, M.D.
Gary B. Seltzer, Ph.D.
Carol Farb Fishbein, M.S.W

Acknowledgments

This book grew out of work on an RSA Innovative and Experimental grant awarded to Memorial Hospital of Rhode Island, which is affiliated with Brown University. We wish to thank our project officers, Toby Holland and Betsy Bush. Their support, guidance, and facilitation within the Department of Education enabled us to complete our project goals and to write this book.

There were many other people at Memorial Hospital who were instrumental in the completion of this work. In particular, we want to thank Elaine Rasmussen and Lorraine Laramee for their administrative support. A special thanks is extended to Virginia Turcotte who typed and retyped the manuscript and to Maureen MacNamara whose keen organizational and personal skills kept our projects going and our spirits elevated. Also, we thank Don Wineberg and Cary LaCheen, both of whom did the early research and drafting of material for this book.

In addition, we extend our appreciation to Dr. John Whyte for his critique of the chapter on Organic Mental Disorders: Dementia, to Dr. Mary Howell for her comments on the chapter on Mental Retardation, and to Dr. George C. Branche for his review of the chapter on Cardiopulmonary Rehabilitation.

We wish to express our appreciation to members of our families for their support throughout this lengthy process.

Finally, we are indebted to Frances S. Sherwin for her help in organizing and editing the manuscript and Rosemary Meinzer for additional typing, which helped move this work to fruition.

Contents

CHAPTER 1
Introducing a Functional Approach to Primary Care

As the proportion of elderly people in the population continues to rise, medical attention will focus increasingly on individuals who survive with persisting, chronic illnesses. As Lehmann[5] states:

> Whereas previously acute and contagious disease prevailed, at the present time chronic illness . . . is dominant. Whereas previously the patient, in the majority of cases, either died or recovered fully, now a large number of patients have to adapt to a life with a chronic disease and often have to adjust to long term functional loss.

More than 10% of the total noninstitutionalized civilian population of the United States have functional limitations that interfere with their ability to perform a major activity, such as maintaining a job, doing housework, or attending school.[13] In the United States, 85% of those over 65 years of age are reported to have at least one chronic condition,[14] and nearly 50% of those 85 years old or older report some activity limitation due to chronic disease.[13]

A few leaders in the fields of medical education and gerontology have examined the impact of functional limitations on the quality of life of persons with chronic illnesses. However, traditionally, medical education has focused on the curative aspects of the disease process—the diagnosis and treatment of an organic impairment. Although such an approach may be satisfactory for treating patients with acute conditions, it is inadequate when caring for patients with chronic ones. Patients with chronic conditions are frequently burdened with persisting medical problems and accompanying physical and functional limitations. Chronic impairments may interfere with the ability to perform many normal activities of daily living, including personal care, household tasks, childrearing, and vocational tasks. Medical care of the chronically ill patient,

1

therefore, must be based on long-term management. Attention must focus not only on the acute, episodic medical problems, but on the functional consequences of the disease as well.

Physical medicine and rehabilitation is the medical discipline that specializes in treatment of the patient with long-term illness. The specialist in this field is known as a *physiatrist*. For the most part, the physiatrist treats patients who have dysfunctions due to disorders of kinesis—disorders of movement and mobility typically associated with muscle weakness or paralysis, restriction of freedom of movement, instability of movement, pain that interferes with physical functioning, or absence of a part of a limb. Although the physiatrist directs attention primarily to diagnosis, evaluation, and therapy of pathological conditions of the neuromusculoskeletal system, he also tries to alleviate the effects that the specific impairment may be having on the whole person. Therefore, a significant portion of the physiatrist's attention is directed toward restoring and maintaining the optimum functioning of the individual with disabilities.

The physiatrist specializes in rehabilitation and long-term care of persons whose functional performance is limited. However, since persons who need rehabilitation often are seen by other than physiatrists and in general hospitals, at least initially, and since the number of physicians in the United States who are certified in physical medicine and rehabilitation is limited,[8] it is important to train other groups of physicians to manage patients with these needs. Further, because the basic concepts and techniques of rehabilitation medicine can be applied to other health fields, they should become an essential part of the armamentarium of all physicians, especially those providing ambulatory health care.

There are many comprehensive texts on primary care and rehabilitative care in outpatient settings written from different perspectives from this one. The intent of this book is to provide a bridge between the two fields of practice governed by principles of care advocated by both. It is designed specifically to broaden the perspective and skills of physicians in areas traditionally overlooked in the medical school curriculum.

Physical Medicine and Rehabilitation: An Overview

Rehabilitation involves the restoration and maintenance of a patient's physical, psychological, social, emotional, and vocational abilities. Medical rehabilitative interventions are usually directed toward the consequences of disease and injury. Rehabilitation focuses on re-educating the patient who is experiencing chronic health problems, such as stroke, spinal cord injury, cardiopulmonary impairments, or multiple sclerosis and on helping the patient to adapt to a lifestyle that is realistic, given the patient's residual functional capabilities. Rehabilitation medicine also encompasses the consequences of abnormal development—either congenital or occurring early in life—that is, in the process of "habilitation." Examples of disease processes requiring habilitative techniques include cerebral palsy, spina bifida, sensory deficits, and congenital absence of one or more limbs. In cases such as these, rehabilitation efforts focus on new learning processes as well as restoration.

> Most habilitation clients have never lived independent lives. They need to be educated in basic vocational adjustment and to develop fundamental capabilities, knowledge, experiences and attitudes.[1]

Intensive inpatient medical rehabilitation, after transfer from an acute hospital service, offers the severely disabled patient an alternative to placement in a nursing home or long-term care facility. The aim is to maximize independence, usually within a period of several weeks of goal-oriented, individualized treatment. The patient with an impairment is helped to perform the necessary activities of daily living, and his ability to communicate and interact with the environment is maximized. A variety of professionals work as a team in order to address the patient's total range of needs. Because it is essential that the patient be an active participant in the therapeutic process, the traditional passive patient–physician role is shunned.

The Overlap of Rehabilitation and Primary Care

Care that is comprehensive, coordinated, and continuous is characteristic not only of primary care but of rehabilitation medicine as well. An examination of the components of primary care will illustrate the overlap between the two disciplines.

Comprehensive Care

Comprehensive care has been defined by Haggerty to include:[3]

> . . . family orientation, combined preventive and curative care; and concern for the psychological, social, educational, recreational and economic factors, delivered by personnel, often in team fashion, with responsibility for the whole area of the health of an individual or family. . . .

Comprehensiveness with respect to rehabilitation medicine involves the length and breadth of care and a teamwork approach. It requires that attention be paid to more than the restoration of function and work capacity in a disabled person, but to interpersonal and family competence as well.[6,15] Prevention, which is also essential to comprehensive care, entails limiting the secondary complications that can develop as a consequence of chronic health impairments. Figure 1-1 illustrates an example of a secondary complication that is the result of inactivity due to bedrest. Secondary complications involve all body systems, including musculoskeletal, cardiopulmonary, gastrointestinal, renal, urinary tract, and neurosensory systems. Comprehensive care of a bedridden patient requires attention not only to the condition necessitating inactivity, but also to the potential side-effects of inactivity.

- Psychosomatic Disturbances
- Change in Sleep Patterns
- Learned Helplessness
- Changes in Self Image

↓Cough Reflex
↓Mucous Collection
Recumbent Position   ↑Work of
↓Bronchiolar Diameter   Breathing

Obstruction of
Air Passage

Atelectasis

Pneumonia,
Bronchitis

Disease Atrophy ➤↓Strength
and Size of Muscle

↓BP ➤ Dizziness
Weakness ➤ ↓Ability to do ADL

Heart Atrophy ➤↓CO ➤SOB,
Palpitations,
Fatigue

↓Appetite
Difficulty Swallowing ➤ Malnutrition

Vitamin/Nutrient
Deficiency ➤ Skin Problems

Constipation

Fecal Impaction

↑Calcium Load
Recumbent Position   Urinary/
Stagnant Urine   Kidney
↓Bladder Emptying   Stones

Indwelling
Catheterization ➤Infection

Kidney Damage/Failure

Wrinkled Sheets
Incontinence ➤ Bed Sores
Pressure

Chronic Sepsis

- Wound Healing
- Infection   Contractures
- Edema   of Joints/Ligaments
- Changes in Collagen
                     ↓Mobility

↓Bone Calcium ➤Osteoporosis ➤ ↑Fractures
↓Mobility

Soft Tissue Deposits ➤ ↓Muscle
Function

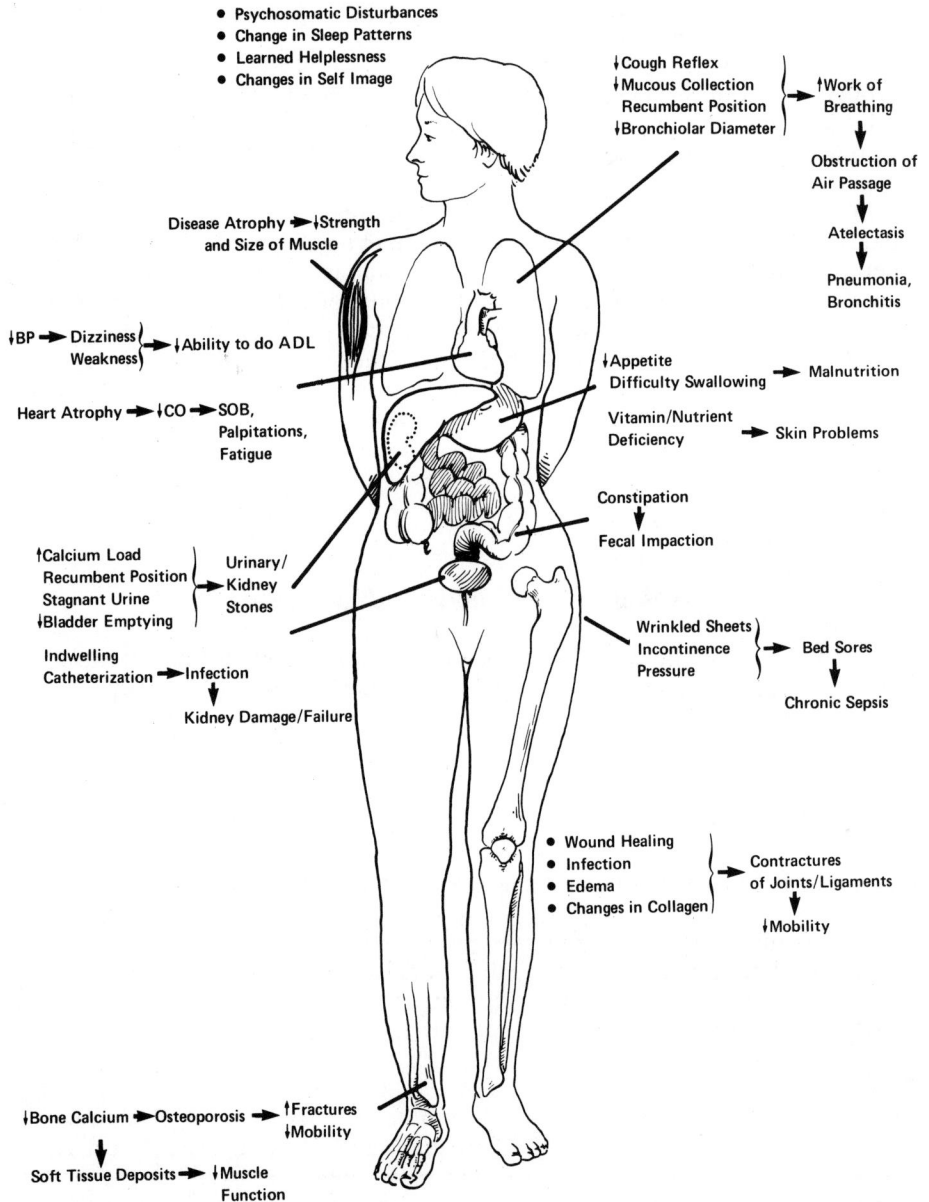

Figure 1-1. Secondary complications due to inactivity and bedrest.[2] (Adapted from Corcoran P: Disability consequences of bed rest. In Stolov W, Clowers M (eds): Handbook of Severe Disability. US Department of Education, Rehabilitation Services Administration, Washington, 1981)

Coordinated Care

Coordinated care is the integration of the various professional services provided through all phases of the patient's treatment plan. Coordination of care is especially important in the practice of rehabilitation, because an interdisciplinary approach is crucial in reducing problems of fragmentation in patient care and assuring a well-balanced assessment of the "total patient." A rehabilitation team includes various kinds of health care personnel including, typically, a physiatrist, a rehabilitation nurse, a clinical psychologist, a social worker, a physical therapist, an occupational therapist, and a speech pathologist. Whenever possible, the patient and significant family members are encouraged to participate in the treatment plan.

Continuous Care

Continuous care involves monitoring a patient's ongoing problems and reviewing and modifying treatment strategies to ensure effective case management. Because rehabilitation addresses problems that require long-term supervision and possible intermittent care rather than short-term, cure-oriented treatment, prevention, patient education, and family education are its hallmarks.

The overlap in practice between rehabilitation medicine and primary care traditionally has been limited to followup care after release from tertiary care institutions. The interplay between these two medical fields also can occur through the identification and management of patients with chronic conditions in *outpatient* primary care settings. For example, rheumatologists treat only 10% of patients with rheumatic disease. The remaining patients who receive care for this condition are treated by primary care physicians.[11] Seltzer and colleagues[10] reported that 20% of the patients seen in a primary care practice had chronic, disabling problems and might have benefited from rehabilitation services. The most common types of problems found in this study were:

1. Neurologic and neurosensory disorders (*i.e.,* paresis, deafness, visual loss)
2. Musculoskeletal disorders (*i.e.,* arthritis, low-back pain)
3. Cardiopulmonary disorders (arteriosclerotic heart disease [ASHD], chronic obstructive pulmonary disease [COPD])
4. Miscellaneous disorders (*i.e.,* macrocytic anemia, hiatus hernia)

As the number of people requiring rehabilitation services continues to rise, there will be a concomitant rise in the major role that primary care physicians play in the long-term care and followup of patients with chronic diseases and associated functional loss. This trend has important implications. First, primary care practitioners will need to be able to assess the severity of disabling conditions and either refer the patient to a rehabilitation specialist, such as a physiatrist, or handle the more limited rehabilitation cases in their primary care settings. The primary care provider will need to be aware of the necessity for providing rehabilitative services to the patient as early as possible in order to minimize or eliminate the potentially devastating physical, emotional, social, and vocational problems that may occur as a result of delay. Also, if the primary care physician has been able to establish trust and rapport, he or she may have an advantage in effecting patients' compliance with therapy regimens. Similarly, the primary care physician's familiarity with other family members may prove advantageous in helping to ease the adaptation process.

Impairment, Disability, Handicap: A Conceptual Framework

It is impossible to approach care of the elderly or chronically ill or injured patient without a knowledge of some basic terminology. In its study of morbidity and mortality, the World Health Organization has been using a numerical system, the International Classification of Disease, to code and classify acute health problems. Only recently, in response to its recognition of the growing importance of chronic health problems in modern medicine, has it developed a set of definitions and classification codes pertinent to chronic illness as well as acute disease. The following descriptive terms, adapted from definitions by the World Health Organization's Classification System on Impairments, Disabilities, and Handicaps,[4] should be part of the working terminology of all physicians.

Impairment

An impairment is any loss or abnormality of psychological, physiological, or anatomical structure or function. There are two points to keep in mind when considering an impairment:

1. An impairment is independent of its etiology; it is not contingent upon whether it is due to a genetic abnormality, a disease process, or an accident.
2. Although a pathology was involved originally, an impairment does not necessarily indicate that a disease is still present.[4] For example, an amputation represents a situation in which the impairment remains although the original disease process may no longer be present.

Disability

A disability is any restriction or lack of ability (resulting from an impairment) to perform an activity in the manner or within the range considered normal for a person of the same age, culture, and education. It is important to note that:

1. A disability may be temporary or permanent; however, although a sickness may be described as a disability of short duration, disability is usually applied to activity restrictions of long or continued duration.
2. The limitation or inability to perform activities expected of the person is usually in the areas of self-care and mobility, recreational, vocational, and economic activities, or interpersonal communication and fulfillment of social roles.

3. Similar patterns of disability may result from different types of impairments and limitations in function. As an example, the inability to do bimanual labor may result from an upper limb amputation or severe rheumatoid arthritis.
4. Not every impairment results in a disability.[16] For example, paralysis of the lower limbs obviously would present a vocational disability for a dancer, but not necessarily for an identically impaired bookkeeper.

Handicap

A handicap is a disadvantage for a given individual, resulting from an impairment or a disability, that limits or prevents the fulfillment of a role that is normal (depending on age, sex, and social or cultural factors) for that individual.

Understanding the term *handicap* involves the following considerations:

1. A handicap is characterized by a difference between what an individual appears able to do and the expectations of the particular group of which he is a member. Various factors may perpetuate and reinforce societal expectations that excuse or prohibit the disabled person from performing activities of which he is capable. Those that excuse the person from functioning in appropriate social roles include misconceptions (especially underestimations) about abilities, refusal to accommodate to an impaired skill level, and unwillingness to allow the person to continue to do those tasks of which he still is capable. Factors that prohibit the person with disabilities from functioning in appropriate social roles include lack of job opportunities and unavailable social support systems.
2. The state of being handicapped is strongly influenced by existing societal values and institutional arrangements.[4] Inaccessible public buildings, lack of wide door bathrooms, lack of accessible public transportation, and negative public attitudes toward those with noticeable impairments are examples of environments that handicap a person. They represent the further difficulties that society imposes on an individual with disabilities through its architecture, its communication levels, and its attitudes.[12] Yearwood[18] cites an observation of the National Center for Health Statistics that at least 67,900 Americans who suffer from limiting conditions would benefit from a more accessible environment.

Disability Models

The disability models of Nagi[7] and Wood[17] provide the conceptual foundation for the functional approach used in rehabilitation medicine.

Nagi model

    Pathology⟶Impairment⟶Functional limitations⟶Disability

Wood model

    Disease or disorder⟶Impairment⟶Disability⟶Handicap
    (Intrinsic)⟶(Exteriorized)⟶(Objectified)⟶(Socialized)

The models developed by the two authors differ in several respects, but they share a number of important features. In their use of the terms *impairment, functional limitation, disability,* and *handicap,* both models attempt to demonstrate the influences of personal, environmental, and social factors on limitations in task and role performance. Implicit in both models is the value of functional assessment, in addition to diagnosis, in order to understand fully the consequences of the illness on the patient's daily life. It should be noted, however, that the concepts of impairment, functional limitation, disability, and handicap are not necessarily linear or mutually exclusive, but rather are overlapping. The case of a cashier whose face was badly burned in a fire illustrates the interrelationships. The disfigured face did not in any way affect this person's ability to perform her job; however, society's negative reaction toward obvious physical disfigurement prevented her from being hired in any job involving public contact. In this instance, an impairment (burned face) produced a handicap (negative social attitudes preventing employment), which in turn produced a disability (inability to perform as a cashier).

The Functional Approach

Pathology and *impairment* typically are defined by laboratory tests or clinical examinations and observations and are treated with pharmacologic, surgical, nutritional, or other medical therapeutics. On the other hand, *disability* and *handicap* require assessments of the personal and social consequences of the pathological condition(s), which are not routinely addressed by traditional clinical medicine. In carrying out treatment strategies, traditional clinical medicine frequently fails to recognize that persons limited functionally by chronic illness or injury, who can no longer perform tasks and fulfill social roles (important sources of self-esteem), often deteriorate. The *functional approach* to chronic illness focuses on the patient's ability to perform and to fulfill appropriate social roles. Functional loss or a reduction in the fulfillment of social roles is determined in patient and family interviews or by observing the patient during activity. Treatment plans then focus not only on resolving medical problems, but on social, psychological, and environmental problems as well. By addressing the patient's disabilities and handicaps, the care provider hopes to enhance the patient's ability to function more independently and thereby to achieve a better quality of life.

Table 1-1 presents a model for systematically evaluating a handicapping condition or disease. The model provides the basis for defining the various levels of disablement—including relevant types of examination and associated data assessments—as well as strategies for treatment. Although not inclusive, this table helps to delineate differences between traditional pathology-oriented methods and functional performance-based methods. Table 1-2 shows a functional approach to evaluation and illustrates the relationships between the concepts, clinical manifestations, and treatment responses for a common chronic illness. Rheumatoid arthritis is used as the example.

The functional approach model for rehabilitation medicine provides a strategy for addressing many of the chronic health problems seen in outpatient care. High-quality patient care should include:

1. Promotion of health and prevention of disease and injuries
2. Diagnosis and treatment of specific disorders
3. Assessment of the consequences of disease or injury, including determination of chronic impairment, disability, or handicap
4. Alleviation of the long-term disadvantage imposed by disease or injury by restoring and maintaining function at an optimal level, thereby enhancing quality of life

Although typical history-taking techniques and laboratory tests may permit physicians to achieve the first two items included as part of high-quality patient care, they do not permit them to achieve the third and fourth. For example, accurate assessment of the range of motion and muscle control of an arthritic patient will not reveal that patient's actual performance of daily activities. The patient's willingness to perform functional tasks in spite of the pain is as important as the ability to move in ways requested during a clinical examination.[9]

The functional approach focuses not only on the disease, but also on the disease consequences, by examining the patient's ability to perform and the ease with which he performs a number of activities of daily living that are expected of

TABLE 1-1   Means to Define, Assess, and Treat Pathology, Impairment, Disability, and Handicap, Using the Handicapping Condition/Chronic Disease Model

	Defined by	Database Assessment & Documentation	Treatment
Pathology	Histopathology Biochemical abnormality	Laboratory procedure	Drugs Surgery Nutrition (protein, vitamins, minerals)
Impairment/ Functional Limitations	Symptoms and signs of somatic, mental, or emotional deficit	Static observations Clinical exams and dynamic tests	Restorative therapies Orthotics Prosthetics
Disability	Performance or behavioral losses	Dynamic observations Interviews (distinguish capacity versus actual)	Counseling Environmental adjustments
Handicap	Reduction in expected social role performance, such as work or independent living Limitation of recreational and leisure time activities	Administrative and case management	Balance personal, social, and environmental interactions Team orientation

TABLE 1-2   Means to Define, Assess, and Treat Pathology, Impairment, Disability, and Handicap of Rheumatoid Arthritis, Using the Handicapping Condition/Chronic Disease Model

	Defined by	Clinical Manifestation	Treatment
Pathology	Histopathology Biochemical abnormality Physical abnormality	Synovitis Vasculitis	Anti-inflammatory drugs Surgery: synovectomy; joint replacement
Impairment/ Functional Limitations	Signs Symptoms	Joint swelling, pain, instability Muscle weakness General fatigue Limited motion Deformity	As above, plus: Physical therapy Occupational therapy Braces/splints
Disability	Inability to perform tasks	Reduced walking Decreased ability to elevate body Decreased ability in self-care	As above, plus: Counseling Environmental adjustments
Handicap	Reduction in expected social role performances	Job loss Changes in sexual attitude/function Change in role as wife/husband	As above, plus: Social service Community resources

an able-bodied person. The functional approach identifies the patient's deficits as well as his or her remaining capabilities and assets. Factors contributing to the functional limitations in task performance, which have been identified, include the relevant diagnoses; anatomical, physiological, psychological, and mental deficits; capability to perform social roles; family and social support systems; and environment. The influences of these various components are analyzed and treatment intervention is planned with the goal of restoring functioning and independence as much as possible. If the functional limitation cannot be changed, intervention focuses on alternative means of meeting daily needs, such as devising another method of performing the task or arranging for a family member or outside agency to perform the task. Finally, prescriptive services such as pharmacologic agents, restorative therapies, appliances and devices, housing or environmental modifications, and community-based services, are considered. The criteria for employing prescriptive services are whether they are appropriate to the enhancement of health, psychosocial status, and vocational functional status.

The functional approach we are advocating in this book should not be considered the province of rehabilitation medicine physicians only, but should underlie the practice of most physicians. It is especially appropriate to integrate the functional perspective of rehabilitation into primary care, because it can help physicians to identify patients easily who are in need of rehabilitative services. After screening and assessing the patient, followed by planning and carrying out treatment, repeated assessments of functional status over time can serve to enhance the effectiveness and efficiency of treatment. The functional approach also can help primary care physicians prevent functional limitations through early identification of impairments likely to reduce functional capacity. By developing treatment plans which address problems that the patient views as most limiting the primary care physician can improve compliance and thereby enhance the patient's quality of life.

TABLE 1-3.   The Functional Approach to Medical Care and the Disablement Model

Organ Level	Person Level	Societal Level
Pathology	*Behavioral*	*Role Assignment*
Conditions		
Anatomical, physio-logical, mental, and psychological defi-cits	Performance deficits within the physical and social environ-ments	Environmental defi-cits influenced by social norms and social policy
Determine	Contribute to	Create
Key Terms		
Impairment ⟷ (Organic dysfunction)	Disability ⟷ (Difficulty with tasks)	Handicap (Social disadvantage)
Limitations		
Demonstrating skills	Performing tasks	Fulfilling social roles
Analysis		
Selected diagnostic descriptors	Selected performance (behavioral) de-scriptors	Selected role de-scriptors

Functional Assessment of Abilities and Activities

Interventions		
Medical and restor-ative therapy	Adaptive equipment and reduction of physical and attitu-dinal barriers	Supportive services and social policy changes

All needing long-range coordination to improve and maintain functioning

(Granger CV, Gresham GE (eds): Functional Assessment in Rehabilitation Medicine. Baltimore, Williams & Wilkins, 1984)

Relationship of the Functional Approach to the Disablement Model:

A schematic representation of the functional approach and its relationship to the disability models previously described is presented in Table 1-3. The upper half of the table (Conditions and Key Terms) illustrates the three levels of concern—the organ level, the person level, and the societal level. The organ level of the disability model is defined by *impairments*—physical and mental deficits. For many people an impairment causes an inability or difficulty in performing daily living activities and thus leads to *disability*. Disability occurs at the person level and represents performance deficits. *Handicapping* conditions are at the societal level. These are imposed upon the individual by society and prevent the individual from fulfilling social roles.

The lower half of the table (Analysis and Interventions) depicts the functional assessment approach to disablement levels. The focus of functional assessment is performance. Three descriptors are used to account for deficiencies in performance: diagnostic (due to an impairment), behavioral (due to disability consequences), and role (due to difficulties in fulfilling social roles).

A functional assessment (discussed in Chap. 2) provides a systematic inventory of the activities the individual is capable of or has difficulty performing. Analysis may reveal reversible disability and indications for restorative therapy or disability that cannot be accounted for by impairment alone. If the impairment does not account entirely for the disability, it is necessary to identify other intervening factors. The ultimate goal of a functional analysis of task performance is to identify unmet medical, psychosocial, and environmental needs and to intervene appropriately to achieve optimal function and enjoyment of life.

Summary

Greater longevity and decreased mortality from disease have increased the number of people with chronic illnesses and problems amenable to rehabilitation interventions. Since these problems may be present in any type of practice, it is the premise of this book that most physicians, but especially those involved in primary care, should be exposed to the techniques and concepts of rehabilitation medicine.

In this chapter we have presented the holistic approach of rehabilitation medicine to long-term patient care. We have explored the characteristics rehabilitation medicine has in common with primary care medicine, namely, comprehensiveness of care, coordination of care, and continuity of care. We have defined the terms *impairment, disability, handicap,* and *functional approach,* and we have provided a diagrammatic representation relating functional assessment to the disablement model. Physicians who are aware of these concepts and make a conscious and consistent effort to apply them may improve the quality of life for their patients.

In the following chapters, we consider the role of the interdisciplinary team in medicine, methods of neuromusculoskeletal, sensory, and affective examinations, as well as the treatment and management of common, chronic illnesses and impairments due to injury. In Chapter 2, we discuss the tool of the functional medical approach—the functional assessment.

References

1. Bitter J: Introduction to Rehabilitation, p 3. St Louis, CV Mosby, 1979
2. Corcoran P: Disability consequences of bed rest. In Stolov W, Clowers M (eds): Handbook of Severe Disability. Washington, US Department of Education, Rehabilitation Services Administration, 1981
3. Haggerty R: Does comprehensive care make a difference? Introduction: Historical perspectives, Am J Dis Child 122:467–468, 1971
4. International Classification of Impairments, Disabilities and Handicaps. Geneva, Switzerland, World Health Organization, 1980
5. Lehmann J: Patient care needs as a basis for development of objectives of physical medicine and rehabilitation medicine teaching in undergraduate medical schools. J Chronic Dis 21:3, 1968
6. Lindenberg R: Work with families in rehabilitation. Rehab Counsel Bull, p 67, Sept 1977
7. Nagi S: Disability Concepts and Prevalence. Presented at the First Mary Switzer Memorial Seminar, Cleveland, OH, May 1975
8. Roeback G, Randolph L, Mead G, Pasko T: Physician characteristics and distribution in the United States. Chicago, AMA, 1984
9. Rusk H: Rehabilitation Medicine. St Louis, CV Mosby, 1977
10. Seltzer G, Granger C, Wineberg D: Functional assessment: Bridge between family and rehabilitation medicine within ambulatory practice. Arch Phys Med Rehabil 63:453–457, 1982
11. Seltzer M, Sherwood, C: Family Practice and Rehabilitation: A Review of the Literature. Manuscript RSA Grant No. 44–p–81442/1, Brown University and Pawtucket Memorial Hospital, 1980
12. Wilke H: The Caring Congregation. Quarterly Periodical of The Hearing Community 2(3), 1981
13. US Dept. of Health, Education and Welfare. Washington, US National Health Survey Current Estimate, Series 10 #139, p 24, 1978
14. US Dept. of Health, Education and Welfare: As cited in LaRose A, Bank L, Jarvik G, Herland MJ: Health in old age: How physicians' ratings and self-ratings compare. Gerontology 34(5):687, 1979
15. Versluus H: Physical rehabilitation and family dynamics. Rehabil Lit 41(34):58, 1980
16. Whitten E (ed): Pathology, Impairment, Functional Limitation and Disability: Implications for Practice, Research, Program and Policy Development and Service Delivery. Report of the First Mary E. Switzer Memorial Seminar, Cleveland, Ohio, May 1975. National Rehabilitation Association, 1980
17. Wood P: Classification of impairments and handicaps. Geneva, World Health Organization, 1975
18. Yearwood A: Being disabled doesn't mean being handicapped, Am J Nurs 80(2):299, 1980

Additional Readings

1. Branch LG, Katz S, Kniepmann K, Papsidero JA: A prospective study of functional status among community elders. Am J Public Health 74:266–268, 1984
2. Fagan T, Wallace A: Who are the handicapped? Personnel and Guidance J 58(4):215, 1979

3. Katz S, Branch LG, Branson MH, Papsidero JA, Beck JC, Greer DS: Active life expectancy. N Engl J Med 309:1218–1224, 1983
4. Licht S (ed): Rehabilitation and Medicine. Baltimore, Elizabeth Licht, Waverly Press, 1968
5. Mackey F: Rehabilitation goes beyond diagnosis and cure. Hospitals, 54:32, October 16, 1980
6. Materson R: Physical medicine and rehabilitation for the medical practitioner. In Practice of Medicine, Chapter 20. Hagerstown, Harper & Row, 1978
7. Sherwood S, Greer DS, Morris JN, Mor V: An Alternative to Institutionalization: The Highland Heights Experiment. Cambridge, MA, Ballinger, 1981
8. Stolov W, Clowers, M (eds): Handbook of Severe Disability. US Dept. of Education Rehabilitation Services Administration, 1981
9. Wood P, Badley E: People With Disabilities—Toward Acquiring Information Which Reflects More Sensitively Their Problems and Needs. New York, World Rehabilitation Fund, 1980
10. Yates G: Rehabilitation and the general practitioner. J Roy Coll Gen Pract 17:292, 1969

CHAPTER 2

The Functional Assessment

Incorporation of Analysis of Functional Limitations into the Routine History Interview and Physical Examination

As a stethoscope is the primary instrument for a cardiologist, a functional assessment is a necessary tool for rehabilitation specialists and other physicians using the functional approach to medical care. A significant proportion of patients seen in primary care settings have health problems that limit functional performance, but outpatients do not routinely receive functional evaluations. We suggest that every primary care physician ask each patient with a chronic health condition a basic set of functional screening questions covering his self-perceived general health status, as well as an assessment of the degree of difficulty he experiences in the performance of representative personal care, household, vocational, transportation, and leisure-time activities.

A functional assessment determines as accurately as possible how a patient with a chronic health condition functions in everyday life, that is, his ability to perform the tasks of daily living and to fulfill the social roles expected of a physically and emotionally healthy person of the same age and culture. The emphasis on social roles and tasks performed is extremely important. Researchers recently have reported that personal attitudes, social status, and participation in social activities are as important to a person's perception of his health as the medical and physiological factors physicians typically consider in a health evaluation.[2]

The chronically ill patient's impairments may improve, stabilize, or continue to progress toward an even greater degree of disability. It is important, therefore, for the physician to monitor these patients periodically to identify potentially disabling factors. It is necessary to understand the consequences of the disease and its treatment on the patient's social well-being and not merely to treat the organ impairment only. In other words, one can not presume to know just how the social performance of an individual has been affected by knowing only the organ impairment. Six key social roles have been identified by the World Health Organization as indicative of the patient's actual state of well-being. These social roles are orientation, self-sufficiency, mobility, social integration, economic sufficiency, and occupation. Persons with similar organ impairments have widely divergent social role profiles. Only by determining what tasks and activities a person performs can we translate from impairment to fulfillment or lack of fulfillment of expected social roles.

The functional medical examination provides a means to analyze the consequences of organ system impairment on the natural skills that a person employs to perform the tasks of daily living. Functional limitation is a term used to describe a decrement or loss of a natural skill that is a consequence of disease, injury, or birth defect affecting a body part. The functional examination permits us to intervene appropriately to help the patient function as optimally as possible and to perform his or her social roles.

By considering diagnostic and laboratory data in the context of the information obtained through a functional assessment, all of the patient's needs can be analyzed systematically with a view to achieving a fulfilling and satisfying life. Also residual deficiencies and remaining capabilities are identified, and treatment can be planned and carried out accordingly. This chapter presents a sample functional assessment screening form and discusses its rationale and application in the primary care setting.

The functional examination may indicate any of the following:

1. Further examination or diagnostic workup
2. Pharmacologic or nutritional treatment
3. Surgical correction
4. Restorative therapies
5. Prosthetic or orthotic fitting
6. Psychological or social adjustment
7. Patient and family education
8. Bioengineering and environmental adaptation

General Guidelines

A functional assessment instrument should permit an appraisal of the long-term chronically ill patient at periodic intervals. This will facilitate appropriate matching of services with needs, as those needs may change over time. An initial assessment can be used to determine a patient's baseline level of functioning. Repeated assessments at prescribed intervals can be used to compare and monitor a patient's progress during treatment.

Most functional assessments include indices of both personal care and role functioning. Some global characterizations such as personal attitudes, functional levels, living styles, work potential, and support systems of individuals needing long-term medical care are necessary. A functional assessment thus provides an overview of how functional limitations are incorporated into the life of the person who has them.

A sample functional assessment screening questionnaire (FASQ) is presented in Figure 2-1. It has intentionally been formulated to be both brief and direct, allowing it to be administered and analyzed quickly, within the confines of a usual medical appointment schedule.

The functional assessment screening questionnaire (FASQ) presented in this book is designed to be self-administered by the patient. The assessment form can be filled out while the patient is in the waiting room or examination room, with little guidance from auxiliary personnel. The literature is supportive of the reliability of self-administered questionnaires in health-care settings. The sample questions provided in Figure 2-1 can be presented as is or can be incorporated into a regular health history form, which might include information regarding the patient's demographic characteristics, financial coverage, pertinent medical history, and any other background material desired by the physician. The self-assessment method is efficient both for the patient and for the doctor, who then has an accessible pool of pertinent information to which he can refer during the examination. The self-administered form encourages the patient to pinpoint areas of greatest difficulty. Furthermore, patient participation in history taking encourages a more active role in the patient–physician relationship. Finally, although physical examinations normally evaluate what a patient is capable of doing, self-assessment questionnaires are particularly valuable in assessing what a patient actually does do outside the confines of the examination room.

Analysis of results from the FASQ allows the physician to interpret (1) the patient's relative state of well-being versus his social handicap by the number of tasks with which the patient is experiencing difficulty according to the categories of activity, (2) the patient's perception of his health in relation to the number of tasks with which he is experiencing difficulty, and (3) the functional limitations and skill deficits that are contributing to disability. The physician who knows the functional limitations can confirm by examination the relative degree of disability attributable to impairment. Then the physician assesses how much other causes, such as the environment, psychological factors, unrealistic expectations, or inappropriate social pressures or barriers, contribute to disability. Thus treatment can be directed toward those factors that are responsible for disability, and the effort can be focused on interventions most likely to produce the desired results of improving the patient's health, well-being, and social role performance.

Figure 2-2 shows the relationships between tasks on the FASQ and the World Health Organization social role expectations.

The guidelines that follow serve to explain to physicians and other health professionals the rationale for the questions asked on the FASQ and also may be used to provide additional explanation to patients on how to complete the form.

Functional Assessment Categories

The FASQ includes four questions about the patient's general state of health as he perceives it and fifteen specified tasks and activities during which the patient

Name:_____ Age:____ Number:_____ Date:_____

Please check the column (either excellent, good, average, poor, or very poor) which best describes your health state as described in questions 1 through 4.

	E X C E L L E N T	G O O D	A V E R A G E	P O O R	V E R Y P O O R
In comparison with others of your age, how well do you feel in terms of:					
1) Your general state of health?	5	4	3	2	1
2) Your ability to be active?	5	4	3	2	1
3) Your ability to do *needed* things?	5	4	3	2	1
4) Your ability to do *desired* things?	5	4	3	2	1

For each of the activities listed below, please check the column that best describes the degree of difficulty you have, if any, in trying to perform each one. As a guideline:

EASY: You have no difficulty performing the task.

SOME: You have some difficulty performing the task, but you can still manage it well enough

A LOT: You are still able to perform the task, but you do it with considerable difficulty

UNABLE: Although you attempt to perform the task, it is too difficult

NOT APPLICABLE: Someone else in the household does this task, or else it does not get done

Tasks and Activities	Degree of Difficulty				
	E A S Y	S O M E	A L O T	U N A B L E	N O T A P P
(P) Cut toenails	( )	( )	( )	( )	( )
Get up from a low seat	( )	( )	( )	( )	( )
Climb stairs	( )	( )	( )	( )	( )
(I) Wash windows and walls	( )	( )	( )	( )	( )
Shop for groceries	( )	( )	( )	( )	( )
Handle finances	( )	( )	( )	( )	( )
(L) Play sports	( )	( )	( )	( )	( )
Converse	( )	( )	( )	( )	( )
Be socially active	( )	( )	( )	( )	( )
(O) Concentrate	( )	( )	( )	( )	( )
Sit for long periods	( )	( )	( )	( )	( )
Stand for long periods	( )	( )	( )	( )	( )
Reach, grasp, pinch	( )	( )	( )	( )	( )
(T) Drive an automobile	( )	( )	( )	( )	( )
Ride a bus	( )	( )	( )	( )	( )

Comments: _____
_____

Figure 2-1. Functional Assessment Screening Questionnaire (FASQ).

FASQ Tasks	Key WHO Social Roles					
	Orient	Self-suff	Mobility	Soc Integ	Econ	Occup
Personal Care	X	X	X			
Cut toenails						
Up from low seat						
Climb stairs						
Instrumental (house)	X	X	X			
Wash windows/walls						
Shop						
Handle finances						
Leisure	X		X	X		
Play sports						
Converse						
Social activities						
Occupational	X		X		X	X
Concentrate						
Sit for long periods						
Stand for long periods						
Reach, grasp, pinch						
Transporation	X		X	X	X	X
Drive an automobile						
Ride a bus						

Figure 2-2.   Relationship between tasks on the FASQ and the WHO social role expectations.

may experience some degree of difficulty. The patient rates general health as either excellent (exce), good, average (aver), poor, or very poor (vpoo).

Self-Rating of Health and Functioning

The first four questions on the screening form elicit information about the patient's perception of his own general physical abilities compared to the abilities of others of the same age.[1] The answers to these questions may alert the physician to the need to probe further into specific task areas (detailed in the section that follows). These four questions can be helpful when inconsistencies between task performance and attitudinal responses emerge. Consistently favorable answers in the general health section, in combination with several severe functional limitations (as indicated by the physical examination findings and responses to the activities questions on the form), may reflect an optimistic outlook. An astute physician can capitalize on these positive attitudes when determining treatment strategies. On the other hand, a patient having few functional limitations, but reporting a negative subjective health assessment, should alert the physician to the possible presence of social and psychological problems or the need for a counseling referral.

Difficulty in Task Performance

The second section of the form is the activities assessment. On this section the patient is asked not only whether he is able to perform the function, but also how difficult it is to perform the task. The question is asked in this way in order to identify functional limitations as they develop and before they result in irrevocable limitations in task performance.

It has been determined empirically that patients in a primary care setting commonly report having difficulty performing the tasks in this sample FASQ.[4,5] These carefully selected items are helpful in identifying reduced functional capacity before it progresses to the stage of more severe disability. The information these items provide may be a clue that a particular organ system involved in the performance of activities necessary to daily living should be investigated. Measures of specific task ratings are generally more reliable than measures of broad and complex activities.[3] Although a broad array of specific items within a functional category may serve to increase accuracy of response, an assessment proposed for clinical use must be brief to be practical. A functional assessment form might include substantially more task questions than this one contains (*e.g.,* a patient's ability to cook, dress, do childcare, read a book, listen to music, and so on), but our research has shown that an increase in the number of questions is unlikely to provide additional useful information. For example, inquiring about difficulty in dressing might reveal problems in manual dexterity or upper limb and neck control; these same systems, however, are already assessed in tasks listed in the abbreviated functional assessment form presented. Thus the suggested FASQ task items represent a minimum number of life activities that provide a maximal return of information for physicians to use when assessing early functional loss. Individual physicians should feel free to supplement this FASQ with additional tasks or activities that would clarify a patient's functional status or be more appropriate to the particular clientele being served.

Task difficulty is rated by the patient as: EASY to perform, SOME difficulty experienced in performing the task, A LOT of difficulty experienced in performing the task, or UNABLE to perform the task. Sometimes patients do not perform a specific activity for reasons other than disability. For example, patients may not wash walls and windows because their spouses always do it. In this case, a reply of NOT APPLICABLE (NOT APP) should be selected. An answer of UNABLE should be registered only when the patient actually has enough difficulty to make it impossible to perform, not because he chooses not to perform it.

The letters in parentheses to the left of the items listed, which spell PILOT vertically, are a mnemonic representing five categories of activity—P for personal care activities, I for instrumental (household) living activities, L for leisure and social activities, O for occupational activities, and T for transportation activities.

Personal Care

The section on personal care measures the range of tasks a person performs in relation to his own body. As with questions in each of the other categories, the inquiries reveal whether the individual is able to perform specific tasks in order to handle customary social roles; indirectly they assess also the musculoskeletal, neurological, and sensory systems necessary for proper performance. For instance, getting up from a low seat requires low-back flexibility, whereas cutting toenails requires trunk control and manual dexterity. Difficulty with tasks in this section may indicate potential problems in fulfilling social roles that require mobility and physical independence.

Instrumental (Household) Activities

This section measures mobility around the house and assesses the patient's responses to the instrumental demands of living independently. Because the tasks in this section require both planning and physical movement, difficulties with them may indicate impaired functioning of either kind. Difficulty in the performance of tasks in this area may pinpoint problems in fulfilling social roles requiring mobility, adequate cognitive skills, and maintenance of one's personal care or household environment.

Leisure Activities

The section on leisure activities measures the ease with which the patient pursues activities that maximize the quality of life. Negative responses to these questions may indicate impaired cognitive or sensory functioning or psychological difficulties such as depression or anxiety. Difficulty performing leisure activities may reflect inability to fulfill social roles, that is, to participate in and maintain social relationships (social integration) or to receive and respond to environmental signals (orientation).

Occupational Activities

The purpose of the occupational tasks section is to ascertain the patient's ability to perform many of the sustained movements required on the job and to function for prolonged periods outside the home. Concentrating on a task, sitting, standing, and manual dexterity are basic skills required for most vocational pursuits. Difficulty in performing these activities signals the likelihood of problems in fulfilling economic roles.

Transportation Activities

Availability of transportation (and the ability to use it) is essential to the performance of tasks in many social situations. These abilities increase one's potential to interact with a wide circle of people, to travel to work, and to engage in leisure-time activities. Transportation problems may hamper the effective pursuit of social integration and economic self-sufficiency.

Scoring the Functional Assessment

The number of responses at each level of difficulty can be tallied to provide a quick overview of the patient's general functioning ability. A large number of responses checked in the EASY column indicates that the patient's impairments are not disabling and that the patient is able to function at a normal or near normal level. On the other hand, many UNABLE replies indicate severe functional limitations, which should cue the physician to investigate relevant physical, emotional, and cognitive systems.

Use of the FASQ in Identifying
System Impairments

By identifying body parts or systems that may be affecting performance of each task, the FASQ can help direct the physician toward possible problems during the physical examination. This process can be facilitated by the inclusion on the FASQ form of functional systems, which help to identify the anatomical, sensory, and mental systems that contribute to the performance of the listed tasks. In order to examine system impairments, the physician should transfer the patient's self-reported data obtained from the form illustrated in Figure 2-1 to the form illustrated in Figure 2-3. In addition, each of the listed tasks presented in Figure 2-3 shows the approximate energy consumption in metabolic units or METS. This measure of energy consumption permits the physician to estimate the patient's level of physical conditioning according to the nature of the tasks being performed on a daily basis. An example is shown in Figure 2-3.

Below the functional systems heading are two letter headings which designate the anatomical, sensory, and mental systems involved in performance of those tasks listed on the form.

(Up) Upper limbs and neck	Neuromusculoskeletal impairments
(Ma) Manual dexterity	
(Lo) Lower limbs and trunk	
(Sp) Speaking and writing	Communication impairments
(Se) Seeing and reading	Sensory impairments
(He) Hearing	
(St) Stamina	Cardiopulmonary impairments
(Co) Cognition/mental status	Cognitive impairments
(Af) Affective/emotional status	Affective impairments

For each activity addressed in the FASQ, the functional systems denote, by means of parentheses or brackets, which body systems or skills are involved in performance. Primary skills involved in the successful performance of each task are denoted by brackets. For example, "cut toenails" requires use of the upper limbs and neck (Up), manual dexterity [Ma], lower limbs and trunk control (Lo), and seeing (Se). Manual dexterity, indicated by brackets, is identified as the primary skill required for cutting toenails. The other skills indicated by parentheses under the appropriate headings are identified as needed but are less crucial functional systems.

If a patient reports trouble cutting toenails, the physician checks the brackets and parentheses under the systems likely to be deficient in performance of the activity. After all tasks have been assessed and the appropriate brackets or parentheses have been checked, the physician can perform thorough examinations organized around those affected areas. In the following chapter basic examination techniques are provided for assessing the major systems involved if functional performance is limited. In subsequent chapters other examination techniques, considerations, and management suggestions are discussed for common chronic diseases.

Functional Tasks	Energy Cost in METS	Functional Systems								
Ease versus Difficulty		Up	Ma	Lo	Sp	Se	He	St	Co	Af
P _ Cut toenails	1-2	( )	[ ]	( )		( )				
_ Get up from a low seat	2-3			[ ]				( )		
_ Climb stairs	4-5			[ ]				[ ]		
I _ Wash windows and walls	5-6	[ ]	( )	( )		( )		( )		
_ Shop for groceries	4-5	( )	( )	( )	( )	( )	( )	( )	[ ]	( )
_ Handle finances	1-2		( )			( )			[ ]	( )
L _ Play sports	7+	( )	( )	( )		( )		[ ]		
_ Converse	1-2				[ ]		[ ]		( )	( )
_ Be socially active	3-4	( )	( )	( )	( )	( )	[ ]	( )	( )	[ ]
O _ Concentrate	1-2					( )	( )		[ ]	[ ]
_ Sit for long periods	1-2			[ ]						
_ Stand for long periods	3-4			[ ]				( )		
_ Reach, grasp, pinch	2-3	[ ]	( )	( )						
T _ Drive an automobile	2-3	( )	( )	( )			[ ]		( )	( )
_ Ride a bus	4-5	( )	( )	( )	( )		[ ]		( ) ( )	( )

____Task Score, of which
____Tasks are easy (grade 4) and
____Tasks are not applicable (grade 0)

Figure 2-3. Functional Assessment Screening Questionnaire (FASQ).

Application of the Functional Assessment

A functional assessment assists the primary care physician in three important ways by:

Providing a systematic and consistent method for analyzing functional deficits and developing a patient problem list

Determining clinical care outcomes by comparing measures of function before and after treatment interventions

Assuring that a program of care addresses issues that are most likely to maximize the quality of life for the disabled individual

In summary, use of the FASQ provides a quickly arrived at, preliminary overview of the patient's disability by focusing on types and extent of activity restrictions. It also provides a basis for estimating the patient's general level of physical conditioning according to the levels of energy customarily expended. The functional systems series offers a list of possible physical and mental factors contributing to a patient's inability to perform. Each is valuable in evaluating the extent of disability; together they are the basis on which the physician organizes a systematic and focused physical examination that allows him to use time efficiently. A case history follows to illustrate the application of the functional assessment in primary care.

Case History

Mrs. CJ is a 76-year-old widow with a history of osteoarthritis and mild hypertension. During a routine quarterly blood pressure check, she related to her physician, Dr. M, the existence of a persistent pain in both shoulders of 4 to 6 weeks duration. She had no recall of any precipitating incident nor any previous history of similar shoulder pain. In response to his questioning, she reported problems with raising her arms, for example, when she tried to groom her hair or reach kitchen shelves. Hot baths provided only temporary relief.

Dr. M ordered x-rays of the shoulders and suggested Mrs. CJ refrain from stressing her shoulders, take daily aspirin, and get extra rest. He asked her to return in 2 weeks to discuss the results of her x-rays.

When she returned to the physician's office as scheduled, Mrs. CJ was still in pain. Dr. M informed her that, as he had expected, the x-rays showed minor arthritic changes. He injected her shoulders with a local steroid, which brought her some relief. Several weeks later, however, the patient returned to Dr. M's office seeking injections again. She continued to return for injections at shorter and shorter intervals. After 6 months, Mrs. CJ's daughter, distressed at her mother's continuing pain, convinced her mother to see another physician, Dr. R.

Dr. R had Mrs. CJ fill out a functional assessment screening questionnaire while she was in the waiting room. Her replies are duplicated in Figure 2-4.

Subjectively, Mrs. CJ felt that, compared with others her age, her health and ability to be active were average or better than average; she noted, however, that her ability to do needed and desired things was poor.

In the functional tasks section of the FASQ, Mrs. CJ indicated impaired function in a large number of activities, including stairclimbing, that required use of the lower limbs as well as the upper limbs. Dr. R elicited the fact that Mrs. CJ lived alone in a second floor walkup apartment. Lately she found it difficult to climb the stairs and was able to leave her apartment only once each day, which was unusual, as previously she had been a vigorous and active woman. She indicated wistfully that although in the past she had frequently visited her sister, who lived nearby, her visits had dwindled to once a week. Also, she had become dependent on her daughter to do her grocery shopping, since walking about the store and carrying groceries up the stairs exhausted her. Although she had always been a meticulous woman, she was finding it increasingly difficult to maintain the apartment and to entertain her few close friends. She said to the physician, "Don't ever get old. It's really tough when you get to be my age." Encouraged by the physician's interest, she told him of her fears of losing her independence and possibly having to go to a nursing home.

Dr. R noted on the functional systems survey that Mrs. CJ's most troublesome areas involved upper limbs, lower limbs, and stamina. He performed a thorough examination of her extremities, including range of motion, muscle strength, reflex, and sensory testing. He noted that proximal muscle groups were weak and painful with motion. When Mrs. CJ walked across the room, he noted that her gait was unsteady. He examined her heart and lungs and watched her do some simple movements. When asked, Mrs. CJ denied any

Name: Mrs. C.J.   Date: October 19, 1981

	EXCE EDED	GOOD OR DE	AVE RAGE ER	POO ROO R	VPOO P O O
In comparison with others of your age, how well do you feel in terms of:					
1. Your general state of health?	5	X	3	2	1
2. Your ability to be as active?	5	4	X	2	1
3. Your ability to do *needed* things?	5	4	3	X	1
4. Your ability to do *desired* things?	5	4	3	X	1

Health score: 11/20

		Functional Tasks	Energy Cost in METS	Functional Systems								
Ease versus Difficulty				Up	Ma	Lo	Sp	Se	He	St	Co	Af
P	3	Cut toenails	1–2	( )	[ ]	(X)		( )				
	2	Get up from a low seat	2–3			[X]				( )		
	3	Climb stairs	4–5			[X]				[ ]		
I	0	Wash windows and walls	5–6	[ ]	( )	( )		( )		( )		
	3	Shop for groceries	4–5	(X)	( )	(X)	( )	( )	( )	(X)	[ ]	( )
	4	Handle finances	1–2		( )			( )			[ ]	( )
L	1	Play sports	7+	( )	( )	(X)		( )		[X]		
	4	Converse	1–2				[ ]		[ ]		( )	( )
	3	Be socially active	3–4	( )	( )	(X)	( )	( )	[ ]	( )	( )	[X]
O	4	Concentrate	1–2				( )	( )			[ ]	[ ]
	3	Sit for long periods	1–2			[X]						
	2	Stand for long periods	3–4			[X]				( )		
	3	Reach, grasp, pinch	2–3	[X]	( )	( )						
T	0	Drive an automobile	2–3	( )	( )	( )		[ ]			( )	( )
	3	Ride a bus	4–5	( )	( )	(X)	( )	[ ]		(X)	( )	( )

38 Task score, of which
   3 Tasks are easy (grade 4) and
   2 Tasks are not applicable (grade 0)

Figure 2-4. Functional Assessment Screening Questionnaire (FASQ).

recent visual symptoms such as loss of vision or double vision. Finally, Dr. R ordered x-rays of the hips, blood work, and urine testing and asked the patient to report back in 5 days for the results.

When Mrs. CJ returned, she was told that the blood work showed a slight rise in the erythrocyte sedimentation rate and a slight drop in the hemoglobin level. X-rays showed mild degeneration of the hip joint. Dr. R concluded that Mrs. CJ suffered from a systemic problem—polymyalgia rheumatica—which he treated with a low dose oral prednisone. Because of the recent deterioration in the patient's social roles, Dr. R suggested that she should neither rest excessively nor be given anxiolytics to mask her problems, but should be encouraged to continue her social relationships. He referred her to a local senior citizen's center and talked with her about their group shopping sprees and volunteer assistants. He also suggested she consider moving to a first floor apartment.

Subsequent visits demonstrated that the patient experienced a diminution of symptoms and a return to previous levels of functioning, including line dancing. Within 3 months after her initial visit to Dr. R, Mrs. CJ had moved to a ground floor apartment and had resumed frequent social visits. A vast improvement in personal functioning is documented by a subsequent FASQ completed 1 year after treatment by Dr. R, as shown in Figure 2-5.

This case history clearly illustrates the difference between a traditional pathology-oriented approach to clinical care and a functional approach. The first doctor focused only on the patient's presenting complaint and thus treated only a

Name: Mrs. C.J.   Date: September 24, 1982

	E G A P V
In comparison with others of your age,	X O V O P
how well do you feel in terms of:	C O E O O
	E D R R O

1. Your general state of health?		5 X 3 2 1
2. Your ability to be as active?		X 4 3 2 1
3. Your ability to do *needed* things?		X 4 3 2 1
4. Your ability to do *desired* things?		X 4 3 2 1

Health score: 19/20

		Functional Tasks	Energy Cost in METS	Functional Systems								
		Ease versus Difficulty		Up	Ma	Lo	Sp	Se	He	St	Co	Af
P	4	Cut toenails	1–2	( )	[ ]	( )		( )				
	3	Get up from a low seat	2–3			[X]				( )		
	4	Climb stairs	4–5			[ ]				[ ]		
I	0	Wash windows and walls	5–6	[ ]	( )	( )		( )		( )		
	4	Shop for groceries	4–5	( )	( )	( )	( )	( )	( )	( )	[ ]	( )
	4	Handle finances	1–2	( )				( )			[ ]	( )
L	4	Play sports	7+	( )	( )	( )		( )		[ ]		
	4	Converse	1–2				[ ]		[ ]		( )	( )
	4	Be socially active	3–4	( )	( )	( )	( )	( )	[ ]	( )	( )	[ ]
O	4	Concentrate	1–2					( )	( )		[ ]	[ ]
	4	Sit for long periods	1–2			[ ]						
	3	Stand for long periods	3–4			[X]				( )		
	4	Reach, grasp, pinch	2–3	[ ]	( )	( )						
T	0	Drive an automobile	2–3	( )	( )	( )		[ ]			( )	( )
	4	Ride a bus	4–5	( )	( )	( )	( )	[ ]		( )	( )	( )

50 Task score, of which
11 Tasks are easy (grade 4) and
2 Tasks are not applicable (grade 0)

Figure 2-5. Functional Assessment Screening Questionnaire (FASQ).

local symptom. The second doctor, approaching the assessment process from a functional perspective, evaluated the patient's current functioning across the entire spectrum of activities that make up a lifestyle. In the process, he ascertained that decreased functioning was not localized to the shoulder region alone, but included other body systems as well. He uncovered fears, anxieties, and decreased social interactions and was sensitive to their importance in the patient's life. In his treatment plans, the functionally oriented physician concentrated on treating not only the patient's physical impairment, but also the resulting disabilities. The functional approach permitted the patient to return to a level of performance that was not achieved by traditional medical measures. As physicians increasingly take into account function as part of the diagnostic process, they are likely to include functioning issues as part of their treatment formulation and patient management plans.

Summary

This chapter emphasizes the important role functional assessment can play in providing comprehensive medical care. The assessment is a method for evaluating a patient's physical and emotional health by measuring the degree of difficulty and dependence he is experiencing in the performance of selected tasks representative of skills needed in the successful fulfillment of basic social roles: mobility, orientation, social integration, and physical and economic self-sufficiency. The patient's ability to fulfill appropriate social roles is crucial to mental and physical health.

The FASQ, intended to be administered by the patient, includes questions that reveal functional status in five areas of activity: personal care, instrumental (household) living, social interaction and leisure, occupation, and travel. In addition, it includes items related to self-perceived notions about the patient's general state of health as compared with others of the same age.

A tally of the replies with respect to degree of difficulty for each task is a highly efficient way to obtain an overview of a patient's level of functioning. The screening questionnaire, used in conjunction with a functional systems examination, which charts the anatomical, emotional, and cognitive areas involved in the performance of each assessed skill, is an efficient method to evaluate areas producing the most difficulty for the patient and to identify the effects of illness on a patient's lifestyle. Applications of the functional assessment are listed, and a case history is presented to illustrate the benefits to be derived in the primary care setting.

References

1. Berki SE, Ashcraft ML: On analysis of ambulatory utilization: Investigation of roles of need, access, and price as predictors of illness and preventive visits. Med Care 17:1163–1181, 1979
2. Graney M, Zimmerman R: Causes and consequences of health self-report variations among older people. Int J Aging Hum Dev 12(4):291, 1980–81

3. Kerner J, Alexander J: Activities of daily living: Reliability and validity of gross versus specific ratings. Arch Phys Med Rehabil 62:161, 1981
4. Seltzer GB, Granger CV, Wineberg DE: Functional assessment: Bridge between family and rehabilitation medicine within ambulatory practice. Arch Phys Med Rehabil 63:453–457, 1982
5. Seltzer GB, Granger CV, Wineberg DE, LaCheen C: Functional assessment in primary care. In Granger CV, Gresham GE (eds): Functional Assessment in Rehabilitation Medicine, pp 289–304. Baltimore, Williams & Wilkins, 1984

Additional Readings

1. Alexander J, Willems E: Quality of life: Some measurement requirements. Arch Phys Med Rehabil 62:261, 1981
2. Anaisson A, Rundgren A, Sperling L: Evaluation of functional capacity in activities of daily living in 70 year old men and women. Scand J Rehab Med 12:145, 1980
3. Granger CV: Functional assessment and the long term patient. In Kottke FJ, Stillwell GK, Lehmann JF (eds): Krusen's Handbook of Physical Medicine and Rehabilitation. Philadelphia, WB Saunders, 1982
4. Jette A: Functional status index: Reliability of a chronic disease evaluation instrument. Arch Phys Med Rehabil 61:395, 1980
5. Kane R et al: Outcomes of care in an ambulatory primary care population. A pilot study. J Community Health 1(4):233, 1976
6. Kaufert J et al: Assessing functional status among elderly patients. A comparison of questionnaire and service provider ratings. Med Care 17(8):807, 1979
7. Katz S et al: Studies of illness in the aged. The index of ADL: A standardized measurement of biological and psychosocial function. JAMA 185(12):914, 1963
8. LaRue A et al: Health in old age: How do physicians' ratings and self-ratings compare? J Gerontol 34(5):687, 1979
9. Lawton MP: The functional assessment of elderly people. J Am Geriatr Soc 19(6):465, 1971
10. Maddox G, Douglass E: Self-assessment of health: A longitudinal study of elderly subjects. J Health Soc Behav 14:87, 1973
11. Moore J: Functional disability of geriatric patients in a family medicine program. Implications for patient care, education and research. J Fam Pract 7(6):1159, 1978
12. Moore J, Filenbaum G: Changes in functional disability of geriatric patients in a family medicine program: Implications for patient care. J Fam Pract 12(1):59, 1981
13. Moore J, Goldstein Y: Functional disability of elderly family medicine patients in acute care hospitals and nursing homes. J Family Med 10(1):105, 1980
14. Slater S, Sussman M, Stroud M III: Participation in household activities as a prognostic factor for rehabilitation. Arch Phys Med Rehabil 51(10):605, 1970
15. Stewart A, Ware J Jr, Brook R: Advances in the measurement of functional status: Construction of aggregate indexes. Med Care 19(5):473, 1981

CHAPTER 3
A Functionally Oriented Examination of the Patient

Use of the FASQ in the Physical Examination

The Functional Assessment Screening Questionnaire (FASQ) (discussed in Chap. 2) offers a consistent means of measuring the degree of activity limitation a patient is experiencing and pinpointing areas of dysfunction. If, for example, the patient reports on the FASQ that he is having difficulty getting up from a low seat, climbing stairs, and standing for long periods, but has no problems with reaching, grasping, pinching, or being active socially, the physician should suspect lower limb (Lo) dysfunction or weakness and focus the examination on this anatomical area. If, on the other hand, the patient consistently reports a lot of difficulty with FASQ items requiring manual dexterity (Ma), the physician should look for metacarpal and interphalangeal joint inflammations or weakness, or paralysis of the hand muscles. Once activity restrictions involving major anatomical areas are identified, brief but specific physical examinations can be directed toward precise diagnoses. Functional status can be monitored over a specified period of time by periodic re-administration of an FASQ, thereby helping to determine the effectiveness of treatment.

Despite finding an impairment on physical examination that could possibly interfere with an activity, it is important to note whether the patient is having difficulty with that activity. The dynamics of this seeming contradiction should be analyzed in the light of the patient's response to the four general health questions. A patient who has positive feelings about health and well-being, despite the presence of anatomical deficits, may not require much direct medical intervention. On the other hand, the patient who has negative feelings about health and well-being, despite the absence of significant anatomical deficits, may require a great deal of investigation, particularly with regard to psychosocial issues.

This chapter presents a protocol to follow in performing physical examinations relevant to the functional systems. Following a section on testing range of motion is a discussion of muscle testing. Next problems of gait are presented and methods to assess gait are described. Somatic pain and the common neuromusculoskeletal pain syndromes are then described, and examination techniques to identify causes of pain are presented. The chapter concludes with a rather detailed discussion of tests of the functional systems that can be related to the FASQ.

Unlike many other branches of medicine, rehabilitation medicine is highly dependent upon astute, systematic, and comprehensive observations of patient behaviors to assess problems. Although the intention of this chapter is to present typical state-of-the-art functional assessment as authoritatively as possible, the goal of the chapter, rather than being exhaustive, is to give the reader a fundamental approach so that he can apply his highly trained examination skills in settings in which primary care is being provided. In all likelihood the reader will have to go to other sources to expand his knowledge in various areas. The reader is referred to texts by Swezey,[22] Polley and Hunder,[17] or Rosse and Clawson[19] for elaboration on these examination techniques.

Range of Motion (ROM) Examination

The need to follow range of motion closely for patients with certain diseases is readily apparent. Treatment intervention for diseases such as rheumatoid arthritis and ankylosing spondylitis is directly related to the degree of joint mobility. Yet losses in range of motion are easily overlooked in the physical examination, particularly with respect to the hip and the knee. Flexion contractures at these joints may be both painless and insidious if they are secondary to prolonged bedrest or sitting. It is important to assess active and passive range of motion to determine whether or not there is a loss, a discrepancy, or both. In this section of the chapter the basic considerations and methods for examining range of motion during the physical examination will be covered.

Active range of motion is tested first by having the patient attempt to move the joint the full arc. The passive range of motion is tested by the examiner, who moves the joint without assistance from the patient. Normally the ranges of active and passive motion are equal; when they are not, passive range of motion is usually greater and the more reliable indicator of the actual range.[18] If there are any discrepancies between active and passive motion measurements, the physician should be able to identify the reason based on physical findings and supplemented by information obtained from the FASQ and the medical history. Range of motion may be limited by paralysis, inhibition because of pain, or residual joint swelling. When discrepancies arise between active and passive ROM measurements, psychological factors should also be considered.

The goniometer (Fig. 3-1) is the instrument used to measure the degree of movement of the joint. Although they can provide very accurate findings, goniometric measurements are time-consuming and require experience to read. Only some conditions, such as rheumatoid arthritis or ankylosing spondylitis, warrant the degree of accuracy provided by a goniometric measurement to

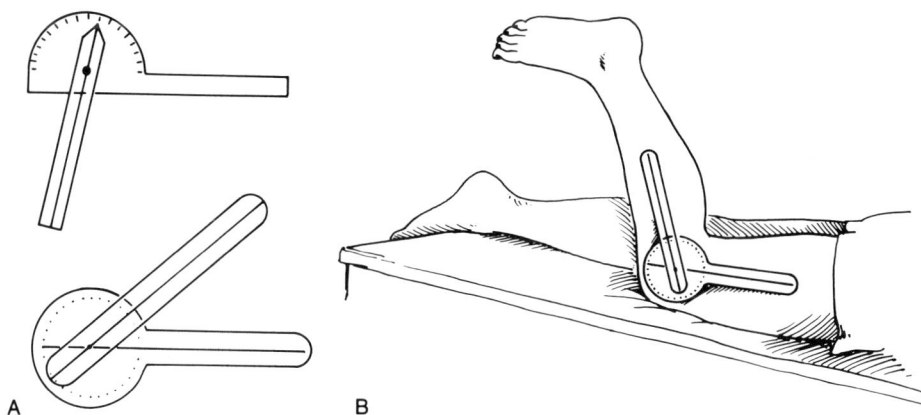

Figure 3-1. *A*. Two examples of universal goniometers commonly used by the clinician. (From Kottke, FJ, Stillwell, GK, Lehmann, JF (eds): Physical Medicine & Rehabilitation. WB Saunders, Philadelphia, 1982[11]) *B*. Goniometric measurement of the knee joint. (From Rusk, HA: Rehabilitation Medicine, p 10. St Louis, CV Mosby, 1977)

monitor ROM. In most instances, approximate values are acceptable. Examiners can use themselves as standards, assuming they have normal range of motion. If necessary, the patient's unaffected side may be used as a control, unless the disease is one that presents bilaterally.

Joint motion may be limited either temporarily (reversibly) or permanently. Polley and Hunder[17] list five possible causes of *temporary* motion limitations. These include: (1) muscle spasm from fear of pain; (2) periarticular stiffness that improves with repeated movements; (3) intraarticular effusion and synovitis; (4) "locking" secondary to loose bodies in the joint, defects or disorders of the meniscus, or malposition of tendons; and (5) fibrous proliferation producing intraarticular or periarticular adhesions, tenosynovitis, or contractures of muscles, fasciae, and tendons. *Permanent* limitations in ROM, according to the same authors, can be due to intraarticular causes (*e.g.,* fibrous or bony ankylosis, destruction of articular surfaces, subluxation), or extraarticular causes (*e.g.,* tightening of the articular capsule, contractures).

Figures 3-2A, 3-2B, and 3-2C present the normal range of motion values for the joints of the upper limb, hand, and lower limbs, respectively, as well as special positioning requirements, when using the goniometer.

Each joint should be observed as it is employed in normal use (anteriorly, laterally, and posteriorly). It should be inspected for deformity, swelling, or redness. It should be palpated for warmth, tenderness, swelling, spongy or firm consistency, and presence of fluid. The joint should be palpated for crepitation while it is moved, first actively by the patient, then passively by the physician. An outline is presented of examination procedures used for the shoulder, hip, and knee, which are affected by various disorders and are commonly associated with limitations in functional performance (Table 3-1, page 36).

Joint Motion Measurements
Upper Extremity

Zero position is supine with feet at right angles, extremities parallel to midline of body and palms facing medially. Measurements are passive to reflect maximum range of motion. When active motion is requested, record in adjacent column. Elbow, knee, and ankle are measured at lateral aspect.

Side		Right			Left		
Examiner							
Date							

Remarks	Motion and Range						
	Shoulder						
(Flex hips and knees to flatten spine)							
Measure from table	Flexion 0 to 180°						
Scapula stabilized laterally/superiorly Elbow 90° rotation 0°	Abduction 0 to 90°						
Abducted to above range. Elbow 90°	Int. Rotation 0 to 60°						
Scapula stabilized antero-superiorly	Ext. Rotation 0 to 90°						
	Elbow and Forearm						
	Extension 0°						
	Flexion 0° to 145°						
Shoulder 0°	Pronation 0 to 90°						
Elbow 90°	Supination 0 to 90°						
(Elbow 90°, Forearm pronated)	Wrist						
Measure on ulnar border for metacarpal III	Extension 0 to 70°						
	Flexion 0 to 80°						
Wrist 0° Measure on dorsum of metacarpal III	Radial deviation 0 to 20°						
	Ulnar deviation 0 to 45°						

A

Figure 3-2.   Sample range of motion charts. *A.* Joint motion measurements, upper extremity. *B.* Range of motion of hand. *C.* Range of motion, lower extremity.

Range of Motion of Hand							
Right ( )				Left ( )			
Date							
Examiner							
	Normal Range	Passive	Active	Passive	Active	Passive	Active
	Ext/Flex						
Thumb							
MCP	(10)/60						
IP	(10)/80						
Index							
MCP	(20)/90						
PIP	0/100						
DIP	(20)/70						
Middle							
MCP	(20)/90						
PIP	0/100						
DIP	(20)/70						
Ring							
MCP	(20)/90						
PIP	0/100						
DIP	(20)/70						
Little							
MCP	(20)/90						
PIP	0/100						
DIP	(20)/70						
Tip to metacarpal head in cm. and ring size of PIP		Tip to MC Head	Ring Size	Tip to MC Head	Ring Size	Tip to MC Head	Ring Size
	Index						
	Middle						
	Ring						
	Little						
Angle of I & II metacarpals (thumb web)							
60°	Radial abduction						
	Palmar abduction						

B

Figure 3-2 *(continued)*

Range of Motion of

Lower Extremity

Zero position is supine with feet at right angles, extremities parallel to midline of body and palms facing medially. Measurements are passive to reflect maximum range of motion. When active motion is requested, record in adjacent column. Elbow, knee, and ankle are measured at lateral aspect.

Side	Right			Left		
Examiner						
Date						

Remarks	Motion and Range						
	Hip						
(First measure extension bilaterally) (Pelvic motion marks end point)							
Opp. hip and knee held flexed to hold spine flat	Extension 0°						
Opp. hip held as measured above to hold spine flat	Flexion 0 to 130°						
Opp. leg abducted 20°	Adduction 0 to 20°						
	Abduction 0 to 45°						
Opp. hip and knee flexed to flatten spine. Hip 0° Knee 90°	Int. Rotation 0 to 45°						
	Ext. Rotation 0 to 45°						
Maximum intermalleolar distance hips 0°							

c

Figure 3-2 *(continued)*

Manual Muscle Strength Examination

A manual muscle strength examination is performed to identify weak muscles and, if they are weak, to measure the degree of weakness. This examination is indicated if deficits in body or limb movements are observed, and if the patient complains of neuromusculoskeletal pain. Muscle strength testing serves a number of purposes: First, it serves as a diagnostic tool; second, as a means for determining the amount of residual functional capacity that might be used to perform the activities of daily living; third, as an aid in determining the prognosis

Knee											
	Extension 0°										
Hip flexed	Flexion 0 to 140°										
Ankle (Align with bottom of foot and midleg)											
	Plantar Ext. 0 to 45°										
Knee 0°	Dorsiflexion 0 to 20°										
Knee 90°	Dorsiflexion 0 to 20°										
Foot (Align with ball of foot and parallel to leg)											
	Inversion 0 to 40°										
	Eversion 0 to 30°										
Miscellaneous (Pelvic motion marks and point)											
Opp. leg flat on table	Hamstring length- Straight leg raising 0 to 90°										
Prone Hip 0°	Quadriceps length- flexion of knee 0 to 90°										

C

Figure 3-2 *(continued)*

of diagnosed conditions; and fourth, when repeated periodically, as a method to monitor the effectiveness of treatment.

An examination of muscle strength is carried out by the examiner first placing the limb in the position to be tested and then applying manual force to displace the limb. The patient is instructed to maintain the original position. The examiner observes the point at which the patient can no longer do so. Muscle strength is graded on a scale from five to zero. Five is normal, and zero indicates no evidence of muscle contraction. A rating of three represents less than normal strength, that is, the patient is able to maintain the position against a force no greater than the weight of gravity. Table 3-2 summarizes the muscle strength grading system.

TABLE 3-1　Outline of Examination Procedures for the Shoulder, Hip, and Knee

Palpation	Motion	Special Maneuvers
Shoulder		
Sitting Deltoid Trapezius Supraspinatus fossa Infraspinatus fossa Synovial membrane 　and joint fluid Coracoid process Bicipital groove Subacromial space Supraspinatus tendon	*Sitting or Standing* Observe scapulohumeral rhythm, 　flexion, and abduction ranges *Supine* Stand on right side for right scapula Stabilize the scapula with the left 　hand for all motion except flexion Move humerus in flexion, abduc- 　tion, internal and external rotation 　positions *Note*: Scapular motion indicates the 　end point (except when testing 　flexion, which is evaluated as 　combined scapulohumeral and 　scapulothoracic motion).	*Sitting* Pull and push humerus 　for subluxation
Hip		
Supine Anterior aspect Greater trochanter Gluteus medius Gluteus maximus	*Supine* Abduction—keep hips extended Flexion—flex one hip at a time 　while maintaining opposite hip in 　extension Rotation—keep hips extended, 　knees flexed over end of table Extension—keep hips flexed to 　flatten lumbar spine, buttocks at 　end of table, then extend one hip 　at a time *Note*: Pelvic motion delineates 　endpoint.	*Standing* Trendelenburg test
Knee		
Sitting, Leg Pendent Collateral ligaments Joint line Popliteal space Synovial membrane *Supine, Knee Extended* Synovial membrane Fluid wave Patella ballottement 　(click)	*Supine* Move leg to full extension and 　flexion During movement, palpate for 　crepitation	*Sitting, Leg Pendent* Push and pull proximal 　part of leg (cruciate 　ligaments) *Sitting, Leg Relaxed, Extended* Lateral stress applied 　for medial collateral 　ligament; medial 　stress applied for 　lateral collateral 　ligament *Supine or Prone* Rotary stress for torn 　meniscus (also 　checked in prone 　position)

TABLE 3-2   Grades for Muscle Strength Testing

5	Normal	Completes range of motion against full manual force
4	Good	Completes range of motion against some manual force
3	Fair	Completes range of motion against gravitational force only
2	Poor	Does not complete range of motion unless gravity is eliminated
1	Trace	Minimal evidence of muscle contraction
0	Zero	No evidence of muscle contraction

Abbreviated and Screening Muscle Strength Tests

Two shortened versions of muscle strength tests are presented in Tables 3-3 and 3-4. Both are diagnostic tools easily administered by a primary care provider. The first, the abbreviated muscle strength test, is a guide to a sequence for testing selected muscles. The second, the screening muscle strength test, is outlined more succintly than the first, but serves as a reminder to examine range of motion of joints, sensibility, balance and coordination, and reflexes in the full evaluation of the patient. When either test reveals muscle weakness, the patient should be followed up by a physiatrist or a physical therapist who performs detailed muscle strength testing. Forms for recording group muscle strength of upper and lower limbs are shown in Figures 3-3 and 3-4.

The primary care provider who uses one of the shortened muscle strength tests should keep a number of considerations in mind.

1. These shortened versions of muscle strength testing have some limitations. In the interest of brevity, only certain motions and muscles have been selected for testing, and compromises have been made in selecting

(Text continued on page 42)

TABLE 3-3   Abbreviated Muscle Strength Test

Observations	Motion
Observe anteriorly, posteriorly and laterally	
Disrobing	
Observe any abnormal or trick substitution movements	
Stance	
Observe symmetry and asymmetry of general body contour and limbs	Have patient elevate arms overhead; look for smooth rhythm between scapula and humerus
Look for evenness of shoulders and pelvis bilaterally	Have patient alternately stand on one leg; see if pelvis drops on opposite side (positive Trendelenburg sign denoting weak hip abductors)
Look for signs of atrophy, hypertrophy, or joint contracture	Have patient balance on one leg and rise up and down on toes 10 times; repeat with opposite limb to test for plantar flexor muscle weakness
Observe for scoliosis	

Continued

TABLE 3-3   *Continued*

Observations	Motion
Gait	
Observe swing and stance phases	Have patient turn 180 degrees; note width of base of support—see if it widens more than 2″ from midline when turning
Listen for auditory cues such as uneven cadence, foot slap, etc.	
Note symmetry or asymmetry of gait. Look for excessive or diminished components of the normal gait	Have patient walk on heels
	Inability to sustain weight due to weak dorsiflexors is observed in a foot slap (or foot drop in more severe cases)
Observe degree of arm swing	Have patient step up and down, alternating legs, on a chair with an 18-inch seat (be sure to offer protection against falling or striking an overhead object); difficulty or unsteadiness suggests weakness of hip or knee extensors
Sitting	
Observe neck flexors and abdominals	Have patient place chin on chest and hold against a gentle upward push against the forehead; test strength of neck flexors while palpating tension of abdominal muscles; patient is not to use hands for support
Observe cranial muscle functions	Test the following cranial nerves: facial nerve (frontalis, orbicularis oculi, zygomaticus, orbicularis oris); oculomotor nerve (three recti, interior oblique, ciliary); trochlear nerve (superior oblique); abducens nerve (lateral rectus); hypoglossal nerve (genioglossi), spinal accessory nerve (upper trapezius)
	Test shoulder abduction and adduction (arm at side), external rotation, elbow flexion and extension, supination, thumb and finger flexors and thenar and hypothenar muscles
Observe upper limbs	Perform arm drift test:
	Have the patient sit and raise arms forward to 90 degrees at the shoulders with elbows extended, wrists neutral, and digits extended with palms up; have patient maintain the hands, with eyes closed, about 12 inches apart and parallel with the floor. A positive sign for "drift" is indicated if the patient cannot hold the position for 15 to 30 seconds (the elbow begins to flex or the forearm pronates; drift is an early sign of hypotonia)
Observe lower limbs	Test hip flexion and internal rotation, knee flexion, foot dorsiflexion and eversion, and toe extension and flexion.

TABLE 3-4   Screening Muscle Strength Test

Principle	Test

In testing for weakness the examiner must provide an appropriate and adequate challenge without overchallenging or causing the patient discomfort.	Erect
	  Walk on heels
	  Balance on either foot and rise on toes of either foot
	  Step up on chair
	  Elevate arms (view from behind)

Check	Sitting—Cranial nerves and trunk
	  Facial (frontalis, orbicularis oculi, zygomaticus, orbicularis oris)
	  Extraocular movements

If patient is completely disrobed, examiner should observe:
  General contour of body and limbs (symmetry and asymmetry)
  Scoliosis
  Level of shoulders and pelvis
Range of motion of major or pertinent joints (limbs and spinal), straight leg raise (SLR)
Sensory evaluation with Romberg (single leg)
Gait (arm swing, limp, width of base)
Walk tandem
Atrophy, fasciculation, muscle tone
Deep tendon reflexes, Babinski, other
Position sense in toes if lower limb weakness is present
	Tongue
	  Neck flexors and abdominals
	Sitting—Upper limbs
	  Shoulder hiking (trapezius) elevation
	  Shoulder abduction/external rotation
	  Shoulder adduction (arm at side)
	  Elbow flexion and extension
	  Forearm supination
	  Wrist extension
	  Finger and thumb flexion
	  Finger and thumb adduction
	  Thenar and hypothenar opposition
	Sitting—Lower limbs
	  Hip flexors
	  Hip internal rotators
	  (toe flexors and extensors, palpate extensor digitorum brevis—EDB)

If Joint Abnormality Is Present	
Observe joint as it is employed in stance and gait (anteriorly, laterally and posteriorly) Inspect for deformity, swelling and redness Palpate for heat, swelling (consistency and fluid), tenderness, and crepitation Have patient move segment actively Record range of motion If active motion is restricted, move the distal segment passively, stabilizing the proximal segment Compare passive range of motion with active range of motion Grade muscles that are concerned with that particular joint Special maneuvers for particular joints in appropriate sequence	

Muscle Strength Test of Upper Extremity

5	N	Normal	Considered normal for age, size, sex of patient.
4	G	Good	Complete range of motion against gravity with some resistance.
3	F	Fair	Complete range of motion against gravity.
2	P	Poor	Complete range of motion with gravity eliminated.
1	T	Trace	Slight contractility. No joint motion.
0	O	Zero	No evidence of contractility.

S–Spasm   C–Contracture   P–Pain   R/S–Range/strength grade

Side	Right				Left			
Examiner								
Date								
Neck								
Flexion								
Extension								
Rotation								
Shoulder								
Scapula elevation								
Scapula depression								
Flexion								
Extension								
Adduction								
Abduction								
Internal rotation								
External rotation								
Elbow and Forearm								
Flexion								
Extension								
Pronation								
Supination								
Wrist								
Flexion								
Extension								
Radial deviation								
Ulnar deviation								
Fingers								
Flexion								
Extension								
Adduction								
Abduction								
Opposition (thumb)								

Figure 3-3. Muscle strength test of upper extremity.

Muscle Strength Test of Lower Extremity

5	N	Normal	Considered normal for age, size, sex of patient.
4	G	Good	Complete range of motion against gravity with some resistance.
3	F	Fair	Complete range of motion against gravity.
2	P	Poor	Complete range of motion with gravity eliminated.
1	T	Trace	Slight contractility. No joint motion.
0	O	Zero	No evidence of contractility.

S–Spasm   C–Contracture   P–Pain   R/S–Range/strength grade

Side	Right				Left			
Examiner								
Date								
Trunk								
Flexion								
Extension								
Rotation								
Hip								
Hiphiking								
Flexion								
Extension								
Adduction								
Abduction								
Int. Rotation								
Ext. Rotation								
Knee								
Flexion								
Extension								
Ankle and Foot								
Flexion (dorsal)								
Extension (plantar)								
Inversion								
Eversion								
Toes								
Flexion								
Extension								

Figure 3-4. Muscle strength test of lower extremity.

test positions. Results may be invalidated by several conditions, such as deformity, limited joint motion, pain, or limited patient cooperation. In addition to muscle strength testing, a comprehensive evaluation of motor function must include other tests, such as range of motion, coordination, deep tendon reflex testing, pathologic reflexes, and sensation (especially position sense of the toes).

2. Accessible muscles and tendons should be observed and palpated, if feasible—at rest and during contraction—for tension and muscle mass.
3. Performance should be compared bilaterally.
4. The patient should begin with the less vigorous tests first.
5. The examiner should employ leverage so that the patient, not the examiner, is operating at a mechanical disadvantage. The examiner will then be able to concentrate on evaluating the patient's strength, rather than on expending efforts to overcome it.
6. A consistent pattern of testing should be developed.
7. The examiner must provide an appropriate and adequate challenge without overchallenging or discouraging the patient, or causing the patient discomfort.

The abbreviated and screening muscle strength tests can be performed in 3 minutes or less with great accuracy. Both tests are intended to be used as quick guides for evaluating potential problem areas noted on the FASQ. They are good screening items in that they enable the examiner to identify proximal versus distal weakness, to observe muscles innervated by each of the major nerve groups, and to test the frequently impaired segments. These tests provide an overview of functional skill levels of the face, trunk, upper limbs, and lower limbs.

Both tests are based on the principles of observation (including inspection for deformity, swelling, and redness) and examination for motion, warmth, consistency, or swelling (including muscle strength testing and palpation of muscles and joints during movement, when appropriate). Special maneuvers (*e.g.*, tests for Trendelenburg's, Tinel's, and Phelan's signs) often are employed to evaluate specific nerve or muscle group functioning.

Common Pitfalls in Muscle Testing

Common pitfalls in muscle testing are usually due either to the examiner's failure to appreciate some of the underlying concepts of muscle strength testing (*e.g.*, substitution, synergism), or to his failure to perform a thorough and careful physical examination.

Substitution in this context is the use of a muscle or muscles other than the one(s) normally used to perform a movement. Because the movement is produced, the examiner may miss underlying weakness. For example, if the muscles that initiate abduction of the right shoulder are weakened, the patient may initiate abduction instead by suddenly deviating his trunk to the right side. As another example of substitution, if the ankle dorsiflexor (anterior tibialis muscle) is weakened, a patient may utilize the long toe extensors rather than the anterior tibialis to dorsiflex the ankle. Many faulty evaluations and misdiagnoses are due to the physician's failure to detect substitutive movements.

To avoid assessing the strength of a muscle improperly, the examiner must be aware of certain principles. The long axis of the fibers of the muscle being tested must be in alignment with the direction of forces across the joint; otherwise substitution may occur if that muscle is weak. For example, if a patient with a weak deltoid muscle elevates the arm to 90° abduction with the forearm supinated, the combination of external rotation and supination places the long head of the biceps brachii in alignment with the shoulder motion, and it may function as an abductor. A deltoid muscle that is less than antigravity strength would seem to be stronger than it really is, if supination is allowed; thus the muscle that could serve as a substitute (in this case, the biceps brachii) must be kept out of alignment with the motion by keeping the forearm in pronation. Similarly, the hip abductors (gluteus medius and gluteus minimus) could be assessed inaccurately if the hips are tested for abductor strength in the sitting position. Flexion of the hip allows the gluteus maximus (hip extensor) and tensor fasciae latae to act as hip abductors. Hip abduction should be tested with the patient in a supine or side-lying position.

Another common error in testing muscle strength is failure to palpate the muscle and its tendon during contraction. As a consequence, the examiner may attribute strength it does not have to a muscle, because other muscles are performing the desired motion. An example is the assumption that the upper trapezius muscle is strong if a patient can shrug or elevate his or her shoulder against resistance. Other muscles (levator scapulae, rhomboids, serratus anterior) can substitute for the upper trapezius to perform this maneuver. The examiner must palpate the upper trapezius muscle to determine whether this muscle is elevating the shoulder against resistance.

To avoid misinterpretation when substitution is occurring, the examiner must remember to position the patient so that synergistic muscles are least likely to assist in the movement under consideration. As an example, in testing to determine the antigravity status of hip extensors with the patient supine, the knee should be flexed to diminish the hip extensor effect of the hamstrings.

Another common pitfall in muscle testing is the failure to differentiate between normal and abnormal patterns of motion. For example, when observing a patient's gait, an examiner may neglect to observe a diminution (which can signal muscle weakness) in the normal reciprocal patterns of motion in the upper limbs. This diminution can also be a sign of upper motor neuron disease, limitation in range of motion of the upper limb, or a painful upper limb.

Failure to evaluate a muscle through a complete range of motion (ROM) may result in erroneous examination findings. Regarding a gastrocnemius–soleus muscle group as normal simply because the patient can walk on his toes is a case in point. These muscles could be very weak, and yet the patient could still walk on his toes by using peroneals and long toe flexors to maintain plantar flexion (a substitutive maneuver). The best test for normal power of this muscle group is to ask the patient to stand on one leg and come up on the forefoot slowly, approximately ten times. Another example that illustrates the importance of complete ROM testing involves the quadriceps muscle. Reporting that a quadriceps muscle is normal because it produces a great deal of tension in a position of partial knee flexion may prove erroneous. A quadriceps mechanism may appear strong in a position of partial knee flexion, but may be weak in the last few degrees of extension due to vastus medialis weakness. On the other hand, a misdiagnosis in the other direction may result from assuming that a quadriceps is weak because a patient is unable to extend the knee completely in the sitting position, when actually tight hamstring muscles prevent complete extension. To assure an accurate assessment, the patient should be placed in the supine position to identify the factor that is preventing complete extension of the knee.

Failure to stabilize proximal segments is another common pitfall in testing muscle strength. Both substitution and faulty identification of muscle weakness result. For instance, erroneous results may be obtained if the examiner reports that the abductor of the hip is below antigravity strength in the sidelying test position, when stabilization of the pelvis is inadequate. In this instance, the hip abductors may be of antigravity strength or better, but the lateral abdominal musculature may be insufficient to stabilize the pelvis, causing the limb to drop toward the examining table. Thus the pelvis must be stabilized manually by the examiner.

Gait Examination*

In the general practice of medicine, the physician often arrives in the examining room to find the patient sitting or lying disrobed on the examination table. He leaves prior to the patient's dressing, and there is little specific analysis of the patient's gait. Critically viewing the patient walking, however, is a procedure that will have rich rewards for one assessing the neuromusculoskeletal system.

Two simple principles should be considered when examining a patient's gait: First, gait is ordinarily an automatic sequence of limb segment motions and muscle activity. The patient usually is paying attention to where he is going, but is not thinking about the exact coordination of limb segment motions and muscle activities necessary to get there. Injury to the neuromusculoskeletal system partially removes this automatic sequencing and replaces it with a slower and less coordinated system. The net result is the loss of a perfectly smooth translation of the body from one place to another in a rhythmic fashion; instead, movement develops which is either asymmetric or lacks smoothness. Second, the center of gravity in the body of the average adult remains within a square approximately 2 inches wide and 2 inches high during normal ambulation. The center of gravity shifts from side to side, and also rises and falls; it is at its lowest point when the weight is equally distributed between the limbs (double stance), and at its highest point during unilateral stance. Normally stride lengths are approximately equal, as is stride time (the length of time spent on one stance leg). Smooth transition through space with minimal vertical deviation is the most energy-efficient method of walking. Jerky or abrupt movements require considerably more expenditure of energy and are usually not utilized by the body unless there is some significant abnormality.

The portions of the gait cycle have been named to provide a means of

---

* This section on gait examination has been adapted from Physical Medicine and Rehabilitation for the Medical Practitioner by Richard S. Materson, M.D., Chapter 20 in PRACTICE OF MEDICINE, Vol 1, Hagerstown, Harper & Row, 1978.[13]

describing abnormalities accurately (Fig. 3-5). The single forward step has been divided into a series of timed movements, which can be observed in slow motion. The step sequence begins with the heel strike of the limb that has just swung forward. The sequence is heel strike, foot flat, heel off, knee bend, toe off, toe clear, and heel strike. The single forward step may also be divided into a stance phase (approximately 45% of the time necessary to take a step) and a swing phase. During the stance phase the foot is on the ground, and during the swing phase it is moving forward for the next step. To shift from the swing phase to the stance phase, the foot must accomplish a remarkable deceleration when the heel of the rapidly swinging leg hits the ground: dorsiflexor muscles of the foot must lengthen smoothly to allow the foot to become flat without slapping; weight will be nearly fully borne on the stance leg, and the ankle and knee of the stance leg must stabilize at the same time so that the torso may balance on the stance leg. Then, the ankle and toe plantar flexors must push firmly into the ground. The weight-bearing line progresses forward from the heel, along the fifth metatarsal, and then from the metatarsal head to the great toe, as the body is propelled forward in pushoff. Once it is off the ground, the limb must re-accelerate. Adequate hip flexion, knee flexion, and ankle dorsiflexion must be maintained in order for the toe to clear.

The examiner should note that the heelstrike is smooth and without a thud. Weight from the opposite side should be accepted smoothly on the stance limb. A foot slap between the heelstrike and the foot flat phases suggests weakness of the muscles innervated by the peroneal nerve. Normally during the midstance phase, the body conserves excess rise of the center of gravity by maintaining a progressive flexion of the knee of approximately 15°. A *stiff knee gait* may be due to weakness of the quadriceps or hip extensor. *Weakness of the plantar flexors* of the toes and foot can produce an abnormal pushoff phase. *Hip flexor weakness* frequently is indicated by a backward lurch of the trunk (and a forward lurch of the pelvis) at the beginning of the swing phase, resulting in a lordotic gait. If an isolated hip extensor is weak (*gluteus maximus weakness*), gait is characterized by a sudden backward lurch of the trunk and pelvis just after the heelstrike on the affected side and, simultaneously, an apparent forward protrusion of the affected hip due to continued trunk motion. The knee in gluteus maximus weakness is tightly extended during midstance, since flexion at the knee would allow flexion at the hip, which cannot be tolerated by the weak hip extensor. Some of the more common abnormal gaits are presented in Table 3-6 on page 60.

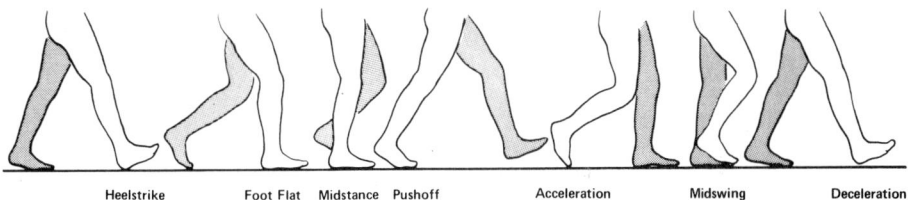

| Heelstrike | Foot Flat | Midstance | Pushoff | Acceleration | Midswing | Deceleration |

Figure 3-5. Portions of the gait cycle. (Adapted from Hoppenfeld, S: Physical Examination of the Spine and Extremities, p. 134. NY, Appleton-Century-Crofts, 1976[9])

A *gluteus medius gait* is typified by certain characteristics. If the limp is uncompensated during the stance phase, the pelvis tilts downward from the stance limb, resulting in an apparently overly long swing leg, which requires exaggerated hip and knee flexion on the opposite side. If this limp is compensated, a very different gait results. During the stance phase on the involved side there is a lurch of the trunk toward the affected side. Despite this, the opposite hip drops, but to a less marked extent than is characteristic of the uncompensated gluteus medius gait. Because of the lateral bending of the trunk over the affected hip, the shoulder on the affected side appears to dip markedly.

Some gait disorders are readily apparent to the observer. For example, the combined gluteus maximus and gluteus medius gait of the patient with Duchenne type muscular dystrophy results in a *waddling gait*. Such patients are usually characterized by a compensated gluteus limp, or a trunk lurch over the affected side, with each step. At the same time, because of hip extensor weakness, they attempt to keep the center of gravity behind the axis of rotation of the hip joint, resulting in exaggerated lordosis.

The *ataxic or unbalanced gait* also is readily discernible because the base of the gait is overly wide, the stride length is uneven, the stride times are unequal, and the body flails about to retain balance. A smooth, wide-based gait is sometimes observed in patients whose cerebellum is intact, but whose posterior columns or sensory afferents are impaired; eye closure significantly aggravates the posterior column type of gait deficit. When the ataxia is of cerebellar origin, sound cues and visual correction become less useful to the patient, and there is a varying width of the base of gait and minimal correction.

Parkinson patients typically exhibit retropulsion (movement backward prior to forward motion), often accompanied by a festinating gait (small steps without adequate foot pickup, progressing in speed so that the patient has difficulty stopping) or a shuffle. Bradykinesia and rigidity are manifested by paucity of arm swing and facial expression.

A *steppage gait* commonly is seen in patients who have paralysis of the peroneal innervated muscles. Their gait is characterized by drop foot, exaggerated hip and knee flexion, and toe strike prior to heel strike. A weakness (rather than paralysis) of the peroneal innervated muscles results in a foot slap (described earlier) due to the decreased ability of these muscles to let the forefoot down gently following heel strike.

Finally, in disorders of joints resulting in pain, an *antalgic limp* to avoid pain is not uncommon. The timing of such a limp is related to the maximal stress during weight-bearing through the joint. Careful observation of the weight-bearing limbs during the various walking maneuvers is helpful in diagnosing arthritis of the hip, knee, or ankle.

Observation of discrepancies between functional performances of walking and voluntary muscle strength grades are also quite helpful in diagnosing weakness due to a psychological conversion reaction. An understanding of the roles of various muscle groups in the different phases of gait enable the examiner to know which muscles are involved when he observes a specific deviation in gait. Furthermore, an examiner who observes a discrepancy such as that of a patient who is able to flex or extend his hip or his knee while walking, but who is unable to extend his hip or knee when requested to do so, may suspect that psychological factors are operating.

In summary, common causes of a gait disorder are:

1. Musculoskeletal (discontinuity, malalignment, limitation of motion)
2. Pain
3. Vestibular disturbance
4. Cerebellar ataxia
5. Motor unit weakness
6. Upper motor neuron spasticity or weakness
7. Hyperkinesia or dyskinesia
8. Parietal lobe dysfunction producing spatial disorientation
9. Dyspraxia or apraxia
10. Conversion reaction

Somatic Pain

There are four types of somatic pain:[15,16,21,23,24] local, transmitted, referred, or central. The origin of *local pain* is a local stimulus associated with or responsible for tissue damage, which may be manifested by tenderness of a structure, swelling, redness, or heat. An example is pain resulting from a direct injury such as a hammer blow to a finger. *Transmitted pain* follows a neural pathway, and the affected sensory segments may be tender; swelling may be present, but usually redness and heat are not. Transmitted pain implies proximal involvement of a sensory neural structure. An example is pain from pressure on a nerve root caused by a herniated disk. *Referred pain* follows an aborted neural pattern; there is no tenderness unless the sympathetic nervous system comes into play. Sometimes a somatic sensory structure is directly involved; frequently, however, the origin of the sensory irritation may lie within a visceral structure, with corresponding sensory representation along the somatic neurosome. An example is pain felt in the left shoulder or upper limb due to myocardial infarction. *Central pain* may be a "stored" sensation that originally arose from a peripheral stimulus, but can no longer be relieved by a nerve block. An example is pain that persists from an attack of herpes zoster long after the herpetic lesions have healed. Central pain also occurs following a stroke, if the infarction has involved the thalamus.

To evaluate pain, the history needs to include: (1) location, (2) character, (3) severity, (4) circumstances of onset and duration, (5) time–intensity pattern, (6) aggravating factors, (7) alleviating factors, (8) nature of resultant disability, and (9) associated somatic and psychological reactions.

Psychogenic accompaniments of pain may include: (1) exaggeration of pain of somatic origin, (2) induced muscle tension associated with anxiety, and (3) regional distribution of pain unrelated to anatomic neural patterns. The individual with pain who also has a troubled life situation may display one of several forms of psychiatric syndromes. These include a psychophysiologic musculoskeletal reaction—a somewhat intense involuntary muscle spasm in reaction to pain; a psychoneurotic conversion reaction—stress is emotionally expressed as a somatic disturbance; a compensation neurosis—a patient receives secondary gain, such as monetary compensation, for displaying disability; and syndromes characterized by depression, malingering, and attention-seeking behaviors.

Because pain is a highly subjective symptom that is not dependent upon a particular condition of tissue pathology, long-term chronic pain of undetermined origin can present significant diagnostic dilemmas. Further, because pain is subject to great differences of individual perception, even varying at different times with the same individual, it is necessary to assess the psychological component of the perception of pain and to look at the effects of chronic pain on the individual's behavior and interpersonal relationships. Although it is likely that long-term pain has some psychological component, the ways in which it is expressed and the functional significance of that component are highly variable.

Despite treatment, pain may persist. The chronic pain syndrome (CPS),[1,2,8] now regarded as an entity in itself, can be recognized by a number of features: (1) Patient complaints are out of proportion to the physical, laboratory, and x-ray findings; (2) chemical dependency is common; by definition, however, since the pain is chronic, past treatment that relied upon drugs and surgery for "cure" has been unsuccessful and, is therefore, inappropriate; (3) depression, anxiety, and even hostility are common emotional overtones; (4) pain dominates the lifestyle, and (5) pain becomes a way to manipulate close family members and others in the environment.

There are several seemingly unjustifiable reasons for pain to persist: First, the physician may obtain an incomplete history by failing to elicit all of the relevant somatic, psychological, and environmental factors. Psychogenic overlay or compensation factors and other sources for secondary gain may be missed. Second, the physician neglects to perform range of motion examinations, or does not palpate involved joints and muscles, thus overlooking important physical findings. Erroneous localization of the source of pain as well as misdirected treatment therapies may result. Inappropriate prescriptions for physical therapy, useless nerve blocks or local injections, as well as misuse of traction and manipulative methods may all contribute to frustrating the physician in his efforts to relieve the patient's pain. Finally, pain may persist for no apparent reason because of the physician's failure to relate pain circumstances to an individual's total range of physical impairments and functional limitations. By administering the FASQ prior to performing a musculoskeletal screening examination, the physician may be able to pinpoint trouble spots and be alert to possible psychogenic sources of pain. For additional information about back pain, see Chapter 12.

Features of Common Neuromusculoskeletal Pain Syndromes

Subdeltoid Bursitis

The bursa is located under the deltoid muscle and the acromion of the scapula and above the supraspinatus tendon. Although not normally continuous with the joint capsule, the bursa may have become so as a result of preceding trauma or degenerative changes. The lesion begins with compression of the supraspinatus tendon between the greater tuberosity of the humerus and the acromion process of the scapula when the arm is elevated. Eventually a tendinitis results. The tendon may calcify and when it ruptures, the contents of the inflamed tendon are released into the bursa, producing a foreign body reaction, pain, and swelling. The pain, which may or may not be localized in the region lateral to the deltoid muscle and which ranges from mild to very severe, is aggravated by motion, particularly abduction. Swelling may or may not be apparent. Radiographs may reveal the associated amorphous calcium deposit in the supraspinatus tendon.

Treatment to avoid stiffness of the joint is based upon a balance of principles of rest (particularly the avoidance of extremes of motion) and gentle (initially pendular) range of motion exercises. Either superficial heat or cold is indicated for pain relief, as are analgesics or antiphlogistics (*e.g.,* salicylates, aspirin, or nonsteroidal, anti-inflammatory agents). Deep heat may make the pain worse in the acute stage. Injection of a solution of Xylocaine and Decadron can relieve the pressure by mechanical lysis, but also can act pharmacologically to relieve pain and inflammation. The eventual goal is to increase range of motion progressively by means of circumduction exercises and to maintain the muscle tone of the shoulder muscles. Extremely vigorous activity and competitive sports should be avoided until the inflammation has subsided significantly.

Lateral Epicondylitis of the Humerus (Tennis Elbow)

Strain of the tendon of origin of the finger and wrist extensor muscle, near the lateral epicondyle of the humerus, produces this condition. A site of inflammation develops, presumably induced by chronic or unaccustomed stress. Pain is reproduced through motions that require wrist or finger extension, particularly when resistance is applied. Hammering, woodchopping, gardening, and various other hand activities can cause epicondylitis. Occasionally calcification at the tendon of origin may develop, but radiographs rarely reveal calcification at the site.

Treatment is based upon avoiding stressful or strong gripping movements and using analgesics, anti-inflammatory agents, and local heat. Occasionally, in order to reinforce rest, a splint may be required temporarily. Some patients respond well to local injection of a steroid, whereas others may require a surgical procedure. Often patients respond well to a program of progressive resistance exercises to the wrist and finger extensors, despite the fact that initiation of such a program may be uncomfortable for the patient at first.

Carpal Tunnel Syndrome

Compression of the median nerve within the passage formed by the volar transverse carpal ligament and the carpal bones is the basis of the pain and sensory symptoms of carpal tunnel syndrome. The compression occurs because of conditions that reduce the space for the nerve in the canal or predispose the nerve to injury from the pressure. Conditions that reduce the space include: (1) perineural edema associated with pregnancy or upper limb edema; (2) synovitis (nonspecific, secondary to repeated trauma or use, rheumatoid disease, gout, collagen disease, infections, or postfracture of the wrist); and (3) lesions (such as scarring, tophus, hematoma, bony exostoses from degenerative joint disease or fracture) that occupy the space. Certain neuropathies, which may predispose the nerve to compression, may result from diabetes mellitus, thyroid dysfunction, and certain drug intolerances. The symptoms include pain of an aching nature felt in the volar aspect of the wrist, the palm, or along the path of the median nerve in the forearm. The patient may also feel pain along the arm up to the neck, thus indicating that the pain is not well localized to the median nerve distribution. Tingling and paresthesia may be felt over the median nerve distribution or else may be felt in the whole hand. The thumb, index, and middle fingers are most likely to feel numb. Symptoms characteristically intensify at night or early in the morning; upon awakening, the patient wants to wring and shake the hand to obtain relief. The examiner can reproduce the symptoms of pain and tingling by hyperflexion of the wrist held for a minute (Phelan's sign) or by tapping the median nerve at the wrist at the proximal crease on the radial side of the palmaris longus tendon (Tinel's sign). Weak pinch and thenar muscle atrophy are late signs. Electromyography and nerve conduction testing of the distal segments of the median nerve, the most reliable diagnostic means to determine impaired nerve conduction, are usually performed by a physiatrist or neurologist.

Treatment ranges from benign neglect to surgical decompression through resection of the volar transverse carpal ligament. Local injections of Xylocaine and a steroid preparation may provide temporary relief. Care must be taken to avoid penetration of the nerve. Other treatment modalities include analgesics, restriction of sodium intake, and splinting the wrist at night to avoid hyperflexion during sleep.

Bicipital Tendinitis

Bicipital tendinitis is an inflammation occurring at the site where the tendon of origin of the long head of the biceps brachii passes through the humeral bicipital groove and is surrounded by a synovial sheath continuous with the shoulder joint. The examiner can confirm inflammation of the synovial sheath in two ways: One, by palpating the groove which lies between the greater and lesser tuberosities of the humerus, and two, by having the patient fully rotate the humerus internally by reaching behind the back to touch the opposite scapula.

Treatment includes avoiding extreme or stressed movements of the shoulder while gently preserving range of motion. Superficial heat or cold may be used, along with analgesics and anti-inflammatory agents, in the acute condition. Local injection of Xylocaine and Decadron can be helpful, as can deep heat—particularly ultrasound—if the condition is no longer acute.

Localized Elbow Ulnar Neuropathy (Tardy Ulnar Nerve Palsy)

The symptom of localized elbow ulnar neuropathy is commonly a vague discomfort rather than a frank pain. The discomfort usually includes numbness and tingling along the ulnar side of the hand. This neuropathy is caused by compression of the ulnar nerve as it passes through the olecranon groove of the medial epicondyle of the humerus. The compression may be due to repeated trauma around the elbow, scarring from a previous elbow fracture, or susceptibility of the ulnar nerve because of an underlying neuropathy. Examination may reveal thickening of the ulnar nerve in the olecranon groove and tenderness to palpation. There may be a sensory deficit of the little and ring fingers. Atrophy and weakness of the interosseous muscles are not necessarily late signs. Prolonged or impaired nerve conduction upon testing the elbow segment of the ulnar nerve is the most reliable diagnostic test.

Treatment ranges from avoiding further stress to the nerve, to surgical translocation of the ulnar nerve to the front of the medial humeral epicondyle.

Radicular Pain (Cervical or Lumbar)

Cervical radiculopathy most commonly affects roots C6 and C7 and, less frequently, roots C5 and C8. Lumbar radiculopathy most commonly affects roots L5 and S1 (producing sciatica) and, less frequently, roots L3 and L4 (in a femoral nerve distribution). The specific diagnosis of radiculopathy depends upon the pattern of pain and sensory changes (dermatome pattern), alteration of muscle stretch reflexes, and muscle weakness and atrophy (myotome pattern). Although it is usually unilateral, radiculopathy may also be bilateral. Cervical radiculopathy may coexist with lumbar root pains, as well as with other causes of musculoskeletal pain. Electromyography is a useful test for identifying signs of lower motor neuron involvement indicative of a radiculopathy.

Unless sensory and motor changes are severe, nonoperative treatment is most frequently beneficial. The recommended approaches consist of periods of rest and removal of physical and emotional stress, analgesics and anti-inflammatory agents, support devices such as a cervical collar or lumbosacral support, traction for the cervical spine, graded exercises for mobilization, postural control, and muscle strengthening. For further elaboration on the management of cervical and arm pain or low-back pain, the reader is referred to works by Cailliet on musculoskeletal pain syndromes.[4]

Myofascial Pain (Fibrositis)

Myofascial pain is a ubiquitous condition of young and middle aged adults, more commonly women, between the ages of 20 and 50. Entirely benign, but extremely troublesome for the sufferer, myofascial pain is referred to by several names, including levator scapulae syndrome, scalene anticus syndrome, temporomandibular syndrome, and others. Muscles of the axial skeleton are affected from the base of the skull to the sacroiliac joints, producing almost constant dull, aching pain characterized by periods of sharper exacerbations. Patients sometimes experience inconstant symptoms of numbness and tingling. The pathology is not clear. When symptoms are florid, the examiner, in palpating the muscle, can discern pea-sized to almond-sized "knots," which have a "ropy" texture when the examining finger is rolled over them. Rolling the finger over the knot frequently produces the characteristic jump reaction from the patient as he pulls away from the examiner. Intensification of the symptoms, but not in a consistent time-locked relationship, is associated with episodes of physical or mental stress. For example, if the worsening of symptoms is delayed by 24 to 48 hours after the inciting stress, there can be an enormous degree of confusion when the patient tries to relate an inciting event to the crescendo of symptoms. Frequently the patient becomes aware of the distressful symptoms for the first time after some trauma, such as an automobile whiplash injury. Even though fibrositis is an entirely benign condition, there seems to be no way to bring about a cure; fibrositis runs its own course. However, with massive reassurance the patient can learn to manage life with the condition, if he maintains a judicious balance between rest and activity, occasional use of mild analgesics and anti-inflammatory agents, application of local heat or cold (coupled with muscle stretching and postural correction maneuvers), and the employment of psychological techniques to induce relaxation and reduce the tensions associated with stress.

Relationship of Physical Examination to FASQ Functional Systems

In this section a series of tests is presented, accompanied by an explanation of the significance of each. The decision to administer specific tests depends on findings from the FASQ. The rationale for this decision-making process is described fully in Chapter 2. However, the importance of employing a systematic process, such as outlined below, cannot be overemphasized.

> Neck, Upper Limbs, and Hands
>> Types of Tests
>> Testing Maneuvers
>>> Arm Drift
>>> Range of Motion
>>> Muscle Strength
>>> Reflexes
>>> Sensory
>>> Coordination With the Patient Seated
>>> Pain Responses for Carpal Tunnel Syndrome
> Lower Limbs and Trunk
>> Types of Tests
>> Testing Maneuvers
>>> Balance
>>> Range of Motion
>>> Muscle Strength
>>> Reflexes
>>> Sensory
>>> Coordination
>>> Pain Response
> Speaking and Writing
> Seeing and Reading
> Hearing

Stamina and Endurance
Cognition
Emotional Adaptability

Neck, Upper Limbs, and Hands

Types of Tests

1. Arm drift
2. Range of motion of neck, upper limbs, digits
3. Muscle strength of neck, shoulders, elbows, and forearms, wrists, digits
4. Reflexes
5. Sensory testing of graphesthesia, double simultaneous stimulation
6. Coordination testing of finger-to-nose, rapid alternating hand slapping, fingers-to-thumb
7. Pain responses to Tinel and Phelan maneuvers

Testing Maneuvers

Arm Drift

Test Have the patient who is in a sitting position raise his arms forward to 90 degrees at the shoulders with elbows extended, wrists neutral, and digits extended with palms up. Have the patient with eyes closed maintain the hands about 12 inches apart and parallel with the floor. A positive sign for "drift" is represented by lack of holding the position for 15 to 30 seconds (*e.g.,* the elbow begins to flex or the forearm pronates). The patient should be able to maintain the position even if the examiner taps the suspended arm to displace it a bit.

Significance A positive test is an early sign of hypotonia, which may be the result of subtle damage to proprioception or the motor innervation of the muscles. Hypotonia at times may be due to cerebellar disease or muscular disease. Fine motor/sensory skills may be affected, although gross motor/sensory skills may not.

Range of Motion

Neck Test Have the patient perform the following movements in sequence: (1) touch the chin to the chest, (2) elevate the chin so that the face is toward the ceiling, (3) from the neutral position, turn the chin toward one shoulder and then the other, without elevating the shoulder, and (4) bring each ear toward its respective shoulder, without elevating the shoulder. If restriction is present, gently help each movement manually without forcing movement.

Significance Normal range of motion in the presence of complaints of pain about the neck, upper trunk, or upper limb suggests that there is neither structural change about the facet joints, a significant degree of muscle spasm, nor impingement of a nerve root. Thus, the origin of pain is likely to be benign, rather than one of a more serious nature. Gross motor/sensory and fine motor/sensory skills may be unaffected by limited mobility of the neck.

Upper Limbs Test Use a goniometer to record range of motion according to the accompanying chart (see Fig. 3-2A).

Digits Test Use a goniometer on the dorsal surface of the digits to record range of motion according to the chart (see Fig. 3-2B).

Significance The pain of active bursitis, tendinitis, or arthritis is associated with limitation of the affected joint. Limited joint mobility may be a residual finding from prior episodes of bursitis, tendinitis, or arthritis, with or without appreciable pain. Gross motor/sensory and fine motor/sensory skills may be affected by limited upper limb and digit mobility. Depending on the degree and distribution of limited joint motions, ability to perform functional tasks may be affected very little or a great deal.

Muscle Strength

Neck, Shoulder, Elbow and Forearm, Wrist, Digits Test Test strength against manual resistance of muscle groups and record according to the Muscle Strength Test of Upper Extremities chart (see Fig. 3-3).

Significance Gross motor/sensory skills may be affected by subtle weakness in any part of the neck or upper limbs. Fine motor/sensory skills are usually affected by weakness of muscles of the forearm, wrist, and digits.

Reflexes

Examine reflexes according to Table 3-5.

Significance Reflexes, per se, do not affect the functional response, but are indicators of the state of the peripheral and central nervous systems.

Sensory

Test Graphesthesia and double simultaneous stimulation (DSS) provide the most information on sensation with the least time expended. Graphesthesia is tested by drawing numerals on the tips of the digits with a pencil point while the patient's eyes are closed. DSS is tested using two simultaneous touch stimuli to different locations on the same or different limbs with the patient's eyes closed. In each case the patient is asked to report the locations of the stimuli.

Significance A patient with good range of motion of joints and strength may have marked limitation of function if sensory loss is present. In some cases, this may closely simulate muscle weakness. Graphesthesia and double simultaneous stimulation represent the highest integration of sensory information in the nervous system and, if impaired, may therefore be an early indication of disease of the nervous system. Gross motor/sensory and fine motor/sensory skills may be affected.

TABLE 3-5   Tendon and Other Reflex Tests

Reflex	Location of Tap	Response	Nerve
Upper Limbs			
Deltoid	Near humeral condyle	Abduction of arm	C5,6
Biceps	On tendon	Forearm flexes	C5,6
Brachiorad	On radial insertion	Forearm flexes	C6
Triceps	Triceps tendon	Forearm extends	C7,8
Pron teres	Medial distal radius	Forearm pronates	C7
Fl. car rad	Near radial styloid	Wrist flexes	C7
Finger flex	Finger tendons	Fingers flex	C8
Palmo-mental	Scratch palm	Chin twitches	Release
Grasp	Stroke palm	Grasp	Release
Hoffman	Flick middle finger	Thumb flexes	C8
Lower Limbs			
Adductor	Adductor insertion	Adduction of thigh	L3
Quadriceps	Patellar tendon	Knee extends	L3,4
Medial hams	Inner hamstring tendon	Knee flexes	L5
Lateral ham	Outer hamstring tendon	Knee flexes	S1
Achilles	Triceps surae tendon	Foot plantar flexes	S1,2
Plantar	Scratch lateral sole and across metatarsal heads	Extension of great toe, fanning of other toes, knee flexes	Release
Other Reflexes			
Corneal	Cotton to corn-scl jct	Closure of eyelid	Cr V,VII
Jaw	Slack jaw	Closure of jaw	Cr V
McCarthy	Supraorbital ridge	Lower lid moves up	Cr V,VII
Gag	Touch posterior pharynx	Palate elevates	Cr IX,X
Sternomas/trapezius	Muscle insertion	Contraction	Cr XI
Superfi abd	Scratch abdominal wall	Contraction	T 7–12
Deep abdom	Deep tap to stretch musc	Contraction	T 7–12
Cremasteric	Stroke prox inner thigh	Elevation of testes	S 2,3,4
Anal	Stroke perianal skin	Sphincter contracts	S 2,3,4
Bulbocavern	Stroke dors glans penis	Compressor urethra	S 2,3,4

Coordination With the Patient Seated

Finger-to-Nose Test The examiner places his finger approximately 2 feet from the patient's nose and asks the patient to touch his or her nose and the examiner's finger alternatively as fast as possible. For additional refinement, the examiner's finger becomes a moving target within a radius of about 2 feet from the patient.

Alternate Hand Slapping Test Have the patient slap his knee alternately with the palm, and then the back of the hand, as rapidly as possible. Each strike should make a slight slapping sound.

Fingers-to-Thumb Test Have the patient move his thumb to and fro while tapping the pad of each finger as rapidly as possible.

Significance Disturbances of movement may be caused by lesions of the cerebellum, muscle disease, disease of peripheral nerves, disease of posterior columns, and disease of the frontal and postcentral cerebral cortex. Gross motor/sensory and fine motor/sensory skills are affected by disturbed coordination.

Pain Responses for Carpal Tunnel Syndrome

Tinel's Sign Percuss the volar surface of the wrist at the proximal crease toward the radial side of the palmaris longus tendon. Attempt to reproduce pain or tingling in the fingers.

Phelan's Sign Passively hold the patient's wrists in a posture of full flexion for a full minute. Ask if pain or tingling in the fingers is reproduced.

Significance The pain from carpal tunnel syndrome is frequently misidentified as either due to arthritis of the hand or thoracic outlet syndrome, or else a pinched nerve in the neck. It is an important disorder to identify correctly because confirmation by electromyography and nerve conduction testing is reliable and surgical decompression is effective treatment. The condition affects fine motor/sensory skills, most probably through interference with epicritic sensation, and later through muscle weakness and atrophy.

Lower Limbs and Trunk

Types of Tests

1. Balance by Romberg test, tandem walking, hopping, and stepping up onto a chair seat
2. Range of motion of spine, lower limbs, straight leg raising
3. Muscle strength of trunk, lower limbs
4. Reflexes
5. Sensory testing of toe proprioception, graphesthesia, double simultaneous stimulation
6. Coordination testing of heel-to-shin, rapid toe tapping
7. Pain responses to superficial and deep stimulation

Testing Maneuvers

Balance

Test
1. Romberg test. Have the patient place both feet tightly together with eyes closed, and then test balancing on either foot alone, with slight support to the patient's hand
2. Tandem walking with heel to toe

3. Hopping on either foot, with slight support given to the patient's hand

4. Stepping up and down from a chair seat with either foot

Significance The Romberg test is positive when unsteadiness is increased by closure of the eyes. It is positive when proprioceptive sensation to the lower limbs is lost due to disease, such as tabes dorsalis, subacute combined degeneration, or polyneuritis. Unsteadiness is to be differentiated from cerebellar disease, hysteria, or normal swaying. Tandem walking, hopping on either foot and stepping up on a chair seat are further tests of balance, to be used with precautions in questionable cases.

Range of Motion

Spine Test Inspect the patient who is in a sitting position from behind and look for asymmetry of shoulder levels, hip levels, or paraspinal prominences. Palpate for paraspinal muscle spasm. Inspect the patient who is in a standing position in a similar fashion and look for differences between sitting and standing. Observe spinal flexion, extension, and lateral flexion while the patient is both standing and sitting. Look for any stiffness or discontinuities of movement.

Significance Normal range of motion in the presence of complaints of pain about the trunk, back, hips, and lower limbs suggests that there is neither lack of structural change about the facet joints, a significant degree of muscle spasm, nor impingement of a nerve root. Thus, the origin of pain is likely to be benign, such as postural strain, rather than serious. Almost all skills, except cognitive/communicative, may be affected by painful and limited mobility of the spine.

Lower Limbs Test Use a goniometer to record range of motion according to the range of motion of lower extremity chart (see Fig. 3-2C).

Significance Neuromuscular and musculoskeletal disorders particularly, but almost any disorder with prolonged immobilization, may result in loss of range of motion. Loss of hip or knee extension, or a tight heel cord producing plantar flexion, are particularly detrimental to standing and ambulation. Walking with a hip or knee flexion contracture can contribute to low-back strain. On the other hand, a stiff hip, knee, or ankle that is stable, fixed in a functional position, and not painful may not limit functional performance in a major way. A knee fixed in extension, however, can limit transferring skills.

Straight Leg Raising Test With the patient lying supine, gently raise one leg, passively keeping the knee fully extended. The end-point of movement is marked by pain that prohibits further elevation or an indication of motion of the pelvis. At the end-point of movement, a sharp motion to dorsiflex the ankle confirms a positive test if the patient feels additional radicular pain. Test each leg separately.

Significance This maneuver places a stretch on the lumbosacral nerve roots and is a test to confirm the presence of nerve root irritation as a possible contributing cause for a painful back and leg condition.

Muscle Strength

Trunk, Hip, Knee, Ankle and Foot, Toes Test Test strength against manual resistance of muscle groups and record according to the accompanying chart (see Fig. 3-4).

Significance Gross motor/sensory, transferring, fine motor/sensory, or cognitive/motor skills may be affected by weakness of the lower limb.

Reflexes

Tendon and Other Reflex Tests Examine reflexes as in Table 3-5.

Significance Reflexes, per se, do not affect the functional response but are indicators of the state of the peripheral and central nervous systems.

Sensory

Test Toe proprioception, graphesthesia, and double simultaneous stimulation (DSS) provide the most information about sensation with the least time expended. Graphesthesia is tested by drawing numerals on the dorsum of the foot with a pencil point while the patient's eyes are closed. DSS is tested using two simultaneous touch stimuli to different locations of the same or different limbs with the patient's eyes closed. In each case the patient is asked to report the stimuli.

Significance A patient with good range of motion of joints and strength may have marked limitation of function if there is sensory loss, which may closely simulate muscle weakness. Graphesthesia, DSS, and proprioception represent the highest integration of sensory information in the nervous system and, if impaired, may be an early indication of disease of the nervous system. Functional skills may be markedly affected by sensory loss; thus, it is important to ascertain the integrity of sensation as well as motor function of the lower limbs.

Coordination

Heel-to-Shin Test While the patient is supine, not seated, ask him or her to slide the heel of one foot smoothly up and down the anterior edge of the shin several times.

Toe Tapping Test While the patient is seated, ask him or her to rest the heel on the floor and raise and lower the forefoot rapidly to produce a short series of taps.

Significance Disturbances of movement may be caused by lesions of the cerebellum, muscle disease, disease of peripheral nerves, disease of posterior columns, and disease of the frontal and postcentral cerebral cortex.

Pain Response

Superficial Test Use a pin prick to determine superficial pain sensation.

Deep Test Pinch the Achilles tendon with gradually increasing pressure to determine deep pain sensation.

Significance Since in the course of ordinary standing and walking, the lower limbs must absorb stress and are subjected to injury, it is important to ascertain protopathic protective sensation. Insensitive ulcers on the plantar surface of the foot can cause prolonged and expensive disability. Some highlights of the more common abnormal gaits are presented in Table 3-6.

Speaking and Writing

Test Language consists of listening, reading, speaking, and writing, each of which is integrated with the others and with other conscious experiences in what may be called "symbolic formulation" or a central language process. Language that involves receiving and transmitting is processed by Wernicke's and Broca's areas of the brain. Impairment of this integrative process affecting the ability to handle language is known as aphasia. Aphasia is to be distinguished from dysarthria, which is a motor defect in articulation, and from apraxia, which is an impairment of volitional activity, in particular, a discrepancy between speaking performance and other language performances.

Different forms of aphasia are distinguished according to characteristics outlined in Table 3-7.

Significance It is important to determine whether a communicative deficit is due to impairment of one or more of the modalities of language encoding or decoding, a mental processing problem such as confusion or dementia, a mechanical problem such as dysphonia or dysarthria, or a hearing problem. Precise diagnosis, including the type of aphasia, if present, is necessary for appropriate corrective measures and appropriate management of any associated disability—particularly since any communicative disorder can be very frustrating to the patient and family members in striving to maintain life roles.

Seeing and Reading

Test Visual acuity is the principal determinant of a person's ability for seeing and reading. Visual acuity is tested separately for each eye for distant and near vision using the appropriate charts. Gross visual field testing is done most commonly by confrontation during which the examiner faces the patient being tested. A simple method for recording the results of testing follows:[12]

Normal	No loss of visual field or acuity
Grade 1	Lenses required, or mild corrected visual deficit (better than 20/50); able to read standard newspaper print
Grade 2	Corrected acuity about 20/50 or worse; magnifying lenses or large print necessary for reading
Grade 3	Corrected acuity about 20/100 or worse; essentially unable to read
Grade 4	Legal blindness; corrected acuity 20/200 or worse

TABLE 3-6   Common Abnormal Gaits

Gait	Characteristic Presentation	Associated Pathology
Regal, lordotic	Shoulders and upper torso tilt backward while pelvis tilts forward; coupled with long pronounced arm swings.	Muscular dystrophy (muscle fibers affected)
Propulsive, festinating	Short, quick steps with progressively increasing speed; may run into wall or fall due to inability to stop abruptly or change direction easily.	Parkinson's disease (or other basal ganglia diseases)
Steppage	Foot drop, exaggerated hip and knee flexion, and toe strike prior to heel strike.	Paralysis peroneal innervated muscles
Trendelenburg	Pelvis drops on side opposite to the weakened weight-bearing extremity.	Weak hip abductors
Short leg	Moderate inequality compensation involves pelvis drop on affected side, elevation of shoulder on the normal side, and dipping of shoulder on the side of the shortened limb. Exaggerated flexion of opposite hip, knee, and ankle may be exhibited. Severe inequalities may be compensated by walking on toes with shorter limb.	Unequal leg length
Triceps surae	Pelvis drops on the same side as weakened weight-bearing extremity.	Weak plantar flexor
Waddling	"Drunken sailor" look.	Bilaterally weak hip abductors; bilaterally dislocated hips
Spastic	Scissoring or circumducted gait.	Hemiparesis; diplegia
Ataxic	Dysmetria and lack of coordination with wide-based, staggering (or jerky) gait, flailing of body to retain balance.	Cerebellar dysfunction; posterior column impairment
Gluteus maximus	Backward lurch of trunk and pelvis after heel strike on affected side, accompanied by forward protrusion of affected hip.	Hip abductor (gluteus maximus) weakness
Gluteus medius	In uncompensated limp: During stance phase, downward tilt of pelvis causes leg swing that is too long; results in exaggerated hip and knee flexion on opposite side. In compensated limp: Trunk lurches toward affected side during stance phase, accompanied by slight drop of opposite hip and marked dipping of shoulder on affected side.	Hip extensor (gluteus medius) weakness

Significance The impairment of blindness is especially overwhelming when combined with a limiting neuromusculoskeletal impairment, thus taking away an important means for compensatory adjustment in personal, instrumental, mobility, leisure, economic, or vocational roles. Many patients with visual deficit have low-grade vision and are not totally blind. Certain low-vision aids can be quite helpful in promoting maximal functioning. For a comprehensive discussion of the problems of visual impairments, see Chapter 13.

Hearing

Test Screen hearing by bringing a watch from beyond the auditory range into the zone of hearing and ask the patient to indicate when he first hears the sound. The Rinne tuning fork of medium pitch (C = 256 vibrations per second) test must be used. The normal person hears the tuning fork better by air conduction (AC better than BC). If the person has obstructive deafness, bone conduction is better than air conduction. If the person has nerve deafness, the normal relations are kept in the deaf ear. Weber test: If the base of the tuning fork is placed on the middle of the forehead of a person with nerve deafness, the person will hear the fork better in the normal ear. If the fork is placed in the middle of the forehead of a person with obstructive deafness, the person will hear the tuning better in the deaf ear. If the person has obstructive deafness and the tuning fork is placed on the mastoid process of the deaf ear and compared with a normal ear, for example, the examiner's, the person will hear the tuning fork in the deaf ear longer than in the normal ear. Using the same test, if the person has nerve deafness, he will hear the tuning fork longer in the normal ear than in the deaf ear. If hearing is impaired, the electric audiometer is used and an audiogram is made to test hearing sense accurately.

Significance The importance of hearing loss is commonly underestimated, and the diagnosis of hearing loss is easily overlooked in young children and older people. The psychological isolating effects of hearing loss can be devastating. Therefore, early detection can prevent significant disability in both younger and older patients. For a comprehensive discussion of the problems of hearing impairments, see Chapter 14.

Stamina and Endurance

Stamina and endurance, which are related to capacity for low-resistance, high-repetition activities, implies adequate systems for aerobic metabolism, hence, cardiopulmonary fitness. Walking, jogging, bicycling, and swimming are among the most popular recreational methods for increasing and sustaining cardiopulmonary fitness, that is, stamina and endurance. Walking at the rate of 3 miles per hour for 5 minutes is equal to a distance of approximately one quarter mile.

The rate of work, which is power, is expressed in kilocalories per minute. One Kcal per minute is approximately the basal metabolic rate for an average sized adult (70kg). One Kcal correlates to about 6 liters per minute of pulmonary ventilation at rest. For many people a work rate greater than 5 Kcal per minute usually results in the accumulation of an oxygen debt and a rise in the serum lactic acid level. Five Kcal per minute is about the maximum one can maintain for several hours. It is this physiological fact that probably sets the limit on light industrial work or comfortable walking speed (Tables 3-8 and 3-9).

TABLE 3-7   Forms of Aphasia

	Broca's	Wernicke's	Conduction
Lesion	Frontal lobe	Posterior superior temporal lobe	Arcuate fasciculus
Speech flow	Nonfluent	Fluent (verbal paraphasia)	Fluent (literal paraphasia)
Comprehension	Good	Poor	Good
Repetition	Defective, but better than speech	Poor	Poor
Naming	Defective, but better than speech	Defective, but better than repetition	Fair
Reading	Good, or difficulty with comprehension	Poor	Good comprehension Cannot read aloud
Writing	Defective	Jibberish	Defective, but improves if trained
Praxis	Defective	May be OK	Defective
Drawing	Defective	Defective, but can imitate	Defective
Other	80% have right hemiparesis	20% have right hemiparesis	

Anomic	Isolation	Alexia with Agraphia	Alexia without Agraphia
Form of isolation aphasia Posterior parietal lobe, or may not be localized	Functional separation from cortex	Angular gyrus, parietal lobe	Calcarine cortex and splenium of corpus callosum
Fluent	Fluent only when spoken to	Fluent	Fluent
Good to Fair	Poor	Good, except orally spelled words	Good
Good	Echolalia, repeats songs	Good	Good
Defective	Poor	Often defective	Good
Good	Poor	Poor, except numbers	Poor
Good	Poor	Poor	Good
Good	Poor	Good	Good
Defective	Poor	Defective	Good
	Very rare Typically carbon monoxide poisoning		Right hemianopia

(Adapted from personal communication with N Geschwind and F Benson)

TABLE 3-8   Energy Cost of Light Activities in Adults[5]

Activity	Average Energy Cost (Kcal/min/70 Kg)
Sleeping	0.9
Lying quietly	1.0
Lying quietly doing mental arithmetic	1.04
Sitting at ease	1.2 –1.6
Sitting, writing	1.9 –2.2
Sitting, playing cards	1.9 –2.1
Sitting, playing musical instrument	2.0 –3.2
Standing at ease	1.4 –2.0
Walking, 1 mph	2.3
Standing, washing and shaving	2.5 –2.6
Standing, dressing and undressing	2.3 –3.3
Light housework	1.7 –3.0
Heavy housework	3.0 –6.0
Office work	1.3 –2.5
Typing, mechanical typewriter	1.26–1.57
Typing, electric typewriter	1.13–1.39
Walking, 2 mph	3.1
Light industrial work	2.0 –5.0
Walking, 3 mph (average comfortable walking speed)	4.3

The entire oxygen transport operation is dependent on the body's ability to increase the oxygen supply to meet the demands imposed by dynamic exercise. The maximum amount of oxygen that can be transported from the lungs to the muscles and other tissues is called the maximum oxygen uptake (VO2 max). Except for patients with severe lung disease or for persons exercising at high altitudes, the capacity of the lungs to replenish the blood with oxygen does not limit maximal oxygen uptake. Maximum oxygen uptake, which sets the upper limit of endurance physiologically, is a standard measure of cardiovascular fitness and functional capacity of circulation, not of lung capacity. A decrease in maximum oxygen uptake occurs in persons who lead a sedentary life and is a part of the aging process. Whether this deterioration is noticeably slowed by physical conditioning remains unclear. There are four functional classes and five therapeutic classes of cardiac disease (Table 3-10). The symptom criteria include dyspnea, angina, syncope, palpitations, cold sweat (autonomic), and fatigue. A MET equals one basal metabolic unit (3.5–4.0 ml oxygen/kg/min).

Test Maximum oxygen uptake is measured by performing a series of work tests on a motor-driven treadmill or a bicycle ergometer during which the heartbeat, electrocardiogram, blood pressure, and sometimes the amount of oxygen consumed are monitored. The exercise is made progressively harder, and the uptake of oxygen per minute rises steadily until the maximum uptake (VO2 max) is attained. After this point, most people can still exercise harder, but the oxygen uptake cannot rise higher. However, an increase in workload can be accom-

TABLE 3-9 Approximate Energy Cost of Some Common Vocational and Recreational Activities[3]

Sitting (Light Tasks [1.5 to 4.5 MET's])	*Standing and/or Walking (Heavy tasks)*
Desk work, typing	*[(Average or range of MET's follows each task])*
Driving cars, trucks	Pushing or moving heavy objects—75 lb
Using hand tools, light assembly	(33.8 kg) or more, e.g., moving-van work 8.0
Crane operation	Cutting wood
Working levers	Power saw 2–4
Playing cards, seated games	Hand axe or saw 5–10
Machine sewing	Digging, shoveling 4–8
Flying	Wheelbarrow 4–10
Painting, recreational	Plumbing 3–8
Horseback riding, walk and trot	Snow shoveling 6–15
Golf cart, riding	Lifting and carrying
Fishing from boat, seated	20–44 lb (9–19.8 kg) 4.5
Riding mower	45–64 lb (20.2–28.8 kg) 6.0
	65–84 lb (29.3–37.8 kg) 7.5
Standing (Moderate Tasks [2.5 to 5.5	85–100 lb (38.3–4.5 kg) 8.5
MET's])	Pneumatic tool work 6.0
Standing quietly, working at own pace,	Skating, roller or ice 5–6
light assembly or hand tools	Badminton, competitive 5–7
Scrubbing, waxing, polishing	Tennis, singles 6–9
Assembly or repair of machine parts	Paddle ball, raquetball, squash, handball 7–15
Light welding, woodworking, interior	Skiing
carpentry	Downhill 5–8
Power sanding	Crosscountry 6–12
Stocking shelves	Water 5–7
Light to medium assembly line work	Hunting
Crank dollies, hitching trailers, operating	Small game 3–7
large levers, jacks	Big game 3–14
Wiring house	Swimming 4–8
Bricklaying, plastering, house painting,	Jogging, running 7–15
paperhanging	Basketball 5–12
Hoeing, raking, weeding	
Cleaning windows	
Walking (Light to Moderate Tasks [2.5 to	
5.5 MET's])	
Gas station attendant	
Carrying trays, dishes, etc.	
Walking to 4 mi/h (6.44 km/h) on level	
Billiards, bowling	
Fishing, bait casting and fly with waders	
Shuffleboard	
Volleyball, noncompetitive	
Archery	
Sail small boat	
Dancing	
Gardening	
Golf	
Tennis, doubles	
Calisthenics	
Making beds	
Mowing lawns, cast or power unit	
Table tennis	

(Brammell HL: Cardiovascular diseases. In Stolov WC, Clowers MR (eds): Handbook of Severe Disability. Washington, US Dept. of Education, RSA, 289–307 1981[3])

**TABLE 3-10   The Functional and Therapeutic Classifications of Patients
With Diseases of the Heart of the American Heart Association
(Continuous–Intermittent Permissible Work Loads)**

Functional

	Cont.	*Int.*	*Maximal*
Class I	4.0 cal/min	6.0 cal/min	6.5 METS

Patients with cardiac disease, but without resulting limitations of physical activity. Ordinary physical activity does not cause undue fatigue, palpitation, dyspnea, or anginal pain.

Class II	3.0 cal/min	4.0 cal/min	4.5 METS

Patients with cardiac disease resulting in slight limitation of physical activity. They are comfortable at rest. Ordinary physical activity results in fatigue, palpitation, dyspnea, or anginal pain.

Class III	2.0 cal/min	3.0 cal/min	3.0 METS

Patients with cardiac disease resulting in marked limitation of physical activity. They are comfortable at rest. Less than ordinary physical activity causes fatigue, palpitation, dyspnea, or anginal pain.

Class IV	1.0 cal/min	2.0 cal/min	1.5 METS

Patients with cardiac disease resulting in inability to carry on any physical activity without discomfort. Symptoms of cardiac insufficiency or of the anginal syndrome may be present even at rest. If any physical activity is undertaken, discomfort is increased.

Therapeutic

Class A   Patients with cardiac disease whose physical activity need not be restricted in any way.

Class B   Patients with cardiac disease whose ordinary physical activity need not be restricted, but who should be advised against severe or competitive efforts.

Class C   Patients with cardiac disease whose ordinary physical activity should be moderately restricted and whose more strenuous efforts should be discontinued.

Class D   Patients with cardiac disease whose ordinary physical activity should be markedly restricted.

Class E   Patients with cardiac disease who should be at complete rest, confined to bed or chair.

plished through a process known as oxygen debt, which is a temporary physiologic adjustment to extraordinary work.[6]

The measurement of heart rate and the heart rate times the mean arterial pressure (double product) are simple measurements. For a given individual at a given time, these correlate with other work measurements and should be used when oxygen uptake studies are impractical.

Significance Decreased stamina may be due to a wide range of causes: reduced cardiopulmonary reserve, severe anemia, pain or discomfort that limits activity, depression/poor motivation/anxiety, prior inactivity/deconditioning, dehydration/electrolyte imbalance, poor nutritional state, subtle neuromuscular loss, etc. A common sign is for the pulse rate to rise disproportionately to the expected amount of work output. Using all clinical data available, patients with heart disease should be classified as to functional and therapeutic classifications of the American Heart Association, according to Table 3-10. For a comprehensive discussion of the problems of cardiopulmonary rehabilitation, see Chapter 8.

Cognition

Test Orientation, registration, attention and calculation, recall, and language are easily tested using the "mini-mental state"[7,18] (Fig. 3-6).

Significance Assessment of a patient's mental status is important for appropriate planning of medical, surgical, or rehabilitative programs, or for environmental support. However, the level of function on a mental status test, per se, should not be used to set limits as to what may be expected of a particular person in a given circumstance such as achievement of independent living goals. Level of mental functioning should be taken into account, however, in providing suitable modification of an intervention in terms of timing and design of support systems. For additional information about organic mental disorders/dementia, see Chapter 15.

Emotional Adaptability

Test Level of anxiety and depression using adaptations of the Philadelphia Geriatric Center and Beck Depression scales shown in Figure 3-7.

Significance Particularly under circumstances of long-term disability, it is most important to be in touch with the patient's mood in order that plans for an intervention or system of support be appropriate. Anxiety, depression, or denial can upset the best laid plans unless the patient's responses are being carefully monitored. Since mood is subjective, it is difficult to use an objective measure with a high degree of reliability, unless the physician has become acquainted with a few assessment tools with which he has become familiar and has learned to interpret.

Summary

Range of motion examination and abbreviated muscle strength screening methods are presented that can be used easily in a primary care setting to identify whether neuromusculoskeletal impairment is causing functional limitations. Common pitfalls in muscle testing, including failure to recognize substitution or abnormal movement patterns, failure to stabilize proximal joints, and failure to palpate during motion or to test a complete range of motion are also discussed. Since abnormal walking patterns often reflect underlying physical limitations, common gait disorders also are discussed.

Maximum Score	Score	
		Orientation
5	_____	What is the (year) (season) (date) (day) (month)?
5	_____	Where are we: (state) (county) (town) (hospital) (floor)?
		Registration
3	_____	Name 3 objects: 1 second to say each. Then ask the patient all 3 after you have said them. Give 1 point for each correct answer. Then repeat them until he learns all 3. Count trials and record. Trials _____
		Attention and Calculation
5	_____	Serial 7's: 1 point for each correct. Stop with 5 answers. Alternatively spell "world" backwards.
		Recall
3	_____	Ask for the 3 objects repeated above. (1 point each.)
		Language
2	_____	Name a pencil and a watch. (1 point each)
1	_____	Repeat the following: "No ifs, ands, or buts."
3	_____	Follow a 3-stage command: "Take a paper in your hand, fold it in half, and put it on the floor." (1 point each).
1	_____	Read and obey the following: Close your eyes.
1	_____	Write a sentence.
1	_____	Copy design.
30	_____	Total score

Assess level of consciousness: _____

          Alert   Drowsy   Stupor   Coma

Instructions for Administration of Mini-Mental State Examination

Orientation

Ask for the date. Then ask specifically for parts omitted, that is, "Can you tell me what season it is?" One point for each correct answer.

Ask in turn "Can you tell me the name of this hospital (town, county, etc.)?" One point for each correct answer.

Registration

Ask the patient if you may test his memory. Then say the names of 3 unrelated objects, clearly and slowly, about 1 second for each. After you have said all 3, ask him to repeat them. This first repetition determines his score (0–3), but keep saying them until he can repeat all 3, up to 6 trials. If he does not eventually learn all 3, recall cannot be meaningfully tested.

Figure 3-6. Mini-mental state.[7,18] (above and top, opposite page)

Attention and Calculation

Ask the patient to begin with 100 and count backwards by 7. Stop after 5 subtractions (93, 86, 79, 72, 65). Score the total number of correct answers.

Recall

Ask the patient if he can recall the 3 words you previously asked him to remember. Score 0–3.

Language

Naming: Show the patient a wristwatch and ask him what it is. Repeat for pencil. Score 0–2.
Repetition: Ask the patient to repeat the sentence after you. Allow only one trial. Score 0 or 1.
3-Step Command: Give the patient a piece of paper and repeat the command. Score 1 point for each part correctly executed.
Reading: On a blank piece of paper print the sentence "Close your eyes," in letters large enough for the patient to see clearly. Ask him to read it and do what it says. Score 1 point only if he actually closes his eyes.
Writing: Give the patient a blank piece of paper and ask him to write a sentence for you. Do not dictate a sentence; it is to be written spontaneously. It must contain a subject and verb and be sensible. Correct grammar and punctuation are not necessary.
Copying: On a clean piece of paper, draw intersecting pentagons, each side about 1 inch, and ask him to copy it exactly as it is. All 10 angles must be present and 2 must intersect to score 1 point. Tremor and rotation are ignored.

Estimate the patient's level of sensorium along a continuum, from alert on the left to coma on the right.

Cutoff point $\Rightarrow$ 24 is not demented, with sensitivity of 87% and specificity of 82%.

Figure 3-6 *(continued)*

Please answer each statement below by a *Yes* or *No*:

	YES	NO
(from PGC—Philadelphia)		
Little things bother me more this year	( )	( )
I sometimes worry so much that I can't sleep	( )	( )
I get mad more than I used to	( )	( )
I take things hard	( )	( )
I get upset easily	( )	( )
I am afraid of a lot of things	( )	( )
(from BDI—Beck)		
I feel sad or blue	( )	( )
I feel discouraged about the future	( )	( )
I feel I have failed more than the average person	( )	( )
I don't enjoy things the way I used to	( )	( )
I feel bad or unworthy a good part of the time	( )	( )
I feel I would be better off dead	( )	( )
I try to put off making decisions	( )	( )

Two or more affirmative answers on the PGC questionnaire are indicative of at least moderate anxiety, and two or more affirmative answers on the BDI are indicative of at least moderate depression.[10]

Figure 3-7. Feelings and Mood Questionnaires.[10]

The process of pain evaluation is reviewed with a description of the different types of somatic pain (local, transmitted, referred, and central) and the pain evaluation history; common reasons for the persistence of chronic pain after treatment, and some common neuromusculoskeletal pain syndromes also are discussed.

Methods have been presented for examining the relevant functional systems—upper limbs and neck, manual dexterity, lower limbs and trunk, speaking and writing, seeing and reading, hearing, stamina, cognition/mental status, and affective/emotional status—in an abbreviated, orderly manner. Use of an examination, directed by findings derived from the FASQ, enables the clinician to concentrate on areas involved in activity restrictions and offers insight into potential physical or psychological etiologies of functional limitations. Results of the examination, coupled with a goal-directed care plan format as discussed in Chapter 4, allow the physician to develop treatment plans for the most deficient areas and facilitate a holistic approach to medical care as advocated by rehabilitation medicine.

References

1. Black RG: The chronic pain syndrome. Symposium on recent developments in anesthesia. Surg Clin North Am 55(4) August, 1975
2. Bonica JJ: Pain. New York, Raven Press, 1980
3. Brammell HL: Cardiovascular diseases. In Stolov WC, Clowers MR (eds): Handbook of Severe Disability, pp 289–307. US Dept. of Education, RSA, 1981
4. Cailliet R: Rene Cailliet Pain Series: Foot and Ankle Pain (2nd ed.) 1983, Hand Pain and Impairment (3rd ed.) 1982, Knee Pain and Disability (2nd ed.) 1983, Low Back Pain Syndrome (3rd ed.) 1981, Neck and Arm Pain (2nd ed.) 1981, Shoulder Pain (2nd ed.) 1981. Philadelphia, FA Davis
4. a. Cailliet R: Scoliosis. Philadelphia, FA Davis, 1975
4. b. Cailliet R: Soft Tissue and Disability. Philadelphia, FA Davis, 1977
5. Corcoran PJ: Energy expenditure during ambulation. In Downey JA, Darling RC: Physiological Basis of Rehabilitation Medicine, pp 185–198. Philadelphia, WB Saunders 1971
6. Dehn MS, Mitchell JH: Exercise. In American Heart Association: The American Heart Association Heartbook, pp 68–84. NY, EF Dutton, 1980
7. Folstein MF, Folstein SE, McHugh PR: Mini-mental state: A practical method for grading the cognitive state of patients for the clinician. J Psychiatr Res 12:189–198, 1975
8. Fordyce WE: Behavioral Methods for Chronic Pain and Illness. St Louis, CV Mosby, 1976
9. Hoppenfeld S: Physical Examination of the Spine and Extremities. New York, Appleton–Century–Crofts, 1976
10. Kane RA, Kane RL: Assessing the Elderly, p 114, p 184. Lexington, MA, DC Health & Co, 1981
11. Kottke FS, Stillwell GK, Lehmann JF: Krusen's Handbook of Physical Medicine and Rehabilitation, 3rd ed. Philadelphia, WB Saunders, 1982
12. Kurtzke JF: A proposal for a uniform minimum record of disability in multiple sclerosis. Acta Neurologica Scandinavica (Suppl) 87, 64, 110–129, 1981

13. Matterson RS: Physical medicine and rehabilitation for the medical practitioner. In Practice of Medicine, Chapter 20. Hagerstown, Harper & Row, 1978
14. Mayo Clinic: Clinical Examinations in Neurology, 3rd ed, pp 222–230. WB Saunders, 1971
15. Melzack R: The Puzzle of Pain. London, Penguin, 1973
16. Merskey H. Pain terms: A list with definitions and notes on usage: IASP Subcommittee on Taxonomy. Pain 6:249–252, 1979
17. Polley HF, Hunder, GG: Rheumatologic Interviewing and Physical Examination of the Joints, 2nd ed. Philadelphia, WB Saunders, 1978
18. Roca RP, Klein, LE, Kirby SM, McArthur JC, Vogelsang GB, Folstein MF, Smith CR: Recognition of dementia among medical patients. Arch Intern Med 144:73–75, 1984
19. Rosse C, Clawson OK: Introduction to the Musculoskeletal System. New York, Harper & Row, 1970
20. Rusk HA: Rehabilitation Medicine, p 10. St. Louis, CV Mosby, 1977
21. Sternbach, RA: Pain Patients, Traits and Treatment. New York, Academic Press, 1974
22. Swezey RL: Arthritis: Rational Therapy and Rehabilitation. Philadelphia, WB Saunders, 1978
23. Travell JG, Rinzler SH. Scientific exhibit: The myofascial genesis of pain. Postgrad med 11:425, 1952
24. Zohn DA, Mennel JM. Musculoskeletal Pain: Principles of Physical Diagnosis and Physical Treatment, Boston, Little, Brown, & Co, 1976

CHAPTER 4
Documenting Functional Assessment in the Medical Record

Administration of the Functional Assessment Screening Questionnaire (FASQ) provides a means to ascertain efficiently a profile of the patient that represents his range of activities. Analysis of the data obtained from the FASQ gives the physician important information about the patient that is fundamental to successful treatment. The FASQ reveals the patient's perception of his own health and provides a picture of his integration. The FASQ identifies also the functional limitations and skill deficits that contribute to a patient's disability. With this background information, the physician can perform a physical examination to confirm the degree to which impairment contributes to disability. In the full diagnostic workup, the physician also will be considering other factors contributing to disability, such as environmental limitations, psychological factors, unrealistic expectations, or inappropriate social pressures or barriers. Treatment plans based on this comprehensive information then can be directed toward preserving and enhancing the patient's health and well-being.

When assessments are conducted periodically over time, trends and changes in functioning are revealed. Such information provides crucial documentation of the improvement, maintenance, or deterioration of a patient's community living skills and the degree to which a sick role is being perpetuated or reversed. The addition of current diagnostic information completes the picture of the course and consequences of chronic health impairment.

The SOAP Note

Information obtained from the functional assessment is readily incorporated into the outpatient medical record by means of the SOAP note. The acronym stands for Subjective data, Objective data, Assessment, and Plan. The SOAP note,[1,2] a protocol for entering progress notes in the medical record, encourages systematic and complete data collection, analysis, and planning.

After the following steps have been completed, the clinician is ready to record the SOAP note.

1. Completing of the FASQ to provide subjective data on perceived health status and levels of difficulty in performing common tasks
2. Scoring the number of tasks performed easily or with difficulty to obtain an overall picture of functioning
3. Using the *functional systems* to identify those conditions that may be contributing to limitations in activity
4. Examining the patient to identify specific problem areas
5. Analyzing subjective and objective data to determine if known and suspected diagnoses account for the activity limitations (if not, other factors are to be considered)
6. Formulating treatment plans focused on needs according to areas of most severe limitation and those amenable to correction

In a standard SOAP note, the *subjective* data consist of the patient's signs and symptoms. This information is derived from patient complaints or comments. *Objective* data are obtained from results of the physical examination, mental status test, laboratory tests, radiologic, electrodiagnostic, cardiopulmonary stress tests, and other diagnostic procedures. Previously documented diagnoses and relevant social history are additional objective data. The *assessment* is an analysis of both subjective and objective data to determine whether the diagnosis is consistent with the patient's symptoms and complaints, or whether additional pathologies, impairments, or environmental factors must be considered. The *plan* consists of investigation of unresolved issues, amelioration of treatable problems, consultation with specialists, and preparation of the patient and family for the necessary adjustments to illness.

Incorporating the FASQ Into the SOAP Note

The SOAP note is well suited for integrating functional assessment into the stream of medical information. The FASQ can be incorporated into the subjective, objective, assessment, and planning sections as illustrated in Figure 4-1 and described in the following paragraphs.

Subjective Data

The first four questions of the FASQ, which measure self-perception of general health, provide a possible score of from 20 to 0 for the SOAP note. The fifteen common task items, which are graded on a four-point scale of difficulty, provide a gross picture of the patient's normal level of functioning for the SOAP note.

Energy expenditure, which can be very important for patients with cardiopulmonary impairments because their physical performances should approximate their physiological potential, is measured by means of a metabolic equivalent number (MET). The higher the MET number, the more strenuous the

Name:_____Age:_____Date:_____

Problem Title: Personal Functioning

Subjective

General Health

	EXCE	GOOD	AVERAGE	POOR	VPOOR
In comparison with others of your age, how well do you feel in terms of:					
1. Your general state of health?	5	4	3	2	1
2. Your ability to be active?	5	4	3	2	1
3. Your ability to do *needed* things?	5	4	3	2	1
4. Your ability to do *desired* things?	5	4	3	2	1

Health Score: _____

Functional Task Grading

4 = EASY: No difficulty performing the task
3 = SOME: Some difficulty performing the task, but can still manage it well enough
2 = A LOT: Still able to do the activity, but has a lot of difficulty attempting it
1 = UNABLE: Although the individual attempts to perform the task, it is too difficult
0 = NOT APPLICABLE: Someone else in the household does this task or else it does not get done

Functional Tasks Ease versus Difficulty	Energy Cost in METS	Up	Ma	Lo	Sp	Se	He	St	Co	Af
P _ Cutting toenails	1–2	( )	[ ]	( )		( )				
_ Getting up from a low seat	2–3			[ ]				( )		
_ Climbing stairs	4–5			[ ]				[ ]		
I _ Washing windows and walls	5–6	[ ]	( )	( )		( )		( )		
_ Grocery shopping	4–5	( )	( )	( )	( )	( )	( )	( )	[ ]	( )
_ Handling finances	1–2		( )			( )			[ ]	( )
L _ Playing sports	7+	( )	( )	( )		( )		[ ]		
_ Conversing	1–2				[ ]		[ ]		( )	( )
_ Participating in social activities	3–4	( )	( )	( )	( )	( )	[ ]	( )	( )	[ ]
O _ Concentrating	1–2					( )	( )		[ ]	[ ]
_ Sitting for long periods	1–2			[ ]						
_ Standing for long periods	3–4			[ ]				( )		
_ Reaching, grasping, pinching	2–3	[ ]	( )	( )						
T _ Driving an automobile	2–3	( )	( )	( )			[ ]		( )	( )
_ Riding a bus	4–5	( )	( )	( )	( )	[ ]		( )	( )	( )

_____Task Score, of which
    _____Tasks are easy (grade 4) and
    _____Tasks are not applicable (grade 0)

Figure 4-1. Problem-oriented (SOAP) note protocol for identifying and meeting patient needs related to difficulties with personal functioning.

Objective   (Pertinent results of history, physical, laboratory and X-ray examinations)

(Se) Seeing and reading	(Sp) Speaking and writing	(He) Hearing
(Ma) Manual dexterity	(Af) Affective (emotional)	(Co) Cognition
(Up) Upper limb and neck	(Lo) Lower limb and trunk	(St) Stamina (CP)

Assessment

Evaluation of whether examination of the functional systems satisfactorily reflects the documented diagnoses and impairments and satisfactorily incorporates the subjective and objective data or whether additional diagnoses or impairments need to be considered. Are subjective and objective data congruent or incongruent?

Plan

(1) Investigation of unresolved issues; (2) amelioration of treatable impairments; (3) rehabilitation medicine consultation if disability is significant; and (4) preparation for personal and community adjustments and community supports. (Does the plan recognize unrealistic expectations, problems of compliance, over or underutilization of health care resources, or difficulties related to stress among family members?)

Evaluator(s)_____

Figure 4-1 (*continued*)

activity (see Chap. 3). Patients reporting consistent difficulty with high MET count activities in the absence of any obvious musculoskeletal or neurological deficits, should be evaluated either for cardiopulmonary deficiencies or psychosocial difficulties. The MET score may also be entered into the SOAP note. The MET system is described in detail in Chapter 10.

The "functional systems" survey discussed in Chapter 2 highlights body systems that may be involved in activity limitations and helps pinpoint areas to be examined more extensively during the physical examination. The brief functional systems chart also helps the physician to consider systems such as vision, hearing, cognition, and affect, which otherwise might be overlooked.

Objective Data

Objective data collected focus the examination on specific areas that may be deficient and cover regions identified by the functional systems chart as being potentially involved in difficulties with performance. Reported difficulties in tasks such as getting up from a low seat, climbing stairs, or standing for long periods of time, for example, would suggest that the examiner undertake detailed examination of the lower limbs and trunk. Recorded objective data on the SOAP note would include, in this instance, the results of muscle strength, range of motion, coordination, sensation, pain limits, and gait evaluation.

Whereas the patient's self-perceived limitations are noted in the subjective section of the SOAP note, the objective section includes a summation of functional capacities and limitations as determined by *physician observation and physical examination*. Areas to be included are: (1) seeing and reading, (2) speaking and writing, (3) hearing, (4) upper limbs and neck, (5) lower limbs and trunk, (6) manual dexterity, (7) stamina, (8) cognition, and (9) emotional adaptation. If obviously inappropriate, the first three areas need not be completed, but they may be of considerable importance if activity is limited because of reduced communication skills. For example, a handwriting analysis may reveal typical Parkinson's micrographia in a patient who has slowed down generally or who falls without explanation. As another example, constructional apraxia may be found in a patient who is forgetful because of an organic brain syndrome. Apparent confusion actually may be due to hearing loss (and thus may represent misinformed responses rather than cognitive dysfunction). In the same vein, clumsiness and tripping—suggestive of muscle weakness and coordination problems—actually may be secondary to visual loss.

Results of the objective examination, including whether the tested systems are within normal limits or are minimally or grossly impaired, should be recorded under their appropriate headings on the SOAP form. For example, under the headings "upper limbs and neck" or "lower limbs and trunk," the examiner may wish to note limited range of motion, increased or decreased reflex responses, muscle weakness or paralysis, fractures, swelling, discoloration, or abnormal movement. If the examiner has to speak excessively loudly for the patient to hear him, hearing reduction should be noted. This information can be augmented by results of tuning fork or other examinations and should be recorded. Similarly, general affect and memory functions should be examined and recorded.

Assessment

The assessment section of the SOAP note provides space to record the results of the analysis of both subjective and objective data. In this part of the SOAP note the clinician should indicate whether the patient's symptoms and findings can be explained by or are consistent with already established deficits and diagnoses. It is especially important when treating elderly, chronically ill, or accident patients, who often have multiple impairments, to assess whether the known or suspected impairments can account sufficiently for the degree of observed limitation of activity; if not, additional impairments and other nonmedical factors should be investigated as potential causes of activity restriction. When the results of such investigations become available, they should be recorded in the SOAP note.

The assessment, in effect, records the analysis of whether there is concordance between the patient's subjective reports, general health outlook, and activity restrictions and the objective findings with respect to impairment and functional limitations identified by medical tests, physician's observations, and physical examination. If there are no apparent inconsistencies between subjective and objective data, the physician will identify the cause of activity limitation and suggest plans either to ameliorate the condition and its detrimental effects, or to adapt the lifestyle if reduction of the problem is not feasible. On the other hand, if there are contradictions between the subjective and objective findings, the physician must consider other causes such as psychological factors, environmental barriers, social handicaps, or whether additional testing and re-examination are required.

Plan

In the plan the physician notes whether, and what kind of, further investigations of unresolved issues are being considered and lists treatable impairments and referrals for consultation with appropriate specialists. The clinician also indicates in the note if the patient and family are prepared for personal and environmental adjustments (should there be significant and persisting disability), and that an investigation into relevant community resources is to be carried out.

A consultation with a physiatrist should be considered whenever a patient has more than some difficulty performing four or more tasks or a major life activity is significantly compromised. The recommendation for this consultation should be in the note. In addition, treatment plans in the note should include referrals, if appropriate, to physical, occupational, and speech therapists, as well as social service, psychiatric services, or other counseling services. If a patient is unable to continue to live at home, plans in the SOAP note should indicate proposed referrals to nursing homes, rehabilitation institutions, hospitals, or other chronic care facilities. Whenever possible, physicians should encourage home care, with assistance from visiting nurses, homemakers, home health aides, voluntary community supports, and other available assistance programs.

When referrals are made to other specialists, it is important that the primary care physician continue to coordinate and monitor management plans. Sometimes the primary care physician takes responsibility for acute illness, the specialist looks after organ-specific disorders, and no one oversees the patient's total care.

Treatment plans should also include health maintenance programs. Medications should be reviewed—especially if drug interaction or cognition are suspected of contributing to functional difficulties. If appropriate, home exercise and dietary programs should be established. A consultation with a nutritionist may be of value in devising a suitable dietary program to meet the patient's needs and preferences. Home and vocational environments should not be overlooked in plans to increase functional capacity; the physician may need to consider the appropriateness of homemaking aides, home elevators, ramps, or other devices. Physical and occupational therapists may be of great assistance in assessing the need for such devices. Prosthetic or orthotic devices, as prescribed by a physiatrist, also may increase functional abilities. In addition, it is important for physicians to be aware of community resources and to make appropriate and timely referrals. Proposed referral should be documented in the case management plan.

The plan section of the SOAP note should also list unresolved issues, including necessary laboratory tests or medical evaluations to confirm or rule out feasible diagnoses not previously considered. A specified amount of time should be noted in the plan for re-evaluation of the patient's functional status.

The functionally oriented SOAP note model described in this chapter, because of the types and items of information recorded, promotes a comparison between functional limitations and available knowledge of organic impairment. Assessment of performance in long-term management of chronically ill persons is crucial to prevent a patient from losing his ability to fulfill expected social roles unnecessarily. Such losses result in needless family and interpersonal stress and reduced personal satisfaction. The functionally oriented SOAP note ensures that issues of personal functioning will be addressed. Additionally, by bringing attention to functional impairments early, the SOAP note format promotes preventive care by highlighting deficits before conditions worsen or proceed to irreversible stages. Finally practitioners, who ask functionally oriented questions and seek relevant treatment goals to maximize functional capacity, may stimulate patients to become more involved in self-health and to think productively about solutions to their own problems.

The following case presentations illustrate use of the SOAP format. The "x's" under the functional systems examination denote the functional systems most likely to be contributing to the relevant activity restrictions based upon examination of the patient.

Case No. 1

JA, a 34-year-old obese, married man, is the father of three young children. He works as an electrician, but has a sporadic work history due to recurrent episodes of acute low-back pain that began when he slipped while on the job 1½ years ago. He also complains of sharp shooting pain from the back to the right lower limb when he reaches forward or upward. He frequently lies down to rest. He says he wants to return to previous levels of activity, which include returning to work and being able to play with his children.

Problem Title: Personal Functioning

Subjective:

General Health

	E X C E	G O O D	A V E R E	P O O R	V P O O
In comparison with others of your age,					
how well do you feel in terms of:					
1. Your general state of health?				2	
2. Your ability to be as active?				2	
3. Your ability to do *needed* things?				2	
4. Your ability to do *desired* things?				2	

Health Score: 8/20

Functional Task Grading

4 = EASY: No difficulty performing the task
3 = SOME: Some difficulty performing the task, but can still manage it well enough
2 = A LOT: Still able to do the activity, but has a lot of difficulty attempting it
1 = UNABLE: Although the individual attempts to perform the task, it is too difficult
0 = NOT APPLICABLE: Someone else in the household does this task or else it does
       not get done

Functional Tasks — Ease versus Difficulty	Energy Cost in METS	Up	Ma	Lo	Sp	Se	He	St	Co	Af
P 1 Cutting toenails	1–2	( )	[ ]	(X)		( )				
3 Getting up from a low seat	2–3			[X]				( )		
3 Climbing stairs	4–5			[X]				[ ]		
I 1 Washing windows and walls	5–6	[ ]	( )	(X)		( )		( )		
0 Grocery shopping	4–5	( )	( )	( )	( )	( )	( )	( )	[ ]	( )
4 Handling finances	1–2		( )			( )			[ ]	( )
L 1 Playing sports	7+	( )	( )	(X)		( )		[X]		
4 Conversing	1–2				[ ]		[ ]		( )	( )
3 Participating in social activities	3–4	( )	( )	( )	( )	( )	[ ]	(X)	( )	[X]
O 4 Concentrating	1–2					( )	( )		[ ]	[ ]
2 Sitting for long periods	1–2			[X]						
2 Standing for long periods	3–4			[X]				( )		
3 Reaching, grasping, pinching	2–3	[ ]	( )	(X)						
T 3 Driving an automobile	2–3	( )	( )	(X)		[ ]			( )	( )
0 Riding a bus	4–5	( )	( )	( )	( )	[ ]		( )	( )	( )

34/60 Task Score, of which
3 Tasks are easy (grade 4) and
2 Tasks are not applicable (grade 0)

Objective

(Se) Seeing and reading   (Sp) Speaking and writing   (He) Hearing

(Ma) Manual dexterity   (Af) Affective (emotional) anxious/depressed   (Co) Cognition

(Up) Upper limb and neck   (Lo) Lower limb and trunk
Negative myelogram
Splinting of back muscles
Straight leg raising 45 degrees
Normal tendon reflexes
No muscle atrophy or weakness   (St) Stamina (CP) endurance poor

Assessment

Diagnosis: Chronic low back pain. Functional status limitations are associated with post-traumatic, chronic low-back pain with obesity. Secondary effects are musculoskeletal stiffness and deconditioning and maladaptive emotional reactions. The patient is in need of a graded mobilization program with increasing activity and appropriate emotional monitoring and support.

Plan

1. Physiatric referral for physical therapy and counseling program for remobilization and education regarding the dynamics of the low-back disorder and the chronic pain syndrome.
2. Nutritional review and weight reduction.

3. Consider psychological or psychiatric consultation in the future if the patient does not make the expected progress over the next 6 to 8 weeks. The psychologist or psychiatrist would consult in collaboration with the physiatric recommendations.

4. Prepare for return to work in the next 3 to 4 months; if not, consider vocational counseling.

5. Follow at 2 to 3 week intervals.

Case No. 2

MV is a 66-year-old foreign-born man with a history of arthritis. He is widowed and lives alone on the first floor of housing for the elderly. He worked in a jewelry factory for 37 years and retired 4 years ago after the death of his wife. He has no other immediate family. He presently complains of periodic pain and stiffness of his neck, ankles, and elbows.

Problem Title: Personal Functioning

Subjective:

General Health

	EXCELLENT	GOOD	AVERAGE	POOR	VPOOR
In comparison with others of your age,	E X C E	G O O D	A V E R	P O O R	V P O O
how well do you feel in terms of:					
1. Your general state of health?			3		
2. Your ability to be as active?			3		
3. Your ability to do *needed* things?			3		
4. Your ability to do *desired* things?			3		

Health Score: 12/20

Functional Task Grading

4 = EASY: No difficulty performing the task
3 = SOME: Some difficulty performing the task, but can still manage it well enough
2 = A LOT: Still able to do the activity, but has a lot of difficulty attempting it
1 = UNABLE: Although the individual attempts to perform the task, it is too difficult
0 = NOT APPLICABLE: Someone else in the household does this task or else it does not get done

Functional Tasks	Energy Cost in METS	Functional Systems								
Ease versus Difficulty		Up	Ma	Lo	Sp	Se	He	St	Co	Af
P 1 Cutting toenails	1–2	(X)	[ ]	( )		( )				
3 Getting up from a low seat	2–3			[X]				( )		
3 Climbing stairs	4–5			[X]				[X]		
I 3 Washing windows and walls	5–6	[X]	( )	(X)		( )		( )		
3 Grocery shopping	4–5	(X)	( )	(X)	( )	( )	( )	(X)	[ ]	( )
4 Handling finances	1–2	( )				( )			[ ]	( )
L 1 Playing sports	7+	(X)	( )	(X)		( )		[ ]		
3 Conversing	1–2				[ ]		[ ]		( )	( )

Functional Tasks	Energy Cost in METS	Functional Systems								
Ease versus Difficulty		Up	Ma	Lo	Sp	Se	He	St	Co	Af
3 Participating in social activities	3–4	( )	( )	( )	( )	( )	[ ]	(X)	( )	[ ]
O 4 Concentrating	1–2					( )	( )		[ ]	[ ]
4 Sitting for long periods	1–2			[ ]						
3 Standing for long periods	3–4			[X]				( )		
3 Reaching, grasping, pinching	2–3	[X]	( )	( )						
T 4 Driving an automobile	2–3	( )	( )	( )		[ ]			( )	( )
0 Riding a bus	4–5	( )	( )	( )	( )	[ ]			( )	( ) ( )

42/60 Task Score, of which
   4 Tasks are easy (grade 4) and
   1 Tasks are not applicable (grade 0)

Objective

(Se) Seeing and reading   (Sp) Speaking and writing   (He) Hearing

(Ma) Manual dexterity   (Af) Affective (emotional)   (Co) Cognition

(Up) Upper limb and neck   (Lo) Lower limb and trunk   (St) Stamina (CP)
   Restricted motion and   Restricted motion in left ankle   Reduced endurance
   pain in left shoulder   Good muscle strength   with prolonged ac-
   and both elbows   tivity
   Good muscle strength

Assessment

   Diagnosis: Mixed rheumatoid and degenerative arthritis. Functional status limitations are mild to moderate, mainly involving upper and lower limb range of motion and endurance secondary to arthritis. If joint restrictions and reduced endurance are dealt with now, future problems in maintaining independent living may be avoided.

Plan

   1. Encourage full range of motion exercises bilaterally for shoulders, elbows, and ankles.
   2. Basic daily exercise program for strengthening the support muscles of the lower limbs, including stair climbing and frequent standing up from a low chair seat.
   3. Walking program to improve endurance.
   4. Re-evaluate in 6 to 8 weeks.

Case No. 3

BT, an 82-year-old widow, was in good health and living independently in a second floor apartment until approximately 1 year ago. At that time she began to experience blurred and progressively reduced vision. She was seen by an ophthalmologist, who confirmed the diagnosis of bilateral cataracts and macular degeneration. Cataract surgery was performed on each eye 8 and 4 months ago. After surgery the patient moved in with a married daughter who "waits on her 24 hours a day," and only leaves for half hour intervals to go shopping. The patient has three other daughters, who live within a 20-mile radius and visit periodically.

Problem Title: Personal Functioning

Subjective:

General Health

In comparison with others of your age, how well do you feel in terms of:	EXCE	GOOD	AVER	POOR	VPOO
1. Your general state of health?			3		
2. Your ability to be as active?				2	
3. Your ability to do *needed* things?				2	
4. Your ability to do *desired* things?				2	

(column headers read vertically: EXCE = EXCEE... E X C E; GOOD = G O O D; AVER = A V E R; POOR = P O O R; VPOO = V P O O O)

Health Score: 9/20

Functional Task Grading

4 = EASY: No difficulty performing the task
3 = SOME: Some difficulty performing the task, but can still manage it well enough
2 = A LOT: Still able to do the activity, but has a lot of difficulty attempting it
1 = UNABLE: Although the individual attempts to perform the task, it is too difficult
0 = NOT APPLICABLE: Someone else in the household does this task or else it does not get done

	Functional Tasks	Energy Cost in METS		Functional Systems						
Ease versus Difficulty			Up	Ma	Lo	Sp	Se	He	St	Co	Af
P 1	Cutting toenails	1–2	( )	[ ]	( )		(X)				
4	Getting up from a low seat	2–3			[ ]				( )		
3	Climbing stairs	4–5			[ ]				[X]		
I 1	Washing windows and walls	5–6	[ ]	( )	( )		(X)		( )		
1	Grocery shopping	4–5	( )	( )	( )	( )	(X)	( )	( )	[ ]	( )
1	Handling finances	1–2		( )			(X)			[ ]	( )
L 0	Playing sports	7+	( )	( )	( )		( )		[ ]		
4	Conversing	1–2				[ ]		[ ]		( )	( )
2	Participating in social activities	3–4	( )	( )	( )	( )	(X)	[ ]	( )	( )	[ ]
O 3	Concentrating	1–2						( )	( )	[ ]	[X]
4	Sitting for long periods	1–2			[ ]						
3	Standing for long periods	3–4			[ ]				(X)		
4	Reaching, grasping, pinching	2–3	[ ]	( )	( )						
T 0	Driving an automobile	2–3	( )	( )	( )			[ ]		( )	( )
1	Riding a bus	4–5	( )	( )	( )	( )	[X]		( )	( )	( )

32/60 Task Score, of which
   4 Tasks are easy (grade 4) and
   2 Tasks are not applicable (grade 0)

Objective

(Se) Seeing and reading Low vision with reduced acuity and visual fields of both eyes	(Sp) Speaking and writing	(He) Hearing
(Ma) Manual dexterity	(Af) Affective (emotional) Reduced ability to concentrate because of emotional distress Expresses feelings of low self-esteem, frustration and helplessness	(Co) Cognition
(Up) Upper limb and neck	(Lo) Lower limb and trunk	(St) Stamina (CP) Low endurance for tasks requiring physical exertion

Assessment

   Diagnosis: Status postbilateral cataract removal and bilateral macular degeneration. Functional status limitations are associated with low vision of sufficient severity to qualify for legal blindness. Secondary effects include depression with low self-esteem and a hopeless outlook. She has given up on attempting to live alone, and the daughter with whom she lives is fearful of leaving her alone for any extended period for concern that she may harm herself. Reduced strength and endurance in the lower limbs is attributable to prolonged sitting and lack of activity. Depressive feelings interfere with ability to concentrate on tasks. The patient has given up on hobbies she enjoyed such as knitting and crocheting.

Plan

   1. Encourage increased independence in personal care and home maintenance skills with daughter(s) available for guidance and support.
   2. Refer to the Association for the Blind for training in performance of activities of daily living with necessary assistive devices.
   3. Refer to occupational therapy for alternative hobby activities.
   4. Contact local library for talking books program.
   5. Encourage increased socialization outside of the home, including daily walking with another person, to prevent musculoskeletal and cardiovascular deconditioning.
   6. Suggest rotation of care responsibilities among other daughters, including transportation to a day care program.
   7. Consultation with a nutritionist to discuss foods that are easy to prepare and eat without sacrifice of quality.
   8. Consider use of antidepressant medication.
   9. Re-evaluate every 2 to 3 weeks.

Summary

In this chapter a protocol for incorporating functional assessment into the outpatient medical record SOAP note is described. The acronym stands for *subjective* data (self-report of general health and activity limitations); *objective* data (laboratory findings and physical examination, with emphasis on the specific functional systems involved in the reported activity limitations); *assessment* (comparison of subjective and objective examination findings to determine whether already established diagnoses can sufficiently account for reported difficulties or whether additional factors must be considered); and *plan* (followup of unresolved issues, referrals to specialists and community support systems, amelioration of conditions causing functional limitations, and preparation of the patient and family for adjustment to chronic illness).

The SOAP note format is shown to highlight the goals of functional assessment by promoting systematic development of a patient problem list that includes limitations in functioning, assessing clinical care outcomes by comparing known or suspected organic impairments with the ability to fulfill expected social roles, and assuring that treatment programs address issues most likely to maximize the quality of life for the disabled individual.

References

1. Weed L: Medical records that guide and teach. N Engl J Med 278:593–600, 652–657, 1968
2. Weed L: Medical Records, Medical Education and Patient Care. Cleveland, Case Western Reserve University Press, 1970

CHAPTER 5

The Physical Modalities

Many functional limitations due to musculoskeletal or neurological deficits, as detected by the FASQ or examination procedures described in Chapters 2 and 3, can be alleviated or even eliminated through the employment of some physical modalities often used in rehabilitation medicine. These modalities, particularly therapeutic heat and cold, hydrotherapy, electrical stimulation, traction, therapeutic exercise, and functional training, are frequently used to relieve pain, reduce muscle spasm or spasticity, decrease joint stiffness, or improve functional performance. The primary care physician should have a working knowledge of these modalities and their benefits, physiological actions, and specific contraindications. The physician's evaluation of the location and severity of the patient's pain are all helpful factors in determining which mode of therapy should be employed. If the primary care physician is uncertain about which method to use or about specific therapy time and amounts, a physiatrist can be consulted or a referral can be made to a physical therapist. If a physical therapy referral is made, the referring physician retains responsibility for the order that is carried out.[19] Appendix 5-1 summarizes the common modalities used in physical treatment, including their primary effects, as well as indications and contraindications for use.

When prescribing physical modalities, four general guidelines should be kept in mind:[19]

1. Application of the modalities requires removal of clothing, draping for privacy and, often, elimination of metals near the treatment field.
2. The simplest modality that can be prescribed should be used.
3. A modality that can be safely used at home is preferable to one that requires office or hospital appointments, provided specific instructions can be given to and understood by the user or treatment provider.

4. If the predicted effect is not achieved within the expected time, either the diagnosis of the condition being treated is wrong, the prescription is wrong, or both.

In addition to any potential benefits derived directly from use of the physical modalities, the physician should also bear in mind the potential placebo effects these therapeutics offer.

There is, in fact, considerable evidence to document the enormous impact of placebo effects on responses to the use of therapeutic modalities, and any statement regarding the effectiveness of a modality on pain relief or improvement in performance of a functional task must be made with full appreciation of the impact of the placebo phenomenon.[28]

Therapeutic Heat

Therapeutic heat, one of the most commonly prescribed physical modalities, can be used both for acute and chronic conditions. Although heat can be provided in several different forms, whether the form is dry, moist, superficial, or deep, its physiological effects as an analgesic, antispasmodic, decongestant, and sedative are the same.

The primary beneficial physiological effects of local heating involve a local increase in temperature and a concomitant increase in local metabolic rate and heat production. An increased blood flow due to arterial and capillary dilation may result, providing improved blood supply both to and from the body part being treated. Additionally, increases in local blood flow may help in resolving chronic inflammatory processes.[10] Local heating also tends to promote a hypalgesic effect by directly affecting pain conduction through the peripheral nerves and free nerve endings, since heat tends to increase the threshold of sensory nerves.[15] Another beneficial physiological effect of heat is a change in the viscoelastic properties of joints. Collagenolysis, which can occur in articular cartilage when the temperature rises above 38°C,[19] may have therapeutic advantages—especially "for stretching tight, thickened joint capsules, scarred synovium and other structures crossing joints, such as a fibrotic muscle."[15] Thus functional limitations due to limited range of motion and joint stiffness may be substantially reduced in collagen disorders such as chronic periarthritis, fibrositis, subacute and chronic bursitis, and chronic inflammatory diseases.[6] Heat also has an antispasmodic effect; this property seems to result from an ability to decrease the activity of gamma fibers in the muscle spindle.[8] Local heating can produce some systemic effects too; for instance, as core temperature increases, reflex vasodilation and sweating occur as the body attempts to maintain homeostasis. Heating the right hand can result in an increased blood flow in distal areas such as the left hand and other limbs;[19,21] the tendency of the body to maintain this kind of equilibrium may be important when distal limbs that could benefit from heat therapy cannot be heated directly (*e.g.*, open sores, metal implants). Some further benefits of local heating include improvement of certain necrotic ulcers and potentiation of the beneficial effects of radiotherapy for carcinomas.[14]

Heating, however, may also have adverse effects. For instance, the rise in capillary blood flow causes an increase in capillary hydrostatic pressure, which can potentiate edema. Additionally, blood flowing through heated areas normally dissipates the heat from the area being treated; if the vascular system is compromised, as in severe arteriosclerosis, heat will tend to accumulate—sometimes to levels which may burn or cause tissue necrosis.[16,19,26] The increased production of metabolites noted earlier, as well as alterations in protein structures due to temperature increases, may potentiate the release of biologically active molecules such as histamines.[20] Membrane permeation properties may also be affected. Bacterial agents that thrive in hot atmospheres may cause a spread of infection when moist heating methods are used, and tumor growth may accelerate with a moderate elevation in temperature.[15]

Materson[19] outlines several points to keep in mind when using therapeutic heat, as listed below:

1. Wood tables should be used rather than metal ones.
2. Infants and geriatric patients tolerate thermal changes poorly.
3. Heat should not be used over anesthetic or hypesthetic areas.
4. Heat should not be used over areas with arterial insufficiency.
5. Heating an extremity in a dependent position should be avoided to prevent an edema increase. Application of heat should be followed by elevation of the limb and exercise.
6. The patient should never be placed on the heating element, rather, the heating element should always be placed on the patient. The addition of pressure alters the patient's perception of heat change and compresses arterial blood supply so that local temperature increases more rapidly and stays higher.
7. Thermal therapy should be followed by some other treatment, such as massage or exercise.
8. Cardiac pacemakers are a contraindication to diathermy.
9. Shortwave diathermy or microwaves should not be used over metal implants in the body; ultrasound, however, can be used over metal implants with some margin of safety.

Heat may be applied superficially by the processes of conduction, radiation, or convection, or it may be applied deeply by the conversion method. Deep heating is also referred to as diathermy. According the Materson,[19] the effect of heating is dependent upon the size of the area heated, the time of the exposure to heat, the rate of temperature rise, and the level of tissue temperature reached. Therapeutic ranges between 41° and 45°C can be obtained, with treatment times varying from a few minutes to 35 to 40 minutes, depending upon the modality used.

Superficial Heat

Conductive heating involves the transfer of heat from a warmer body directly to a cooler body. The rate of exchange is dependent upon the temperature gradient. Common forms of conductive heating include hot water bottles, electric heating pads, warm packs, and paraffin wax baths. All of these modes produce rather superficial heating but are generally safe, simple to employ, and available for home use. Moist heat offers the most satisfactory results for relief from stiffness, swelling, and joint pain.

Hot water bottles release heat rapidly. Even moderately heated bags will dissipate half of their effective heat before reaching the patient.[26] Patients who overheat a hot water bottle in an attempt to compensate for the rapid loss of heating effect are engaging in a dangerous practice unless sufficient insulation is placed between the water at a high temperature and the skin to prevent burns.

Moist wet packs are frequently used in the home, usually made from pre-pared heated towels or, as with a Kenny pack, from a wool cloth heated with water. Steam hydrocollator packs, which retain their heat up to 30 minutes, are effective if a joint is severely involved—especially as an adjunct to warm baths. These packs are available especially for the back, limbs, and neck, but their weight can be uncomfortable and they are impractical for open wounds. Application of hot packs, however, is time-consuming, and much heat is lost in water evaporation.

Paraffin wax baths are a mixture of paraffin and mineral oil, which lowers the melting point of the wax. A limb can be immersed in the bath. Alternatively, the wax can be applied with a brush onto the body part and then removed after 15 to 20 minutes. Paraffin, used most often to heat hands and wrists, has the advantage of being applicable to an elevated limb. But this method is often messy and malodorous, hindering its success in the home.

Electric heating pads usually produce a constant level of heat. It is important not to place any areas of the body on the pad, but rather to place the pad over the area to be treated, since body weight tends to decrease blood flow through the skin adjacent to the pad, and the temperature of the skin may increase to damaging levels.[19] Also, patients should be cautioned about the dangers of falling asleep while using an electric pad. Electric blankets are advantageous as they offer controlled warmth and freedom of movement without the added weight of the moist hot packs.

The greatest disadvantage of conductive heating devices is that they limit the ability to see what is happening during treatment.[19] They can rarely be applied over open wounds, and they provide only superficial heating. Conductive heating devices are beneficial in treating arthritis, subacute and chronic strains and sprains, and muscle tension headaches.[19]

A primary form of *radiant* heating, another means of superficial heating, is the infrared heating lamp, which produces electromagnetic energy in the 7,000 to 12,000 Å range. The quantum energy of this portion of the spectrum causes thermal agitation. Infrared lamps usually are made of incandescent bulbs and built-in reflectors. The pattern of heating is dependent upon the reflector's shape. Treatment time for an infrared lamp is usually 30 to 45 minutes. The intensity of radiation is inversely proportional to the square of the distance of the lamp from the radiating body. Intensity levels, which can be controlled by varying the distance from the heat source, should be kept at a level easily tolerated by the patient.

The advantages of an infrared lamp are its simplicity, its easy use in a home setting, and its ability to heat an elevated limb. Infrared lamps have physiological effects similar to those obtained from conductive heating. On the other hand, incandescent bulbs occasionally (although rarely) break, causing hot shattering glass to fall on the patient. The patient should be discouraged from using the lamp himself because of the danger of falling asleep under it.

Convective heating, the third form of superficial heating, involves the exchange of heat from a flow of warm liquid or a gas moving past the surface of a solid. Molecules closest to the surface of the solid release heat to the solid and then move on. These molecules are replaced by other molecules, which, in turn, transfer their heat.[19] Agitated water baths, such as whirlpool baths, provide both useful heating and beneficial debriding and stimulation effects. These baths are discussed more fully in the hydrotherapy section.

Deep Heating (Diathermy)

Diathermy, or *Conversive* heating, occurs when electrical, electromagnetic, or sound energy is converted to thermal energy. Conversive heating is deep heating and is supplied for therapeutic purposes either by shortwave, microwave, or ultrasound diathermy. Greater penetration of the tissues can be achieved by the use of the various deep heating modalities than by the forms of superficial heating.

Shortwave Diathermy

Shortwave diathermy involves passage of a high frequency oscillation current through the patient, who becomes part of the circuit and is "tuned" for tissues to oscillate at the same frequency as the oscillation circuit of the machine.[19] Currents are applied either by capacitive or inductive application, dependent upon the body area being treated. The greatest heating occurs in the subcutaneous tissues and superficial musculature.[17] Shortwave diathermy is effective only for deep heating when applied over tissue with minimal superficial subcutaneous covering such as the knee, elbow, or shoulder. Medical diathermy should never cause pain or tissue damage. As with other heating methods, shortwave diathermy is unsafe over cardiac pacemakers, metal implants, or the gravid uterus, and for individuals unable to perceive the sensation of heat or those with suspected malignant growths.

Microwave Diathermy

Microwave diathermy involves the conversion of electromagnetic waves into thermal energy. Microwaves are reflected at the body surface and tissue interfaces and are absorbed in tissues with high water content, such as superficial subcutaneous fat and bursae; bone, on the other hand, is not a good absorber of microwaves.[19] The main therapeutic advantage of microwave diathermy is its ease of application—a beam is directed to the area to be treated. Duration of application is usually 20 to 30 minutes. Specific indications for microwave prescription include musculoskeletal conditions such as joint disease, bursitis, tendinitis, or periarthritis of the shoulder. Microwave diathermy is especially good for mild heating and sprains. Contraindications are those common to all heating agents, as discussed earlier. Additionally, microwave treatment should not be employed over bony prominences or edematous tissues. Shortwave and microwave diathermies are used much less frequently than they were 5 to 10 years ago due to the use of alternative treatment methods.

Ultrasound Diathermy

Ultrasound, the most frequently used deep heating method, involves the conversion to heat of acoustic vibrations that are above the audible range of the human ear (17,000 Hz). The ultrasonic frequency used for therapeutic purposes ranges between 0.8 and 1.0 MgHz.[1,19] The beneficial thermal effects are due to alternating compression and rarifaction of tissue spaces. Since ultrasound wavelengths are smaller than many tissue structures, the waves are reflected.

Two advantages of ultrasound are that it allows deeper penetration and it can be used over metal transplants. Selective absorption of ultrasound energy by bone and tissue interfaces occurs, enabling selective heating of joints and periarticular structures.[13,16] Ultrasound is the only source of diathermy capable of effectively reaching the tissues in the hip joints and is vastly more efficient than microwave diathermy in heating the shoulder joints.[19,28]

In addition to the usual therapeutic benefits offered by heat application, when ultrasound is properly applied and followed by stretching, the collagen tissues lengthen more than they do by either heating or stretching modalities alone.[19] Ultrasound is also effective in treatment of calcific bursitis, tendinitis of the shoulder, and painful phantom limbs with postoperative neurofibromas.[13]

Ultrasound equipment for therapeutic use consists of a generator of high frequency current and an applicator (also known as the sound head). The generator produces electrical oscillations at desired frequencies, which in turn cause the transducer within the applicator to vibrate and generate sound waves. The sonic energy is transmitted to the tissue by contact with the applicator face. Application time is dependent upon the thickness of the overlying subcutaneous tissue. Higher doses for shorter periods are required for thin subjects, and longer, lower doses are needed for heavier subjects. Ultrasound is applied in short, rhythmic strokes; if the sound head is allowed to remain stationary, the tissue will heat too rapidly causing a painful or hot sensation, indicative of an ultrasound overdose.[19]

Although ultrasound is believed to be the most effective deep heating source available, its contraindications are the same as those for any other heating modality. The only exception is that ultrasound may be used by individuals with pacemakers and other metal implants. An additional precaution must be taken, however, to shield the eye from ultrasonic radiation if applied to the face, and it should not be used over the gravid uterus.

Therapeutic Cold

Therapeutic cold is used for several reasons in medicine:

1. To stop bleeding and as an anti-inflammatory agent after an acute injury
2. To relieve pain (local analgesic)
3. To prevent edema
4. To relieve spasms and spasticity
5. To produce hypothermia for control of pyrexia

6. To prevent tissue changes and relieve pain due to second degree burns

7. To retard gangrene in an ischemic limb

The physiologic effects of locally applied cold, by lowering tissue temperature, are in general in opposition to those just described for heat application. The specific effects are dependent upon the rate, duration, extent of area of treatment, and degree of temperature reduction.[22] As temperature decreases, vasoconstriction occurs, which reduces local blood flow and decreases intravascular hydrostatic pressure; this tends to reduce edema, decrease lymph production and extravasation of blood cells, and reduce sweating. Enzymatic reactions and metabolic rates within the areas are slowed and significant temperature reduction may induce protein degradation or precipitation. Decreased metabolic activity may be especially important in preserving a limb, the arterial supply of which is threatened. The lessening of local circulation is beneficial in slowing the absorption of poisons, such as insect sting venom. Bradycardia, hypocapnia, and hypotension may also result. All of these systemic effects tend to conserve energy.

After sufficient cooling has taken place, the "hunting reaction" normally occurs. This phenomenon is characterized by periodic spurts of vasodilation (resulting in periodic reddening of the tissues) followed by constriction.[26] Failure to vasodilate may permit the cold to cause local tissue damage. The body is particularly sensitive to changes in its core temperature; if sufficient cold is applied, the "shivering phenomenon" is activated. Shivering tends to raise the core temperature by increasing heat production through involuntary muscle contractions.

Cold application is said to involve four successive sensation stages: cooling, burning, aching, and finally, numbness or analgesia.[26] As with heat, therapeutic cold may affect muscle spindle activity and may delay nerve fiber conduction. In these ways, cold has antispasmodic and pain relief effects. Borenstein and Desmolt[3] found that cold can improve function at the neuromuscular junction in myasthenia gravis. Because vasoconstriction reduces convection through the bloodstream, cold applications are more efficient and tend to last longer than heat applications.[19]

Therapeutic cold may be applied by means of ice packs, cold wet packs, ice baths and vapo-coolant sprays. Cryokinetics, another form of cold therapy, involves the production of analgesic cooling either by immersion of the body part in cold water or ice massage (rubbing of the skin for several minutes with ice), followed by active exercise to mobilize the injured parts. This method is reportedly beneficial immediately following acute strains and sprains, as well as for bursitis and tendinitis. Contraindications to the use of therapeutic cold include labile hypertension, Raynaud's phenomenon, ischemia, cold insensitivity or hypersensitivity (especially in young children and elderly patients), indolent wounds, and vasculitis.

Hydrotherapy

Hydrotherapy is the external use of water for therapeutic purposes. Because of its high specific heat, water is able to absorb and release heat slowly, making it an effective agent for convective heating or cooling.[31] Three properties of water account for its many useful clinical applications—buoyancy, viscosity, and agitation ability.

Buoyancy, of great value in exercise programs for patients who can not bear weight, can be used either to assist or resist movement of the limbs. Exercises can involve a gradation of difficulty, depending on the level of submersion chosen. For example, exercising close to the water's surface provides less resistance (work) than exercising deeper in water. A treatment program for motor weakness may utilize this principle by increasing resistance as the muscle power returns. Also, because buoyancy allows for movement without weight-bearing, hydrotherapy is useful in patients with paresis or joint inflammation.

The viscosity of water can be used therapeutically to provide resistance to motion. Viscosity causes resistance of all movements in all directions within the water—the degree of resistance being dependent upon the movement, shape of the body, and speed.[31] For example, as the acceleration of the body segment increases, resistance also increases, thus preventing rapid or jerky motions. Progressive exercise programming often includes increasing the speed of exercise performance within the water.

Water can also be agitated to provide mechanical stimulation of the skin. This is the mainstay of whirlpool baths and according to Zislis[31] is especially effective in cleansing the skin, promoting debridement to combat infection, and aiding in the healing of chronic wounds or decubitus ulcers.

A variety of methods is available for hydrotherapy treatment. The selection of mode depends largely on the specific body parts being treated. For example, a large tank or swimming pool may be required for patients with multiple joint or lower limb involvement, in order to allow for total body immersion and exercise. Some of the more common modes include cold water baths (to constrict vessels, increase muscle tone, and refresh the patient) and warm water baths (to dilate vessels, increase metabolic rate and relieve pain). Hot sitz baths are especially helpful in relieving the pain of hemorrhoids, dysmenorrhea, coccygodynia, and prostatitis.[23] Whirlpool baths, which agitate water at high temperatures and can accommodate a limb or even an entire body, provide massage, heat, pain relief, debridement, and relaxation benefits. The Hubbard tank is larger and can be used for total body immersion and underwater exercises. However, the cost and time involved in refilling and sterilizing the tank after patient use has rendered it obsolete in many hospitals. Swimming pools are a means to provide generalized conditioning exercises. Progressive resistance swimming programs are easily developed.

In prescribing hydrotherapy, the physician should specify the temperature, duration, and frequency of treatments.

> Factors that affect the results of hydrotherapy include the water temperature itself, the difference between the skin and water temperatures, the methods of application, the suddenness of application, the extent of surface covered, the duration and frequency of the treatment and the weight, age and general condition of the patient.[31]

The prescription should also indicate whether any chemicals, salts, or detergents should be employed and whether exercises should be performed in the water or subsequent to treatment. Specific precautions or instructions, such as watching the patient for circulatory complications, vital signs, or color, and so on, should be included when prolonged hydrotherapeutic measures are prescribed. Once again, a physiatrist can be helpful in suggesting the most efficient treatment procedures.

There are few contraindications for hydrotherapy, although dry gangrene is one exception. Certain precautions should be taken, however, to minimize potential negative effects of water treatments.

1. Tanks must be properly cleaned to prevent cross-contamination.
2. The sedative effects of the warm bath may potentiate a tendency for the patient to fall asleep in the tank and drown, so patients should never be left alone in a bath.
3. Body electrolytes can be lost during hydrotherapy through open skin or burns. The addition of salt to the water can counter this effect.[19]
4. Immersion of the body into water warmer than the skin temperature will cause the body temperature to rise and may produce a fever.
5. Elevation of body temperature can also cause a sensation of weakness. Persons with multiple sclerosis are especially susceptible to this phenomenon.
6. Individuals with compromised circulatory systems must also be watched to prevent collapse, myocardial or cerebral ischemia, or even injury, upon leaving the pool or tank.
7. Many patients enjoy the soothing effects of hydrotherapeutic treatments and may be reluctant to give up treatment sessions, even after the beneficial effects have terminated. Physician intervention may be necessary to rectify this situation.

Ultraviolet Therapy

Compared with the wavelengths of visible light, ultraviolet wavelengths are shorter and their frequency and energy levels severalfold greater. Ultraviolet rays range from 180 to 390 nm. The absorption of quantum energy in this range enables tissues to change their molecular configuration causing electrochemical changes resulting in heat, chemical reactions, or visible light. The photochemical reactions caused by ultraviolet therapy include:[22] (1) erythema, (2) increased skin pigmentation, (3) epithelialization, (4) antirachitic effects (including the conversion of 7-dehydrocholesterol to vitamin D3), (5) bactericidal effects, and (6) neurohumoral effects.

Ultraviolet therapy can be useful in many situations. In dermatology, for example, it has been found to be effective in the treatment of acne vulgaris and psoriasis, and it is useful in treating bacterial infections and other skin disorders.[19] Also it is used adjunctively in routine wound care, especially decubitus ulcers that show indolent healing. The effects of ultraviolet radiation on epithelialization result from an accelerated cell division of the epidermis; excessive exposure may lead to desquamation, which by thickening the skin makes it less sensitive to itching and pressure, thus benefiting persons who wear orthotic or prosthetic devices.[22]

Ultraviolet radiation is provided by special ultraviolet lamps, which are of several different types, including mercury vapor arc lamps, hot or cold quartz lamps, and sunlamps. Dosages for ultraviolet radiation should be prescribed according to the desired effect rather than set by any strict timetable. There is tremendous variation among individuals in response to ultraviolet rays; for example, blondes generally are more sensitive than brunettes, and men usually are more sensitive than women.[23,27] Erythemas are described in several degrees ranging from minimal to third degree (blister forming) reddening of the skin. The minimal erythemal dose (MED) is defined as the timed dose of ultraviolet radiation that will produce a minimal erythema on the patient's skin. This level must be determined for each individual; then, dosage is prescribed in multiples of the MED. Prescriptions for ultraviolet therapy should also indicate the site and frequency of treatment.

Special precautions should be taken when ultraviolet therapy is used. It is essential that the eyes of both the patient and the therapist be shielded, for example with goggles, as eye tissue is very sensitive to radiation, and massive doses of ultraviolet radiation may cause keratinic changes in the cornea or opacification of the lens. When ultraviolet radiation is used to treat superficial ulcers, surrounding skin should be protected in order to avoid tissue injury.

Traction

Properly applied traction can be of considerable therapeutic value in a number of circumstances. A thorough understanding of the underlying biomechanics is necessary, however, and traction applied by an amateur is probably worse than no application.[19]

Traction, the manual or mechanical application of opposing forces to separate articular surfaces or stretch soft tissues,[18] can be applied for brief periods of time, intermittently, or continuously. Manual traction, applied by the therapist's hands, usually involves brief manipulations—often in combination with lateral or rotational maneuvers—for the treatment of acute symptoms.[21] Intermittent traction involves periods of sustained traction followed by periods of withdrawal of the traction tension. The alternating application and withdrawal are achieved by a mechanical device such as a harness. An example of an intermittent regime would be an alternating sequence of traction for 2 minutes and then rest for 30 seconds, until a total treatment time of 20 to 30 minutes has elapsed.[19] Traction commonly is performed once or twice a day. Continuous traction also is applied with a mechanical device, but with no rest periods. Forces in continuous traction are usually kept at a minimal level. One situation in which continuous traction is indicated is in the treatment of severe pain from nerve root compression.[21]

Traction used to relieve pain or immobilize cervical, low back, pelvic, or limb regions, has been shown to be effective in the treatment of patients with cervical pain due to spondylosis, degenerative disk disease, cervical radiculopathy and strain, torticollis, and myofascial pain syndrome.[19] As described by Materson,[19] cervical traction utilizes a head sling with maximum pull felt at the occiput, with the patient in a supine position. Traction forces usually begin at 8 to 12 pounds (comparable with the weight of the head) and are increased slowly, as tolerated, to 25 to 35 pounds if applied intermittently, and at about half that force if applied continuously.

Pelvic traction can be applied through similar means by use of a pelvic harness. Weights are attached to a pulley that hangs over the end of the bed. The body acts as the counterforce. Traction forces for pelvic traction are much greater than for cervical traction; 65 pounds or more can be tolerated by the average patient. When a regular bed is used for traction treatments, the effects of friction and gravity decrease the effectiveness of the traction, causing it to serve mainly as a means of immobilizing the patient in bed. When specially designed traction tables are used, however, effective pull is maintained, enabling a decrease in lumbar lordosis and a gentle stretch to the posterior soft tissues.[19]

Traction also can be applied to limbs to aid in the aftermath of fractures and dislocations. Continuous traction applied to limbs can aid in relieving pain and overcoming muscle spasm, maintaining anatomical alignment, preventing or correcting deformity and securing rest. Traction, applied along with other physical modalities such as heat or ultrasound, may aid in increasing the extensibility of the soft tissues.

Several considerations should be kept in mind when prescribing traction modalities.

1. The usefulness of traction is limited. As Nichols describes:

   The only effects which traction can be expected to achieve are some distraction between vertebrae at the intervertebral disc and apophyseal joints, tensing the longitudinal ligaments of the spinal column (particularly the posterior spinal ligament), and some slight widening of the intervertebral foraminae. These effects can only be expected to occur while the traction is being applied. Continuous traction might be employed also to achieve effective immobilization of a patient in bed.[21]

2. Prescription orders for positioning, amount of force, and duration of treatment may need to be flexible. Traction forces should be of a magnitude that can be well tolerated by the patient and should be decreased or discontinued entirely if the patient complains of pain or discomfort. Also comfortable relaxation contributes to the analgesic effects of traction. The amount of weight that can be comfortably tolerated may vary from patient to patient, and may change, even on a daily basis, within the same patient. Position comfort may similarly vary on a daily basis, thereby necessitating changes in the original orders to allow the therapist latitude in employing the traction.

3. Precautions should be taken to prevent pressure areas on the skin from ulcerating during prolonged traction—an ever-present potential hazard.

4. Traction is contraindicated in cervical myelopathy, secondary to chronic adhesions, and with metastasis to bone. If the patient does not respond to traction within a period of two to three weeks, its use should be re-evaluated and possibly discontinued.

Therapeutic Electrical Stimulation

The beneficial results of electrical stimulation of motor nerves (faradic) or muscle itself (galvanic) is well established in medical therapeutics. Therapeutic stimulation has been used to prevent muscle atrophy, reduce muscle spasms or spasticity, assist venous return and lymph drainage, promote muscle re-education, and decrease a patient's awareness of painful stimuli.

The underlying principle used in the control of muscle spasms or spasticity of muscle by therapeutic electrical stimulation is that electrically produced tetanic muscle contraction fatigues the muscle. Stillwell[24] cites several experiments in which tetanizing stimulation of several minutes duration resulted in relaxation of spasticity for several hours. Stimulation of innervated muscle may also act as an effective muscle pump to promote lymphatic drainage and decrease edema through stimulated muscle contractions. Effective therapeutic stimulation can be as brief as one millisecond.[25]

Therapeutic nerve stimulation has also been shown to be successful in controlling pain. The process used is called transcutaneous electrical nerve stimulation (TENS) and is based on the gate control theories of Melzack and Wall.[20] The rationale for treatment is based upon the principle of counterirritation, which maintains that one can consciously perceive only one sensation at a time;[19] by drawing attention to cutaneous stimuli, deep pain signals can be blocked from the level of awareness. The proposed physiological basis for the counterirritation theory is that the stimulation of large cutaneous, myelinated afferent fibers tends to inhibit, at the spinal cord level, the transmission of impulses carried by the smaller diameter, afferent fibers in the deeper internal structures. Small, battery-operated units provide a high frequency electrical current of varying duration and amplitude through conductors applied to the skin, flooding the area with excitatory electrical signals. These portable stimulators can be carried with the patient and used as necessary. Voltages produce tingling or paresthesia, but not pain. TENS may be of some value when pain relief is not accomplished through traditional therapy and medication. Other therapeutic uses of electrical stimulation include muscle re-education and stimulation of the diaphragm to aid in respiration.

When prescribing electrotherapy, the physician should indicate the intensity and duration of the current. In muscle and nerve stimulation, the precise location of the electrode should be specified. In using all treatment forms, caution should be taken to avoid skin burns. Directions for handling the equipment safely should be available and strictly followed. Electrodes should be safely attached to the patient (*e.g.,* should not cross the thorax) and care should be taken to obtain proper polarity placement of the electrode pads. Cleansing of the skin and well-prepared contact pads may decrease discomfort from the procedure. Electrical therapy is contraindicated for patients with cardiac pacemakers.

Therapeutic Exercise

Therapeutic exercise involves movements that aid in the improvement of musculoskeletal function, correction of an impairment, or maintenance of good health,[12] and may involve programs developed to restore or improve function in one specific muscle group or contribute to a feeling of well-being. An exercise program should always be individualized, considering each patient's needs and physical limitations. In general, the goal of all exercise is to restore, improve or maintain one of the following:

* Range of joint motion
* Muscle strength
* Endurance
* Coordination and speed

Each exercise goal requires different techniques.

Range of Motion (ROM)

Range of motion exercises focus on moving the joint through its usual or normal functional range. This form of exercise is important both in restoring function to a joint, for example, when a contracture or paralysis is present, and in preventing tightness that threatens to restrict activity. ROM exercises are indicated whenever there is a loss or potential loss of the range of motion. Specific additional indications include paresis, subacute or chronic arthritis, and conditions requiring bedrest.[19]

Range of motion exercises can be performed actively, passively, or with assistance. In *active* ROM, movement of the joints is performed and controlled by the patient, using his or her own strength. Active exercises, in general, tend to improve strength and aid in total body conditioning by increasing cardiopulmonary reserves. In *active–assistive* exercises, the patient lacking sufficient strength is helped to complete the range of movement. This type of exercise may be employed, for example, in mobilization of the joints around which there are slight contractures. Active–assistive exercise helps strengthen muscles and aids in establishing coordination patterns. When a patient is unable or advised not to move his or her own joints, the therapist moves the patient's joints through the range of motion routine. This is called *passive* ROM. Passive movement prepares the patient for eventual active exercise by preventing contractures and adhesions, increasing proprioceptive sensation, and stimulating flexion-extension reflexes.[21]

At least once, and preferably twice, daily all joints should be exercised through a full range of motion for three repetitions.[12] Although the ultimate goal is to achieve a full, normal range, exercise should be performed gently, taking care not to exceed by forced means the usual ROM the patient had prior to the present trauma or onset of disease, especially if inflammation or pain exists. Unlike many of the physical modalities previously discussed, exercise procedures can be taught easily to family members who can help the patient at home. When needed, a skilled therapist should be retained if there is acute joint involvement, since too much exercise or improper exercise may impede recovery during the acute stage.[12] Whenever possible, active and active–assistive ROM exercises are preferable to passive ones. A program can be set up with a gradual progression from passive to active ROM.

Stretching is a specialized form of ROM exercise that can be performed either manually by a therapist, mechanically, or actively. The patient uses antagonistic muscle groups to produce the stretching effect. Stretching involves pulling in opposite directions to prevent fasciae, ligaments, and muscles from shortening, and to restore normal ROM when it has been decreased due to loss of soft tissue elasticity. Successful stretching requires daily repetition; gentle stretching over a longer period of time produces better results than brief, vigorous stretches.[21] One practical clinical use of stretching is in the prevention of contractures in Duchenne–Landouzy dystrophy. A study by Vignos[29] showed that patients receiving stretching exercises showed fewer contractures than patients who did not receive them. Common sites of contractures upon which to focus stretching movement include heelcords, hamstrings, and iliotibial bands. Stretching is contraindicated in osteoporosis. Although discomfort may be experienced from stretching soft tissues, stretching should not be painful. Persistent pain or a decrease in range of motion suggests that either the amount of force or the duration of treatment should be decreased. Inflamed joints may not tolerate vigorous stretching. Also stretching edematous tissue, which is more prone to tearing than normal tissue during stretching procedures, may result in residual pain, swelling, and soreness.[12]

Muscle Strength

According to DeLorme,[7] exercises to increase strength require low repetition and high resistance, whereas exercises to increase endurance require low weight and high repetition regimens. Muscle strength involves the maximal tension that can be exerted on a muscle during contraction.[12] Strengthening usually employs *resistive exercise*. In this form of exercise, external resistance, such as a heavy weight, is applied, and the patient is requested to lift a progressively increasing sequence of weights a predetermined number of times. Alternatively, in *regressive resistance exercises* the patient begins by lifting 100% of the maximum weight that it is determined he is able to lift. This amount is decreased in successive exercises. Because fatigue usually increases as exercise continues, regressive resistance exercises may be tolerated better by some patients than others. According to Materson,[19] maximum strength in a muscle is achieved after 12 to 16 weeks of exercising; thereafter, muscle strength can be maintained with exercise sessions every other day. A lapse of as little as 3 or 4 days can result in a loss of strength.

Physiologically, muscle contractions can be classified as either isometric or isotonic. *Isotonic* exercise involves the use of constant tension while muscle length is allowed to change. This is a type of resistive exercise. The technique involves having the patient perform a planned number of movements in resistance to a predetermined weight. *Isometric* exercise increases muscle tension without changing its length. These exercises are often performed when a joint is immobilized, as in a plaster cast, or when joint inflammation is present, as in arthritis. Isometric exercises help increase muscle strength and bulk; in fact, it has been stated that isometric contractions for 6 seconds daily are ample stimulus to increase both these parameters.[19] Isometric movements, however, must be prescribed cautiously in patients with cardiovascular problems, such as uncontrolled hypertension, recent myocardial infarction, or vascular insufficiency, since the isometric technique causes a transient increase in blood pressure. Some patients tend to hold their breath or do a Valsalva maneuver while performing the exercises; such a tendency can be overcome by having the patient count aloud while exercising.

Isokinetic exercises, a variation of isometrics, allow the joint to move at a constant velocity preventing acceleration of the joint which, in turn, increases resistance. Special mechanical devices eliminate the acceleration effects, allowing for a nearly isometric contraction at every degree of range of the joint.[19] Isokinetic exercises, according to Materson, are valuable strengthening methods because the tension they produce in the muscle is greater than the tension present when contractions are allowed to occur with increasing velocity.[19]

Endurance

Endurance exercises, which utilize low resistance (low weight), high repetition methods, may involve 100 repetitions or more of the same exercise each day, until the exercised muscles begin to fatigue. Muscle fatigue is necessary to develop endurance.[12] Whenever possible, exercise programs should encourage the exercise of multiple muscles in the same endurance activity. Jogging, swimming, cycling, rowing, and stairclimbing are examples of exercises that help build endurance. Cardiac patients who participate in such activities, however, must be monitored. Further, patients in poor physical condition may need to begin with short work periods followed by rest periods. Endurance exercises promote increases in circulatory and respiratory capacities. Kottke[12] cites the finding that repeated, prolonged exercise may increase the number of capillaries in a muscle by 40%. The increase in muscle bulk with exercise is partly due to the increased number of open capillaries. Muscle conditioning is associated also with changes in cellular metabolic capacity and storage, including more intracellular lipids and myoglobin.[12] By progressively increasing time periods of fatiguing activity, concomitant with proper rest periods, these changes can occur without any detrimental effects to the cell. Motivation is an important component of endurance activities and should not be overlooked by the physician or therapist.

Coordination

Coordination exercises, based on the axiom, "practice makes perfect," employ repetitious exercises with little or no resistance. Mastering precision of performance is accomplished by combining the activities of several muscles into a smooth pattern. As an activity is repeatedly performed, a habit pattern is developed which enables the patient eventually to perform the activity automatically, with less effort and greater speed than was previously the case. Coordination exercises are progressive; they begin with mastery of the smallest component of a task and gradually increase the complexity of the skill. Maintenance of optimal coordination function requires regular practice and concentration. Coordination exercises are helpful in cerebellar disturbances and muscle re-education. Occupational therapists, as well as physical therapists, are trained to use coordination exercises and activities.

Therapeutic Massage

Massage is often misunderstood or abused. The terms used to describe the various common types of massage include stroking (effleurage), compression (petrissage), and percussion (tapotement).

Stroking

Stroking involves running the hand lightly over the surface of the skin, producing physical and psychological relaxation. It may also palliate pain by heightening the threshold of sensory nerve endings and contribute to a reflex vascular phenomenon.

Compression

Compression includes motions of kneading, squeezing, friction, and skin rolling. This form of massage, helpful in mobilizing tissue fluid by aiding in the return of blood, lymph, and catabolites to the main circulation also is useful in stretching adhesions, for example, in scar tissue.

Percussion

Percussion movements are intended to stimulate. These involve the alternating motions of hacking, clapping, cupping, or fist beating in order to provide a counterirritant vibration. Percussion may aid in improving bronchial drainage by mobilizing pulmonary secretions.

A prescription for massage should indicate that it is to be used in combination with an exercise modality. Therapeutic massage can be sedative or stimulating. The beneficial effects of a systematized massage include:[30]

1. Improvement of circulation and movement of blood and nutritive elements
2. Increased warmth to the skin and improvement in its condition
3. More rapid elimination of waste
4. Dissolution of soft adhesions
5. Reduction of swelling and induration of tissues
6. Loosening and stretching of contracted tendons
7. Soothing of the CNS and peripheral nerves

Massage is useful for reducing swelling and for mobilizing scarred and contracted tissues.[11] Following trauma, massage is useful in reducing edema and swelling. Prolonged use of massage results in skin that is tougher, more flexible, and less sensitive.[30] Specifically, it has been indicated in the preparation of an amputation stump. This allows the skin to be more roughly handled without discomfort and may be helpful for wearers of prostheses.

Therapeutic massage should be applied only by a knowledgeable therapist. Deep stroking involves a knowledge of the directions of muscle fibers and centripetal blood flow. Application of powders, creams or balms can be used during a massage to prevent irritation and allow smooth hand movement over the skin. Massage can be applied manually, mechanically, or with the assistance of a vibrator or a pneumatic sleeve, such as the Jobst sleeve. The sleeve pumps the elevated limb. After pumping, an elastic, custom-fitted Jobst garment can be worn which applies a predetermined pressure to control lymphedema. The combined use of a Jobst sleeve and garment is especially effective after mastectomies or to reduce scar formation in burned areas of the lower limbs.[19] According to Materson, the use of massage as a means of weight reduction or body conditioning by health spas has no medical validity.[19]

Massage is contraindicated in the presence of infection or inflammatory disease, malignancies, hemorrhagic or clotting disorders, thrombophlebitis, or communicable skin diseases. It is also contraindicated in situations in which, for psychological reasons, the patient's dependency on treatment may be increased.

Biofeedback

Biofeedback deals with the modification of neurally controlled phenomena. According to the American Academy of Physical Medicine and Rehabilitation,[1] the concept of biofeedback, as used in the clinical practice of medicine, is limited to the past 15 years, although the behavioral ideas upon which it is based date back to much earlier times.

> . . . the root idea of biofeedback: basically, that ordinarily uncontrollable or autonomic bodily processes—such as the secretions of glands, the activity of visceral, circulatory, and cardiac muscles, and of neural tissue itself—may be susceptible to modification and control via appropriate delivery of significant information or feedback to the individual regarding their occurrence. This information may be delivered in the form of reinforcement that is made contingent upon the achievement of certain specified changes in visceral, circulatory, or neural activity, in which case the resulting modifications tend to be viewed as a form of learning. Or the information may be delivered to the person along with explicit instructions regarding both what it signifies and what the person should try to achieve in the way of modification or control. In this case, the work tends to be viewed in terms of self-regulation.[2]

Self-regulation is the goal of medical biofeedback therapeutics. Biofeedback training involves the use of instrumentation to provide individuals with moment by moment information concerning some biological processes within their bodies, in an attempt to teach control of the process. Control, in this instance, usually refers to an increase or decrease in the desired response. For example, patients have been reported being capable of increasing or decreasing heart rate, skin temperature, muscle activity, stomach acid, and other physiological processes by feedback monitoring.

Information regarding these bodily processes can be presented in any of three modalities: tactile (*e.g.,* vibrations varying in rate), auditory (*e.g.,* tones varying in frequency) or visual (*e.g.,* needles deflecting on a scale). There are three forms of instrumentation currently available:[9] portable units, modular components, and polygraph machines. The latter two types are useful mainly for research purposes. Some of the common portable feedback equipment used clinically includes:[9]

1. EMG (electromyography) machines—designed to detect muscle activity levels, usually using noninvasive surface skin electrodes. EMG is used to treat musculoskeletal disorders, pain syndromes, tension headaches, and hypertension, and to achieve skeletal muscle relaxation and re-education.
2. EEG (electroencephalography) machines—designed to detect and amplify electrical signals generated by the brain and, by using surface electrodes, to make available information regarding the amplitude and frequency of their components. EEG is useful in diagnosing brain tumors and epilepsy and, in conjunction with relaxation training, in treating insomnia, concentration difficulties, pain, seizures, and anxiety.
3. Temperature feedback—designed to measure and display changes in skin temperature from a selected body site; commonly it involves a thermistor taped to the skin. Since an increase in body temperature can reflect relaxation of the sympathetic nervous system, temperature feedback may measure stress. It is also deemed helpful in treatment of migraine headaches and improvement of peripheral circulation in Raynaud's syndrome.
4. Galvanic skin response (GSR)—designed to detect changes in skin resistance or conductance incurred by changes in a patient's emotional state. GSR involves measurement of sweat gland activity and autonomic nervous system activity. It is useful in treating emotional disorders, including phobias, anxiety, and stuttering. Studies have implicated its use in treatment of asthma and impotence as well.

The single most effective biofeedback method has been electromyographic (EMG) monitoring, especially in the reduction of the severity of symptoms following neurological damage.[5] With the assistance of feedback, motor efficiency can be increased to levels not normally possible through the patient's improved muscular control. For example, EMG feedback is used in stroke patients to strengthen the tibialis anterior muscle in an attempt to enhance ankle dorsiflexion and aid in reducing foot drop and gait problems.[5] Brown and colleagues describe the employment of EMG feedback in facial muscle training after damage to the seventh cranial nerve.

As EMG methods have been used to increase muscle control, they are also used to decrease muscle activity when spasticity is present, although this is more complicated than muscle control. Although the effectiveness of EMG feedback in controlling spasticity is not fully established, positive results have been reported in reducing activity in cerebral palsy.[5]

Pain syndromes, including neck pain, low-back pain, myofascial pain syndrome, and phantom limb pain, have also been treated successfully by biofeedback. The patient with one of these disorders uses biofeedback to control pain related to muscle contraction. Biofeedback allows the prediction of contraction and the use of relaxation methods either to prevent the occurrence of pain or to lessen its effects. Other common clinical uses of EMG biofeedback are the reduction of muscular activity in tension headaches, reduction of spasms in torticollis, and increased sphincter control in fecal and urinary incontinence or retention.

The clinical uses of biofeedback are now being reported in cardiopulmonary fields; reports purporting to reduce hypertension and control arrhythmias have appeared; in neurology, claims have been made that epileptic seizures have been controlled.[2] Biofeedback often has been reported to be successful for conditions for which surgical or pharmacological interventions have proven ineffective. Biofeedback, however, is usually considered as an adjunct to conventional methods and not as a replacement for them. Therefore, patients should not be removed from concurrent medication regimens when biofeedback training has produced the desired results, especially in epilepsy, diabetes, and hypertension. Feedback should be performed only by a professional or in conjunction with a professional such as a physiatrist, psychiatrist, neurologist, orthopedic surgeon, psychologist, nurse, or occupational or physical therapist. Biofeedback sessions typically last from 45 to 60 minutes, occurring on a daily or weekly basis. A typical treatment regimen varies from 20 to 30 sessions. The desired changes are apparent after just a few sessions. Followup sessions, however, are useful. Highly motivated patients attain the best results, especially when biofeedback is presented in conjunction with relaxation training.

Summary

In this chapter some of the more common physical modalities used in rehabilitation medicine are presented. The chapter is intended to present an overview rather than offer specific prescription details. Physical modalities may greatly benefit patients with functional limitations as detected in the FASQ. Primary care physicians have an obligation to be familiar with the different types of modalities that exist and to contact a physiatrist or physical or occupational therapist when unsure about specific prescription details or appropriate modalities to be used.

Several physical modalities are discussed in this chapter. Therapeutic heat, including superficial heating methods (e.g., moist heat, heating pads, paraffin baths, and infrared treatments) and deep heating methods (e.g., shortwave, microwave, and ultrasound) are covered. Therapeutic cold methods are also discussed. Three properties of water—buoyancy, viscosity, and agitation—provide the beneficial analgesic and debridement effects of hydrotherapy. The use of ultraviolet radiation for treatment of dermatological conditions is presented. Several forms of massage, therapeutic exercise, stretching, and traction are also addressed. Suggestions for prescription requirements are made and indications and contraindications are discussed for each modality. An appendix is provided summarizing these therapeutic agents.

The informed physician can do a great deal to help improve a patient's function through physical therapy, occupational therapy, and other physical medicine applications. First and foremost, however, a physician must have a good working knowledge of the modalities and a thorough assessment of the patient's functional abilities and physical limitations. The FASQ and thorough SOAP note evaluation are suggested as the most efficient methods for obtaining this information and following the patient's progress after any treatment therapy has been initiated.

References

1. American Academy of Physical Medicine and Rehabilitation: Medical Knowledge Self-Assessment Program in Physical Medicine and Rehabilitation Syllabus. USA, 1977
2. Birbaumer N, Kimmel HD: Biofeedback and Self-Regulation, New York, Lawrence Erlbaum Associates, 1979
3. Borenstein S, Desmedt JE: Local cooling in myasthenia: Improvement of neuromuscular failure. Arch Neurol 32:152, 1975
4. Brown PM, Nashai, F, Wolf S, Basmajian JV: Electromyographic feedback in the re-education of facial palsy. Am J Phys Med 57:183, 1978
5. Cleveland CC: Biofeedback as a clinical tool: Its use with the neurologically impaired patient. In Filskov SB, Boll TJ (eds): Handbook of Clinical Neuropsychology. New York, John Wiley & Sons, 1981
6. Davis JB: Clinical applications of microwave radiation: Hypothermy and diathermy. Bull NY Acad Med 55(11):118, 1979
7. Delorme TL: Techniques of progressive resistance exercise. Arch Phys Med 29:263, 1948
8. Fisher E, Solomon S: Physiological responses to heat and cold. In Licht S, Kamenetz HL (eds): Therapeutic Heat and Cold, Chapter 4. New Haven, Elizabeth Licht, 1965
9. Gardner KR, Montgomery PS: Clinical Biofeedback: A Practical Procedural Manual. Baltimore, Williams & Wilkins, 1977
10. Gucker T: Use of heat and cold in orthopedics. In Licht S, Kamenetz HL (eds): Therapeutic Heat and Cold, Chapter 15. New Haven, Elizabeth Licht, 1965
11. Knapp ME: Massage. In Kottke FJ, Stillwell GK, Lehmann JF (eds): Krusen's Handbook of Physical Medicine and Rehabilitation, 3rd ed, Chapter 17. Philadelphia, WB Saunders, 1982
12. Kottke FJ: Therapeutic exercise. In Krusen FH, Kottke FJ, Ellwood PM Jr (eds): Physical Medicine and Rehabilitation, Chapter 16. Philadelphia, WB Saunders, 1968
13. Lehmann JF: Diathermy. In Krusen, FH, Kottke FJ, Ellwood PM Jr (eds): Physical Medicine and Rehabilitation, Chapter 11. Philadelphia, WB Saunders, 1968
14. Lehmann JF, Brunner AD, Stowe RW: Pain threshold measurements after therapeutic application of ultrasound, microwaves, and infrared. Arch Phys Med Rehabil 39:560, 1958
15. Lehmann JFD, DeLateur BJ: Heat and cold treatment. In Licht, S (ed): Arthritis and Physical Medicine. New Haven, Elizabeth Licht, 1969
16. Lehmann JF, DeLateur BJ: Diathermy and superficial heat and cold reactions. In Kottke FJ, Stillwell GK, Lehmann JF (eds): Krusen's Handbook of Physical Medicine and Rehabilitation. Philadelphia, WB Saunders, 1982
17. Lehmann JF, Masock, AJ, Warren CG, Koblanski, JN: Effect of therapeutic temperatures on tendon extensibility. Arch Phys Med Rehabil 51:481, 1970
18. Licht S: Physical therapy. In Licht S (ed): Rehabilitation and Medicine. Chapter 2. Baltimore, Elizabeth Licht, 1968
19. Materson RS: Physical medicine and rehabilitation for the medical practitioner. In Practice of Medicine, Volume 1. Hagerstown, Harper & Row, 1978
20. Melzack R, Wall PD: Pain mechanisms: A new theory. Science 150:971, 1965

21. Nichols PJR: Rehabilitation Medicine: The Management of Physical Disabilities, 2nd ed. London, Butterworths, 1980
22. Rusk HA: Rehabilitation Medicine. St Louis, CV Mosby, 1977
23. Shestack R: Handbook of Physical Therapy. New York, Springer-Verlag, 1977
24. Stillwell GK: Clinical electrical stimulation. In Licht S (ed): Therapeutic Electricity and Ultraviolet Radiation. Baltimore, Elizabeth Licht, 1967
25. Stillwell GK: Electrotherapy. In Kottke FJ, Stillwell GK, Lehmann JF (eds): Krusen's Handbook of Physical Medicine and Rehabilitation, Chapter 15. Philadelphia, WB Saunders, 1982
26. Stillwell GK: Therapeutic heat and cold. In Krusen FH, Kottke FJ, Ellwood PM Jr (eds): Physical Medicine and Rehabilitation, 2nd ed. Philadelphia, WB Saunders, 1971
27. Stillwell GK: Ultraviolet therapy. In Kottke FJ, Stillwell GK, Lehmann JF (eds): Krusen's Handbook of Physical Medicine and Rehabilitation, Chapter 14. Philadelphia, WB Saunders, 1982
28. Swezey RL: Arthritis: Rational Treatment and Rehabilitation, p 134. Philadelphia, WB Saunders, 1978
29. Vignos PJ: Rehabilitation in progressive muscular dystrophy. In Licht S (ed): Rehabilitation and Medicine. Baltimore, Elizabeth Licht, 1968
30. Wakim KG: Physiologic effects of massage. In Licht S (ed): Massage, Manipulation and Traction. New Haven, Elizabeth Licht, 1960
31. Zislis JM: Hydrotherapy. In Krusen FH, Kottke FJ, Ellwood, PM Jr (eds): Physical Medicine and Rehabilitation. Philadelphia, WB Saunders, 1968

Additional Readings

1. Basmajian JV (ed): Therapeutic Exercise, 3rd ed. Baltimore, Williams & Wilkins, 1978
2. Cremer RK, Perryman PW, Richards PM: The influence of light on the hyperbilirubinemia of infants. Lancet 1:1094, 1980
3. Keefe FJ, Schapira B, Williams RB, Brown C, Surwit RS: EMG-assisted relaxation training in the management of chronic low back pain. Am J Clin Biofeedback 4(2):93, 1981
4. Scott BO: Clinical uses of ultraviolet radiation. In Licht S (ed): Therapeutic Electricity and Ultraviolet Radiation. New Haven, Elizabeth Licht, 1967

APPENDIX 5-1   Brief Outline of Physical Treatment Modalities

Forms	Effects	Indications	Contraindications/ Precautions
Superficial heat			

Dry
  Infrared lamp
Moist
  Hydrotherapy
  Hot pack
  Paraffin bath
	Increases metabolism and circulation superficially
	Analgesia
	Sedation
		Pain, stiffness, spasm
		Preparation for activity
			Arterial insufficiency, heat insensitivity, edema, malignant neoplasm, active TB, hemorrhagic site, gravid uterus, unprotected eye

Deep heat			
Shortwave Microwave Ultrasound	Increases metabolism and circulation in muscles and joints Selective heating at tissue interfaces by ultrasound	Promote deep circulation when active motion is ineffective Neuritis, fibrosis, bursitis, tendinitis	Arterial insufficiency, heat insensitivity, acute inflammation, edema, osteoporosis, gravid uterus Implanted metal (except ultrasound) Must shield eyes
Superficial cold			
Ice pack	Analgesia Vasomotor response Hypothermia Edema reduction Bradycardia Decrease metabolism	Acute inflammation Edema after trauma Pain, spasm Gangrene (prior to amputation)	Labile hypertension, Raynaud's syndrome, cold insensitivity, ischemia, vasculitis, indolent wounds
Hydrotherapy			
Whirlpool Hubbard tank Swimming pool Vapo-coolant spray Sitz baths Hot/cold baths	Mild massage and relaxation (if anxious) Cleansing and debridement Exercise assist Cardiopulmonary responses	Pain, stiffness, spasm Facilitate weak motions Burns, decubiti, strains/sprains	Dry gangrene Profound neurological deterioration with increased core temp. in MS pts. Body immersion may be dangerous to patients with cardiovascular insufficiency

Continued

APPENDIX 5-1   *Continued*

Forms	Effects	Indications	Contraindications/ Precautions
Massage			
Stroking Compression Percussion	Mobilize scars, decrease edema, Mobilize deep structures in joints Desensitize painful neuromas	Burns Toughen amputation stump	Infection with inflammation, malignancies, hemorrhagic disorders, thrombophlebitis, communicable skin disorders Psychological dependence
Ultraviolet			
UV lamp	Conditions skin Tanning Promotes ulcer healing Combats superficial infections	Decubitus or stasis Dermatological conditions (acne vulgaris, psoriasis) Treat skin after cast removal	Advanced heart disease with failure or decompensation Active TB, hyperthyroidism, renal/ hepatic insufficiency May cause itching in diabetics Must shield eyes
Traction			
Manual Mechanical	Separates or aligns bony parts Stretches muscle spasm Pain relief Immobilization	Muscle spasm Subluxed arthritic joints Cervical pain Torticollis Low back pain	Cervical myelopathy secondary to chronic adhesions or bony osteophytes
Electrical Stimulation			
Long duration (galvanic) Short duration (faradic) TENS	Retards muscle atrophy Maintains contractility Exercise when patient is unable due to pain Reduces spasm and spasticity	Denervated muscle Innervated muscle with pain, spasm, spasticity, edema	Poor sensibility Cardiac pacemaker

Continued

APPENDIX 5-1   *Continued*

Forms	Effects	Indications	Contraindications/ Precautions
Therapeutic Exercise and Passive Stretching			
Range of motion active, passive stretching	Preserves range of motion, prevents contracture, elongates short-ened soft tissues	Paresis Arthritis, bursitis, tendinitis Body reconditioning	Caution with pa-tients with cardiac disease Recent myocardial infarction (espe-cially isometrics) Stretching may cause fracture in osteoporosis or tearing of soft tissues in or around joints
Strength isometric isotonic isokinetic	Maintains muscle bulk Increases strength Increases coordina-tion		
Endurance Coordination	Increases cardiopul-monary fitness and stamina		
Biofeedback			
EMG EEG Temperature feed-back Galvanic skin re-sponse Cardiovascular	Control of auto-nomic bodily processes (skin temp., BP, stom-ach acid) Decreases pain Increases/decreases muscle activity Promotes relaxation	Muscle dysfunction Hypertension Anxiety, concentra-tion difficulties Raynaud's syn-drome Migraine headache Skeletal pain syn-dromes Urinary inconti-nence Psychological dis-order Cardiac arrhythmias Insomnia	

CHAPTER 6
The Rehabilitation Disciplines

Comprehensive care, essential both to primary care and rehabilitation medicine, is provided by a variety of rehabilitation clinicians and other health professionals. In short-term inpatient rehabilitation programs and in some outpatient rehabilitation centers the planning, implementation, and evaluation of care are facilitated by a weekly team meeting where the patient's progress is discussed, treatment plans are modified when necessary, and every effort is made to ensure that the total range of the patient's needs is met. The outcome of a team approach has the potential to achieve an effect greater than the sum of individual team members' efforts.

A multidisciplinary team approach is not typical of outpatient primary care. Nonetheless, primary care physicians should be familiar with the kinds of expertise that various professionals can provide and the type of problems they are able to deal with that are frequently encountered in outpatient primary care settings. Many doctors are now forming groups associations that incorporate interdisciplinary exchange as both a common and a necessary part of the treatment plan. Often the hospital in which a physician practices has physical therapy, occupational therapy, and other rehabilitation disciplines available as outpatient services. Also, offices for social workers and home-care planners, who encourage appropriate referrals from physicians, are now included in some medical office buildings.

Chronicity does not mean necessarily that the health condition is static. Physicians periodically evaluate their chronically ill patients and update the plan of treatment following a review of current functional status and important support systems. The FASQ can help physicians to organize this information and alert them to their own professional limitations regarding certain kinds of problems. Medical and nonmedical staff should be involved in solving problems throughout the course of the patient's illness, whenever changing functional status, ineffective treatment programs, or new needs warrant additional attention. For example, the variability of symptoms and the need for flexible treatment plans necessitate an interdisciplinary approach to successful case management of the patient with multiple sclerosis. Various physicians may be required to make the diagnosis and plan ongoing treatment strategies: A neurologist for confirmation of the diagnosis and evaluation of mental status; a urologist for problems of urinary control; a physiatrist for evaluation of spasticity, gait, or need for an orthotic device; an ophthalmologist for evaluation of visual disturbance; and a psychiatrist for evaluation of emotional adjustment. Various nonphysician health professionals also may be required to address problem areas: Rehabilitation nurses can provide bowel and bladder training and assess learning needs; dietitians can offer nutritional counseling; speech–language pathologists can deal with dysarthria and dysphagia; occupational therapists can provide self-help devices so that patients can care for themselves; physical therapists can assist the patient in performing exercises that increase strength, endurance, and coordination, encourage the patient to carry out movements to prevent contractures, and train the patient in techniques to conserve energy; and vocational counselors, social workers, and psychologists collaborate in evaluating and revising work and family relationships. The total treatment plan is directed toward functional improvement.

The following descriptions of rehabilitation professionals provide information about their expertise as well as the referral requirements necessary to provide the comprehensive, continuous, and coordinated care discussed in Chapter 1. We hope that primary care physicians will make efficient use of these professionals to provide the best of care in their ambulatory practices.

Physiatrist

Physiatry, the practice of physical medicine and rehabilitation, is one of the new specialty fields in medicine. The physiatrist has expertise in the techniques of medical examination, diagnosis, evaluation, and treatment of neuromusculoskeletal impairments. The physiatrist's specialized knowledge in pain evaluation, mobility deficits, and muscle weakness is derived from a strong background in anatomy, physiology, and neuroscience. Unlike most medical specialists, the physiatrist is especially trained in the techniques of functional assessment and is likely to pursue a holistic approach to medical care.

> The physiatrist is trained in understanding the physiologic consequences of injury and illness and commonly functions as the medical rehabilitation program manager for patients with moderate to severe disabilities by identifying and activating solutions to the physical, emotional, social, and vocational problems consequent to disease and/or injury.[4]

The physiatrist in a hospital or rehabilitation center coordinates and administers a comprehensive treatment plan in close association with allied health professionals. The physician, acting as "case manager," discusses both the short-term and long-range goals of each patient with the other members of the interdisciplinary team. Since the nature and degree of disability from any impairment frequently vary from patient to patient, the physiatrist considers psychological and environmental factors in addition to pertinent medical conditions. The physician may enlist the services of the social worker, clinical psychologist, physical therapist, or occupational therapist for further confirmation of presumed diagnoses.

Many physiatrists also play a key role as advocates for the cause of the handicapped and disabled. They may be involved in research to improve prosthetic devices, or they may work closely with community groups to increase the availability of housing or educational or job opportunities and to reduce architectural and prejudicial barriers.

The physiatrist's expertise can be a valuable resource for the primary care physician in the ambulatory setting. Physiatrists aid family physicians not only in confirming diagnoses for acute conditions such as carpal tunnel syndrome or Bell's palsy, but also in helping to develop a case management program and followup evaluation for patients with chronic health impairments. Physiatrists' specialized training in the use of physical treatment modalities (*e.g.*, therapeutic hot and cold, hydrotherapy, electrical stimulation, traction, exercise, and biofeedback) to treat neuromusculoskeletal disorders enables them to determine the appropriate physical treatment. Physiatrists' thorough knowledge of the techniques of treatment allows them also to advise the primary care physician about prescribing and the useful time limits for therapy.

If the family physician does not see any improvement following treatment in the persistent weakness or joint dysfunction that seriously limits performance of work, self-care, or other activities, or cannot discover the etiology of the problem, he might refer the patient to a physiatrist. The physiatrist administers specialized electrodiagnostic tests, including electromyography and nerve conduction studies, which may identify problems not detected in the physical examination or which may confirm suspected diagnoses. When indicated, the physiatrist can also help the primary care physician choose appropriate prosthetic or orthotic devices to maximize the patient's ability to function. Finally, the physiatrist may act as an important referral source and can inform physicians and patients about community and rehabilitation programs. When enlisting the consultative services of a physiatrist, the referring physician should include diagnoses, pertinent history, significant laboratory and x-ray results, and current medications. It is also important to inform the physiatrist of the specific functional problems to be addressed.

Rehabilitation Nurse

The rehabilitation nurse, like other nurses, has the primary concern for daily patient care and health maintenance. She differs from acute care nurses in range of activities and areas of expertise and philosophy. Although the rehabilitation nurse frequently provides care in a specialized rehabilitation setting, many aspects of the care, such as bed positioning, exercise, and patient education are preventive. The nurse in the rehabilitation setting encourages the patient to take an active rather than a passive role in the rehabilitation process. A common feature of inpatient rehabilitation is the presence of a primary nurse who has the responsibility for a patient's total nursing needs. This permits greater continuity of nursing care in response to the patient's progress and needs than is achieved in arrangements typical of acute care settings.

One of the rehabilitation nurse's primary functions is to oversee the implementation of many of the programs designed in physical, occupational, and speech therapy. The nurse who is in daily contact with the patient helps him to practice these therapeutic programs and provides reinforcement and additional training in activities such as transfers, ambulation, communication, and self-care. The rehabilitation nurse uses a knowledge of bed positioning and body alignment to prevent bed sores and postural problems, such as drop foot, which frequently occur with poststroke patients. The nurse also uses passive range of motion to prevent secondary impairments of disuse atrophy and contracture. In addition, the nurse is an expert in intermittent transurethral catheterization and stump care. Rehabilitation nurses often serve as teachers for patient and family members in areas such as bowel and bladder training, use of assistive devices, administration of medication, and other aspects of physical functioning.

As the only rehabilitation clinician to maintain 24-hour patient contact, the nurse is able to observe the patient's physical functioning and emotional adjustment closely. If family members are able to visit only during the evening, the nurse may be the primary contact with the family and the only one available to observe family dynamics relevant to discharge planning or necessary long-term adjustments. Hospitalization in a rehabilitation setting is usually more lengthy than hospitalization in an acute care setting. The rehabilitation nurse often plays an important supportive role and serves as an informal counselor to the patient and family.

The rehabilitation nurse also communicates with the other members of the rehabilitation team so that treatment programs can be continued or modified in accordance with the patient's daily progress. The nurse's responsibilities include an assessment of the patient's posthospitalization nursing needs and possibly a recommendation for a visiting nurse referral. After the rehabilitation team members have agreed upon a discharge plan, the physician must provide a summary of the patient's course in the hospital and, if needed, a referral for home nursing care.

A clinical nurse specialist in rehabilitation has a master's degree and is prepared to function as an educator, researcher, program consultant, and change agent. More and more registered nurses are becoming certified in this specialty.

Physical Therapist

The preparation of a physical therapist (PT) includes a strong background in anatomy, physiology, and kinesiology. In addition, the PT is trained to evaluate musculoskeletal disorders and to use physical treatment modalities.

> The physical therapist plays an essential role in the rehabilitation of the physically disabled, and is responsible for evaluation of the physical capacities and limitations, and for administering treatments designed to alleviate pain, correct or minimize deformity, increase strength and mobility, and improve general health.[2]

Physical therapists usually participate in the rehabilitation of patients with stroke, hemiparesis, amputation, joint and neuromuscular disorders, or chronic pain. In some instances, the PT may be able to test pulmonary function and perform cardiac ergometric studies. Physical therapists are skilled in testing the patient's muscle strength, active and passive range of motion, and the ability to stand and maintain balance. They also analyze gait patterns, develop ambulation and stair-climbing skills, supervise exercise programs, and evaluate the usefulness of orthotic and prosthetic appliances.

Restoration of mobility and functioning is the ultimate goal of all physical therapy treatment, that is, to maximize task performance necessary for daily functioning. Treatment regimens should be designed not only to alleviate pain, but to address the underlying problems as well. Massage ordered for the relief of pain, for example, should not be prescribed in isolation, but rather as an adjunct to other methods of treatment such as exercise and postural and gait training, which correct the underlying functional limitation.

Referral information should include the patient's diagnosis, history, and physical findings. All suspected problems and all aspects of them should be detailed, especially any precautions to be observed during therapy. Furthermore, problems or areas to be treated, duration of the treatment period, and treatment goals should be indicated. Whether the physician should specify procedures to be used or the number and frequency of treatments depends upon the physician's familiarity with the techniques of physical treatment. Therapy that continues after maximum benefits have been reached can be harmful, as it tends to keep the patient in a sick role; on the other hand, if treatment is to continue past the period specified by the original order or beyond 30 days, whichever is sooner, the prescription must be renewed. In addition, when the physician is uncertain about a diagnosis or a treatment, he or she can make a referral for an evaluation by a physical therapist, which may clarify the specific nature of the problem or the appropriate treatment regimen.

A number of problems seen by the primary care physician on an outpatient basis can benefit from physical therapy. Potentially debilitating chronic conditions such as low-back pain and arthritis (which are extremely common in outpatient primary care practice) can benefit from exercise, postural retraining, and treatment with physical modalities. These physical therapy methods help to alleviate pain, reduce swelling, and increase range of motion and mobility. Physical therapy is the mainstay of treatment for maintaining maximum mobility and for preventing deformity typical of muscular and neuromuscular conditions such as cerebral palsy, muscular dystrophy, multiple sclerosis, and Parkinsonism. Patients with pulmonary and cardiac problems are also appropriately referred to specially trained physical therapists. Patients who exhibit difficulty in activities such as sitting, standing, walking, and climbing stairs, as revealed by the FASQ, should be referred to physical therapy for evaluation and treatment. Physical therapy can play a very important role as well in the primary prevention of chronic disability. For example, posture and gait retraining of elderly patients can reduce the risk of falls that result in hip fractures. Range of motion exercises can prevent contractures and deformities that often result from fractures or severe burns.

A note of caution: A patient should not be referred to a PT merely to get him "off the physician's hands." The physician must have a thorough understanding of the physical and emotional factors that may underlie the disabling complaint. If the physician does not understand all the interacting dynamic factors, he should consider a referral to a physiatrist or other rehabilitation specialist.

Occupational Therapist

The goal of the occupational therapist (OT) is to help the patient achieve and maintain maximal ability to perform activities important for independence in everyday living. Primarily the OT is interested in the patient's abilities to carry out personal care activities, household tasks, responsibilities of the work place (including skills and work tolerance), and educational and recreational activities.

The preparation of the occupational therapist includes a background in biological sciences as well as fine and industrial arts and crafts and orthotics. Further, OTs have special instruction in helping people with disabilities to learn self-care techniques. They also learn counseling skills for the assessment and improvement of functional limitations.

Armed with this background in physical, psychological, and developmental skills, the OT is capable of assessing and treating the patient with functional deficits resulting from physical or cognitive manifestations of disease, injury, or congenital abnormalities. It has been said of occupational therapy that, "There is no other profession supplementary to medicine so aptly suited to help the patient bridge the gap between physical disability and functional capability."[5]

The occupational therapist is especially knowledgeable about upper limb function because upper limbs are involved in most activities of daily living. Therefore, the OT can be very helpful in evaluating fine motor activity and functional limitation of stroke, multiple sclerosis, other neuromuscular disorders, arthritis, hand injuries, and upper limb amputations. The OT is able to develop exercises and activities to increase range of motion and muscle strength as well. In this respect activities of physical therapists and occupational therapists tend to overlap. Nichols, in differentiating between the two disciplines, notes that "whereas the physiotherapist is concerned with recording the range of strength of the movement, the occupational therapist is more concerned with applied range, strength and coordination in the performance of essential activities."[7] Exercises to improve balance and coordination, training in transfers, fine motor skills, and adapted activities of daily living skills are all important to the occupational therapy regime. Examples of the OT's contribution to the rehabilitation process are teaching a stroke patient how to dress and eat when one limb is paralyzed or retraining an amputee homemaker to prepare food and maintain a household.

Occupational therapists are also skilled in the administration, interpretation, and application of tests to assess vocational and avocational aptitudes. One application of such testing is in the treatment of children with developmental disabilities. The stimulation of skills such as concentration, perceptual abilities, and social interaction may increase the child's readiness for learning. OTs also use aptitude tests to help physically disabled adults redevelop the skills necessary to return to a former occupation or to adapt to the requirements of a new one. They teach work simplification skills and provide orientation training to visually impaired individuals to enhance their adaptation to functional deficits.

An OT assumes a major role in teaching a patient to use adaptive equipment, such as the one-handed shoe tie, elastic stocking, utensil extension handle, or many of the other devices that help people with disabilities function independently. OTs devise assistive devices such as splints for finger, hand, or arm support, which may be major factors in determining whether a patient can return home after hospitalization. The OT can suggest ways to modify the home environment to maximize personal independence. For example, the OT may suggest that countertops be lowered so that they are accessible to individuals in wheelchairs for cooking and other household tasks.

The physician frequently refers to an occupational therapist, as to other therapists, to conduct an assessment and develop a treatment plan. If the physician is unfamiliar with occupational therapy treatment programs, a referral to a physiatrist is in order. A referral to an OT should always include the diagnosis, present physical, mental, and emotional status, treatment program, and desired results. When the physician makes a referral for a specific treatment, as in the case of the arthritic patient referred for splints, the prescription should specify the presenting or suspected problem. Also the referral form should indicate whether the therapy is to be performed in bed or in the occupational therapy department and should include any precautions. The physician should maintain continuing contact with the OT to discuss treatment goals and progress. Therapy is commonly prescribed for a period of 4 to 6 weeks, after which the patient's progress is evaluated. If therapy is to be continued, an additional prescription is required at this time.

Although occupational therapy is often prescribed on an inpatient basis, assessment and treatment are frequently useful in outpatient practice, before problems become acute. Examples of outpatient referral services include: Developing splints to prevent deformities in patients with arthritis or muscular dystrophy; retraining stroke and upper limb amputees who need to improve their functional abilities; and assessing patients with unexplained arm and shoulder pain or generalized weakness or swelling. In addition, occupational therapists assist and treat patients who on the FASQ exhibit difficulty with transfers, personal care tasks, fine motor skills, cognition, or visual–spatial orientation.

Prosthetist and Orthotist

The prosthetist is responsible for designing and fitting replacement limbs. The orthotist designs and fits exoskeletal devices for the limbs and spine to provide support, prevent or correct deformity, and limit or assist motion. Both the prosthetist and orthotist are responsible for taking measurements, designing and fitting the appliance, and providing information to familiarize the patient with use of the device. These specialists are typically in private practice, but some meet with rehabilitation physicians and therapists or serve as consultants in a hospital or specialized clinic.

Both prosthetic and orthotic devices must be prescribed by a physician. For the physician who is not experienced in the evaluation and prescription of these devices, a referral to a physiatrist should be made. A prescription for a prosthetic device should indicate design requirements, including joint mechanism, suspension apparatus, and material to be used in fabrication. An orthotic prescription should specify desired goals for use of the device, location of straps, types of joints, and material to be used in fabrication.

The prescription for an upper limb prosthesis should include information concerning cables, joints, utility hooks, dress hands, and other holding tools. Information concerning the patient's diagnosis, general health, lifestyle, employment, and range of activities is extremely important in order to design a device that will maximize the patient's functional abilities.

Prior to an amputation, a physiatric consultation helps to ensure that the level of amputation being considered is consistent with optimal fitting of a prosthesis. Successful use of a lower limb prosthesis depends in large part on the postoperative regimen to shrink and toughen the stump. Often a shared evaluation by the physiatrist, orthotist, or prosthetist and attending physician is useful in formulating a prescription. The physician should order a thorough program of instruction and should include physical therapy for a lower limb device or occupational therapy for an upper limb device. A followup evaluation by the orthotist or prosthetist, to observe the appliance in use, is helpful in determining the need for modifications, which are often necessary.

The primary care physician plays a central role in the evaluation and prescription of orthotic and prosthetic devices. Early intervention may be crucial for maximum benefit. An order for an arm prosthesis should be given as early as 6 months of age (or when the child is able to sit unattended and begins to have trunk balance) for a child with a congenital upper limb impairment. As a child or teenager grows, the physician should re-evaluate the need for new or revised devices. Patients and family members should be well informed of the benefits and correct use of assistive devices, as well as their limitations.

Prior to an amputation, the physician should provide adequate information to help alleviate anxiety and encourage reasonable expectations. Emotional support from the physician helps the patient and family accept orthotic and prosthetic equipment and facilitates the adjustment process. Use of the FASQ may help to pinpoint environmental modifications that are needed and affective components of the disability. Continued physician contact with other rehabilitation team members assures a coordinated patient care program. Patients and family members also should be encouraged to participate in planning the treatment program. The patient should be referred to social workers and other counseling personnel when necessary, and to home care nurses to achieve maximal adjustment to the prosthetic or orthotic device.

Speech–Language Pathologist

The speech–language pathologist specializes in the physiological and neurological basis of language processing and speech production. The speech–language pathologist, who should be trained minimally at the level of a master's degree, is able to evaluate and treat a variety of communication dysfunctions including speech, vocal, and linguistic disorders. Speech disorders can be caused by a structural deviation (such as cleft palate), head or neck surgery or trauma, sensory or motor deviation (deafness, hearing loss, dysarthria, dyspraxia), or affective disorders. Voice disorders may be caused by paresis or paralysis of the vocal cords, organic disease, or psychogenic factors. Linguistic disorders may be due to hearing loss, central nervous system dysfunction (aphasia, developmental delay), environmental deprivation, or emotional disturbance. Dysphagia (the inability to swallow), frequently seen in neurologic patients, is treated both by speech–language pathologists and by occupational therapists. Speech–language pathologists can provide training in lip reading and other communication skills. Speech therapists are trained also in the general evaluation of hearing impairments, and some have full certification in the field of audiology. Speech–language pathologists work on communication problems stemming from a wide range of etiologies in addition to stroke, including cerebral palsy, multiple sclerosis and other neurological disorders, congenital malformations such as cleft palate, other physical impairments such as otologic impairment, or acquired pathologic conditions due to surgery, tumor, burn, or trauma. Stuttering and language problems of developmentally disabled persons are also treated by speech therapists.

Speech–language pathologists in the hospital setting frequently work with aphasic stroke patients. Because almost one half of stroke patients suffer from some degree of aphasia, speech therapy is an essential part of stroke rehabilitation. Before a referral is made to a speech–language pathologist for a detailed evaluation, the physician should conduct a general assessment of the patient's functioning, including behavioral observations and, when appropriate, computerized tomography of the brain may be helpful. The referral should be made after the patient has stabilized medically, although a prolonged delay in referral may increase the patient's fear, confusion, and feelings of isolation because he may not understand that the communication difficulties are secondary to the stroke. Because the patient's physical condition can change drastically within the first few weeks, an initial assessment is frequently not sufficient. For example, a patient with global aphasia who was not ready for therapy initially may improve to a point at which speech therapy would be beneficial. At the time of the initial referral, the primary care physician should supply information concerning the patient's premorbid hearing, cognitive function, reading ability, and educational level, to enable the therapist to make an accurate assessment of the degree of communication loss.

In contrast to some other rehabilitation interventions, speech therapy is a relatively long-term process, often requiring a minimum of 6 months. The final outcome of speech therapy may be the complete recovery of speech, partial recovery of speech, or the use of a manual system of communication (sign language). Family members need to participate in therapy in order to facilitate the continuation of exercises at home. The primary care physician can ease the adjustment of the aphasic patient through patient and family education that includes accurate information concerning the probability of a lengthy therapy process and the likelihood of total speech recovery.

In outpatient primary care, the physician is likely to confront problems of speech and delays in language development. Early intervention and referral are crucial for maximal success. The child who does not speak by 2 years of age should be referred for an evaluation. Elderly patients with cognitive, memory, or speech problems may be referred for training in lip reading or improvement of communication skills. The primary care physician should be aware of difficulties of speech and communication at any age, as these problems may lead to frustration, depression, and deterioration of family and social relationships.

Social Worker

> There is no discipline better suited to helping patients and their families learn to cope with the social and emotional problems created by disability than social work.[1]

The social worker has a background in family dynamics, social policy, community structure, and human behavior. Although a Bachelor's Degree in social work is available, the Master's of Social Work (MSW) Degree increasingly is required. The completion of 2 years of postgraduate study with emphases on normal and abnormal human behavior, on casework methodologies on research, and on "hands on" field experience are necessary.

The social worker interviews the patient, family members, and other relevant persons in order to obtain an overview of the patient's current social situation leading to psychosocial adjustment. Information is obtained on living arrangements, family relationships, financial status, vocational training, and future goals. The social worker also studies the patient's responses and attitudes toward disability as a means of evaluating the effect of the illness on his ability to function and participate in rehabilitative efforts. The process of evaluation involves an assessment of the patient's physical and mental abilities, cultural values and norms, social interaction skills, and personal expectations.

Social workers help the patient and family identify and cope with losses due to illness. Deprivation due to chronic and disabling conditions can be compounded by loss of bodily functions and independence, emotional composure, job and family roles, status and self-image, as well as future dreams. The social worker can also be an invaluable source of information and referral (for both the patient and the physician) for available community resources.

The social worker in the hospital setting acts as liaison between physician, patients, and community services. For example, a stroke patient may need adaptive changes in the home, financial counseling, homemaker services, or temporary placement in a rehabilitation facility; a new colostomy patient may need regular visits by a visiting nurse as well as a supply of ostomy aids; or a postmastectomy patient may need information about specialized clothing or community support groups. If permanent physical limitation or impending death threaten relationships, the social worker can offer emotional support and intensive counseling to help the patient and family cope and accept what cannot be changed. The social worker can inform the referring physician if there is a need for additional consultative services by other disciplines or outside agencies.

Social workers in outpatient primary care can provide information about community services, insurance coverage, transportation services, day programs, and extended care facilities. Through counseling they can help people cope with the stress and demands of a disabled family member. They can suggest other social supports that would forestall or delay institutionalization. The social worker can help multihandicapped patients by coordinating the various agency services provided. These are just a few examples of a social worker's role in outpatient medical care.

The physician referring a patient to a social worker should include the diagnosis, treatment plans, prognosis, if known, and any background information available. Also helpful are names and relationships of other family members, job title and location, previous medical or psychiatric problems, previously known familial problems, and any significant behavioral problems occurring during the present hospitalization.

Clinical Psychologist

The clinical psychologist has an educational background in the affective, cognitive, social, and biological bases of behavior. He is trained to assess personality, intelligence, behavioral performance, and perceptual-motor function, as well as to provide psychotherapy and counseling. Within the clinical psychology practice model, it is expected that practitioners prepared at the doctoral level are not only clinicians but research scientists as well. Although a Master's Degree in psychology is conferred, most clinical psychologists have completed at least 4 years of postgraduate education and have obtained a Ph.D. or other doctoral degree. A year of supervised postdoctoral practice is required for licensure.

The psychologist in the inpatient hospital rehabilitation setting is often asked to assess the way patients function cognitively and affectively. The psychologist utilizes standardized tests such as the Wechsler Adult Intelligence Scales or other neuropsychological tests to perform assessments. Standardized tests to measure the patient's affective domain are generally less available than intelligence or achievement tests; however, tests such as the Minnesota Multiphasic Personality Inventory (MMPI) are administered to obtain measures in a somewhat objective fashion. Psychologists also evaluate patients on the basis of observations. By these means of assessment, the psychologist is able to participate with the physician and other rehabilitation team members in making a differential diagnosis of organic brain syndrome and affective disorders.

The psychologist plays an important role in helping the patient adjust to chronic illness and disability. The psychologist can treat patients' anxiety related to illness and explore feelings of loss. Long-term adjustment and modification of self-concept, motivation, and social interaction usually are components of the treatment of chronic illness and disability. The psychologist also functions as a consultant to other team members by helping them to understand the emotional distress that patients experience, or that team members experience when treating the patient who is difficult to manage. Furthermore, the psychologist might help a team member develop behavioral programs for patients in order to maximize their performance in therapy.

Referral to a psychologist is appropriate in an outpatient setting for many of the reasons delineated above, such as cognitive testing, affective evaluation, and psychotherapeutic treatment interventions. Referral information should include a description of the presenting problem, allied medical conditions, and other relevant psychosocial information.

It might be appropriate also to involve a psychologist for consultation when implementing a functionally oriented treatment plan. The focus of analysis of a functionally oriented treatment plan is behavior. Behavior is also the key issue addressed by many psychologists in clinical practice. Psychologists can therefore share their expertise in assessing a patient's behavioral reactions to chronic health problems and aid the primary care physician in developing effective treatment programs that focus on increasing functional capacities. The burgeoning field of behavioral medicine has propelled the clinical psychologist into a new treatment role in primary care settings. The clinical use of treatment intervention techniques derived from the experimental analysis of behavior has been applied increasingly to a wide variety of health problems seen in primary care settings. These include smoking behavior, obesity, self-regulation of hypertension, headaches, insomnia, chronic pain, asthma, Raynaud's syndrome, type A behavior, and so on. A functionally oriented treatment plan is likely to dovetail well with behavior modification and behavior therapy techniques because the focus is on behavior and its effect on health and rehabilitation.

Psychiatrist

Psychiatrists are interested in the evaluation and treatment of patients with mental and emotional disorders. Because of their medical school education, psychiatrists are able to assess the biological aspects of mental illness. In particular, psychiatrists can prescribe psychopharmacologic agents to treat psychological disorders.

Patients in the rehabilitation setting are at high risk for severe emotional and mental disorders due to congenital mental dysfunction, head trauma, senile dementia, and other acquired neurological disorders. Some rehabilitation patients are unable to adapt successfully to having a chronic illness or disabling condition. A psychiatrist should be consulted when organic causes are thought to be related to psychological reactions and, in particular, when the psychological reactions are life-threatening. Examples of reactions severe enough to warrant intervention by a psychiatrist include: continuous, uncontrolled hysterical outbursts; aggressive behavior; suicidal tendencies or attempts; and severe, extended depression that interferes with the patient's ability to perform everyday functions or to receive rehabilitation training.

Vocational Counselor

The vocational counselor has a background in vocational guidance, counseling theory, and the medical and psychosocial aspects of disability. Vocational counselors usually work in state vocational rehabilitation agencies, veterans' hospitals, and large rehabilitation centers.

The counselor works toward restoring and developing the disabled person's ability to maintain employment, which is important for independent living, self-esteem, and physical and mental health. To a vocational counselor the medical patient is the client. He administers aptitude tests to determine a person's work potential and assesses the client's interests and previous work experiences by means of discussion with the client. The counselor helps the client identify occupations that are appropriate to his or her individual skills, arranges for training or retraining workshops, contacts potential employers, assesses the work site (arranging for any necessary environmental modifications), and provides ongoing counseling for long-term support. The vocational counselor may refer the client for medical or restorative care, orthotic and prosthetic devices, or other aids. A sheltered workshop may be indicated for the severely disabled person so that he can learn and practice vocational skills in a supervised environment. The vocational counselor may arrange a home evaluation and training in homemaker skills for the individual who wants to live independently or is the primary homemaker. The vocational rehabilitation agency serves as a source of payment for all of these services. In some states vocational rehabilitation also offers orientation and mobility training for the blind.

Many patients with a chronic or degenerative illness can benefit from a vocational counselor's assistance. To be eligible for vocational services the client must be physically or mentally impaired resulting in a disability for employment. There also must be a reasonable expectation that the individual will benefit from the agency's services. Individuals who are currently working but need help to maintain their employment may also be eligible.

Vocational counselors in the hospital setting often receive referrals through the social service, physical, and occupational therapy departments. Physicians refer both inpatients and outpatients directly when a need is suspected. Many clients seeking services independently might benefit from an earlier referral. To help the counselor in the evaluation process, the physician should provide relevant information concerning the individual's medical, neurological, psychological, and educational status. The vocational counselor is responsible for maintaining contact with the referring physician and with the employer after employment has been arranged.

Dietitian

An often overlooked member of the rehabilitation team is the dietitian. This professional can contribute valuable information and skills both to the in-hospital interdisciplinary team and to the primary care physician's ambulatory practice.

A qualified dietitian, one who is certified by the American Dietetic Association, can work in conjunction with the physician to assess the results of the physical examination and blood tests or other laboratory studies to determine whether there is a nutritional disorder or other physical problem interfering with the eating process. In addition to assessment, the dietitian can help the physician to formulate a nutritional care plan—including weight loss programs, counseling, and monitoring of nutritional adequacy.

The dietitian also works in conjunction with other rehabilitation team members. She may collaborate with the occupational therapist, for example, to identify special equipment or utensils that would ease the eating process for disabled people. Difficulties in chewing, swallowing, or handling food may be alleviated by the dietitian's guidance in suggesting easier foods for the person to handle.

> The nutritionist provides assistance in planning for nutritional needs and working out a diet, adjusting size, shape, texture, consistency, color, and form to conform with the handicap.[3]

The dietitian may also assist the social worker in determining ways to overcome problems involving access to shopping, cooking, and eating facilities, or in reducing the economic burden of specialized diets. A knowledge of community resources such as food stamps, Meals on Wheels, The Women's, Infant's and Children's Supplemental Food Program (WIC), as well as federally or locally funded feeding programs, may help persons with limited funds or limited access to transportation resources. Referral of elderly or disabled patients to day care programs can help assure access both to well-balanced meals and to socialization. Dietitians can refer patients for dental services when they observe that dental problems may be interfering with eating a balanced diet. Many dietitians, especially in public health agencies, offer educational programs on nutrition, consumer education, food co-ops, and selection, preparation, and storage of food.

A referral to a dietitian should be made when the physical examination, medical history, or laboratory studies indicate present or potential malnutrition, digestive problems, or that a special diet is required. When making the referral the physician should indicate the diagnosis, significant blood work, radiographic and clinical laboratory results, previously known digestive or dietary problems, and any available information concerning the patient's background, physical or mental limitations, and social support system.

Visiting Nurse

The visiting nurse is an essential link in the configuration of health services for patients with rehabilitation or extended care needs. A visiting nurse provides a full range of nursing services, which include checking vital signs, administering medication, changing dressings, and educating patients. She also provides followup to physical and occupational therapy services by supervising exercise regimens, ambulation, and personal care activities. Services are available to supplement outpatient care in the early stages of recovery from acute illness or on a temporary or extended basis when functional limitations or environmental obstacles prevent the use of outpatient services.

Nursing assistance, nutritional counseling, physical, occupational, and speech therapy, oxygen and intravenous therapy, and social services are often available to the patient by professionals on the Visiting Nurse Association staff. Some Visiting Nurse Associations also offer pediatric services, which include education in proper nutrition, dress, skin care, home safety for young parents, and nursing care for children with acute short-term conditions. Of particular importance regarding rehabilitation is that nursing care is available for children with longer term developmental difficulties. The Visiting Nurse Association also provides home-care assistance for patients who are acutely ill, thus reducing the time necessary for hospitalization. In addition, visiting nurse services may prevent placement in a nursing home by enabling a chronically ill patient to remain in the community while receiving necessary nursing care.

Physicians can request the Visiting Nurse Association's services prior to the patient's discharge from the hospital so as to prevent a delay in the initiation of services. Often the physician writes an order requesting the hospital or rehabilitation center's social service department to make the necessary arrangements. If there is no social service department, if the family requests it, or if the physician observes that it is needed, he can call the VNA directly or send a written request for service. Most hospitals have special discharge planning forms that the physician must complete, indicating the diagnosis, secondary complications, orders for specific nursing care functions or therapy treatment, and desired frequency of services. The physician also should note any special problems or limitations about which the visiting nurse should be aware and should monitor.

Unlike some rehabilitation professionals, the visiting nurse does not need a physician's referral to perform an initial evaluation. Other nurses, social workers, family members, or neighbors may initiate contact with the regional Visiting Nurse Association for an evaluation and, if necessary, immediate care. The visiting nurse will contact the physician with a report of the patient's nursing needs. After two home visits, physician's orders are necessary for continuance of services and Medicaid reimbursement. When treatment begins the nurse sends a written report of the patient's progress to the physician, noting the residual nursing needs, every 4 weeks. Treatment will be provided for the period of time that it is needed or until it is discontinued by the physician.

Homemaker, Home Health Aide, and Personal Care Attendant

Homemakers, home health aides, and personal care attendants provide health care and supportive services to sick or disabled persons in the patient's own home. These service providers play an important role in comprehensive, functionally oriented health care. They help to meet many essential needs of people during acute illness and convalescence after surgery or chronic disability, when assistance is needed with activities of daily living on an extended basis. Services are provided to all ages, from newborns to the elderly, and can be provided for a single individual or an entire family. "Responsibilities range from complicated home management, which requires a variety of skills, to performance of a few simple tasks, such as weekly marketing or housecleaning."[8] Such interventions may prevent or delay institutionalization of functionally-limited individuals and can provide periodic relief from responsibilities for family members and other social support systems.

The *home health aide* (HHA) is trained to provide assistance in personal and household care. Although no educational degrees are required, preparation includes at least 40 hours of classroom study and supervised in-service training. Additional specialized courses may be available to those working with more problematic patients, such as emotionally disturbed, paralyzed, or visually impaired patients. The range of services he provides includes assistance with personal care tasks such as bathing, oral hygiene, hair, back and foot care, checking of vital signs, ambulation, use of prosthetics, braces, and walkers, medication supervision, and active and passive exercise. Help is provided with household tasks such as bed changing, laundry, shopping, cooking, and home management. Some home health aides are skilled in the areas of work simplification, body mechanics, kitchen planning, and use of special equipment. Home health aides are available from Visiting Nurse Associations and public and private home health care agencies.

In the past two decades, third party health insurance has become a major source of funding for home health-care services. Usually the home health-care services covered by Medicare are short-term, skilled services to be used by persons recovering from an acute illness or injury. At present, home health aide services are provided only in addition to skilled nursing care, speech therapy, or physical therapy. Medicare has no coverage for long-term maintenance or preventive home health-care services. Medicaid has more lenient provisions and often will cover home health aide services when required for medical reasons. Private insurance is now beginning to expand its coverage for coordinated home health-care services. The hospital social worker, health insurance information office, or private home health-care agency can help the patient determine eligibility for home health aide services.

Homemakers, who are often mistakenly believed to be identical to home health aides, provide assistance *only* with household tasks. Homemaker chores include shopping and meal preparation, light housekeeping, and laundry care. Although some homemakers may provide minimal assistance to the patient with dressing and eating, many agencies have a strict "hands off" policy regarding any personal care of the patient. Homemaker services are usually available from private agencies. Although a referral may be initiated by the social worker or physician in charge, many private agencies require a close family member to make the necessary arrangements. At present Medicare and most health insurance plans provide no coverage for the home care services provided by a homemaker. In some states Medicaid will pay for these services provided there is documented need indicated by the physician or social worker.

Most home health agencies require a doctor's order before initiating services. Typically physician involvement in home care is greater when acute care patients are being treated at home than when only maintenance or preventive services are being offered. In both circumstances, however, according to Stewart,[8] the physician should play a contributing role in management of home care services, assuming responsibility for seeing that the overall plan of care is appropriate and necessary.

The *personal care attendant* (PCA) is a new category of health care assistant aiding in the physical care of paralyzed and other disabled persons. PCAs perform a variety of duties including bathing, feeding, and hygienic care of the patient, food preparation and light housekeeping chores, transportation assistance, and transfers to and from a wheelchair. There are no formal educational or training requirements; on the contrary, disabled persons hire and train their own PCAs.[6] This has a dual beneficial effect: First, since formally learned methods may not be suitable for all persons being served, the employer is able to train the assistant to meet his individual needs; second, the disabled person is required to manage his own affairs.

Unlike homemakers or home health aides, PCAs usually are not provided by home care agencies. Rather disabled persons must depend upon newspaper ads, "word of mouth," or local rehabilitation agency contacts for names of suitable people. Additionally, Blue Cross and Medicare do not reimburse for these services at this time. Some state vocational rehabilitation agencies provide up to 100% coverage. When such aid is not available, it is often possible for two or more people to share a PCA in order to lessen the financial burden.

Persons interested in obtaining a personal care attendant should contact the local paraplegia association, vocational rehabilitation office, or independent living program. There are approximately 120 independent living programs throughout the United States that teach the disabled person how to employ and train a PCA.

Physician involvement in home health care depends on client needs, agency policy, and the physician. The individual physician's interest in home care influences the extent of involvement, and physicians who care for a number of elderly, disabled or chronically ill clients tend to have more interest and involvement in home health care programs. The same is true for the physician in family practice whose medical care focuses more on the "whole" person or family rather than a particular organ or disease entity. The practice of health care in the home setting is congruent with these physicians' holistic philosophy of medical and health care.[8]

Summary

In this chapter some of the more common rehabilitation disciplines are described. Specific role functions, as well as the suggested nature of information to be included by the physician in a referral, are presented. No attempt is made to discuss all persons involved in the rehabilitative effort of patient care; for example, podiatrists, pharmacologists, art, dance, and music therapists, audiologists, otolaryngologists, and numerous others can play a significant role in the rehabilitation of a single individual. Instead the relationship between medical and allied health specialists working together as a team to provide comprehensive medical care is emphasized.

Although until now the interdisciplinary approach to medical care has experienced limited use in ambulatory settings, it is important for the primary care physician to realize the extensive role rehabilitation specialists may play in facilitating comprehensive and coordinated patient care. Wherever possible, the applications of these special services for outpatient care has been presented. The position advocated in this chapter is that the primary care practitioner has a responsibility to be knowledgeable about other medical and health professionals and to call upon their services in an appropriate and timely manner. In chapters dealing with specific diseases, the roles of various providers in helping the patient with typical problems are discussed.

References

1. Adams DW, Soifer AL: Social Work: An Holistic Approach to Helping Disabled Persons and Their Families. In Browne JA, Kirlin BA, Watt S (eds): Rehabilitation Services and The Social Work Role: Challenge for Change, p 48. Baltimore, Williams & Wilkins, 1981

2. Goldenson RM, Dunham JR, Dunham, CS (eds): Disability and Rehabilitation Handbook, p 737. New York, McGraw-Hill, 1978

3. Goodwin MT, Weisman B: Nutrition and Foods. In Valletutti PJ, Christoplos F (eds): Interdisciplinary Approaches to Human Services, p 193. Baltimore, University Park Press, 1977

4. Granger CV: Manuscript, 1980
5. Nichols PJR: Rehabilitation Medicine. The Management of Physical Disability, p 41. London, Butterworths, 1976
6. Paraplegia Association of Rhode Island, Rhode Island Occupational Information Co-ordinating Committee: Job Opportunity Brief #5263, Providence, RI, 1980
7. Rusk HA: Rehabilitation Medicine, p 46. St Louis, CV Mosby, 1977
8. Stewart JE: Home Health Care, pp 58, 65, 66. St Louis, CV Mosby, 1979

Additional Readings

1. Allgire MJ: Nurses Can Give and Teach Rehabilitation: A Manual. New York, Springer-Verlag, 1968
2. Dana RH: Foundations of Clinical Psychology Problems of Personality and Adjustment. Princeton, Van Nostrand, 1966
3. Dunten WR, Jr, Licht S: Occupational Therapy: Principles and Practice. Springfield, Charles C Thomas, 1957
4. Ferguson EA: Social Work: An Introduction. Philadelphia, JB Lippincott, 1963
5. Garfield SL: Clinical Psychology: The Study of Personality and Behavior. Chicago, Aldine, 1979
6. Holmes MB, Holmes D: Handbook of Human Services for Older Persons. New York, Human Sciences Press, 1979
7. Ince LP: The Rehabilitation Medicine Services. Springfield, Charles C Thomas, 1974
8. Kottke FJ, Stillwell GK, Lehmann JF (eds): Krusen's Handbook of Physical Medicine and Rehabilitation. Philadelphia, WB Saunders, 1982
9. Licht S: Rehabilitation and Medicine. New Haven, Elizabeth Licht, 1968
10. Sand P, Trieschmann RB, Fordyce WE, Fowler RS: Behavior modification in the medical rehabilitation setting: Rationale and some applications. Rehabil Pract Review, 1(2):11, 1970
11. Shestack R: Handbook of Physical Therapy. New York, Springer-Verlag, 1977
12. Shriver DJ, Ranucci, MH: OT: A Reference Handbook on Occupational Therapy. Denver, 1977

CHAPTER 7

Role of the Primary Care Physician in the Functional Assessment of Motor, Cognitive, and Language Dysfunction in Childhood

Michael E. Msall

The systematic approach to developmental problems in childhood and adolescence is crucial for all primary care providers. In order to assess children and young adults functionally, the primary care practitioner must understand the problems associated with cerebral palsy, mental retardation, communication and learning disabilities, sensory impairments, and behavioral disorders,[26,16] these being the major developmental disabilities. This chapter focuses on the importance of a functional assessment as key to identification, habilitation, and management of children with motor, communication, and learning (cognitive) problems.

Functional assessment of adults documents the loss of previous capabilities and helps to devise *re*habilitative strategies; in contrast, functional assessment of children documents skills not previously developed and helps to devise *ha*bilitative strategies to attain those skills for the first time.

One of the earliest signs of developmental disturbance is motor deficit. Cerebral palsy is the most common of the motor dysfunctions and occurs in approximately 1 in 200 live births. Advances in both neonatal and pediatric intensive care have resulted in unprecedented rates of survival,[4,40,50,59,94] and it would seem that infants who are helped to survive in these units would be at a greater risk for developmental disabilities. However, it is important for the primary care physician to realize that over 80% of infants who survive after neonatal or pediatric intensive care do not have significant motor or cognitive limitations.[4,59,50] Twenty percent of these children can have residual motor and cognition problems.[4]

Another sign of developmental disturbance in children is language delay, which includes receptive, expressive, and articulatory disorders. These occur in about 7% to 10% of the general population. One percent of children has a severe language impairment significant enough to interfere with academic development.

Approximately 10% to 20% of children have problems that interfere with learning.[38] Three percent are accounted for by mental retardation, and 5% to 10% by learning disabilities. These learning disabilities often present as language delays.

An estimated 50% of cases of cerebral palsy and 50% of cases with significant mental retardation, defined as IQ less than 50 to 55, have had no known risk factors or etiology.[41,76] Seventy to eighty percent of children with cerebral palsy or significant mental retardation (SiMR) have not experienced prematurity, asphyxia, meningitis, cardiopulmonary arrest, or head trauma.

With so little to go on with respect to etiology or early warning signs, the primary care physician must be prepared to evaluate all infants and children carefully. A systematic assessment of function at appropriate intervals will improve early diagnosis, development of a prognosis, and planning of habilitative interventions.

Rationale for Functional Assessment

A formal system of functional assessment allows the primary care physician to monitor ongoing and motor and cognitive development in children. In addition to monitoring development and recovery of function in children who received neonatal and pediatric intensive care, the primary care physician must have a system for assessing ongoing developmental function for all children. In contrast to disorders in adults, in whom the mode of presentation is that of localizing pathological processes, developmental disorders present as disturbances of motor, communicative, and learning (cognitive) functions. In children at risk but making developmental progress, reassurance and cautious optimism can be expressed to the parents. In children with significant delays, early referral for diagnostic evaluation and habilitation can take place.

Forty years ago Gesell and colleagues introduced a system of milestones to characterize normal childhood neurodevelopment. The milestones are within the domains of gross motor, fine motor, language, problem-solving, and personal or social functioning (Table 7-1). The importance of examining each domain is that often involvement of one signifies that others may be affected. For example, children with congenital rubella may be deaf, mentally retarded, and have cerebral palsy.[27]

Accardo, summarizing Connolly's examination of mentally retarded individuals, found that 10% of the mentally retarded population had cerebral palsy, 3% had hearing impairment, 4% had visual impairment, and 40% had behavioral difficulties.[2] Hagberg, in a separate study of 122 cases of severe mental retardation, found that 18% of these cases had cerebral palsy, and 30% had epilepsy. Hagberg considered 42% of individuals with SiMR to be multiply handicapped.[41]

Crothers and Denhoff have found that children with cerebral palsy are likely to have seizures (33%), cognitive difficulties (approximately 50% to 75%), communicative disorders (70%), hearing impairment (10%), and visual problems

TABLE 7-1   Assessment of Domains of Development

Domain of Development	Type of Behavior	Significance
Gross motor	Head control, rolling, sitting, crawling, walking, running	Often the initial presentation of a developmental disability
Fine motor	Hand function, grasping and manipulating objects	Reflects both motor control of upper extremity and visual perceptual development
Language	Verbal and nonverbal communication, including receptive and expressive language, play, and gesture language	Best predictor of cognition
Problem-solving	Ability to utilize fine motor and cognitive skills to solve practical problem such as puzzles, drawing, and block constructions	Observable—using appropriate materials in office setting. Determines level of independence with respect to caretakers
Personal/social	Interactions between child and other. Child demonstrates social learning and knowledge of rules and expectations governing appropriate behaviors and self-care	Qualitative factor in child development. Reflects complex interaction of parenting, cultural and environmental forces. Basis for learning activities of daily living

(5%).[25,26] More recently, Scheiner and Moomaw examined young blind children and found that 23% had cerebral palsy, 42% were mentally retarded, 33% had seizures, 2% had hearing impairment, and 19% had learning and behavioral difficulties.[80] Because it is probable that motor, communicative, and cognitive deficits may coexist, it is essential that on initial contact the physician begin by addressing all developmental domains for planning and implementing individualized, comprehensive habilitation.

The primary care physician must be able to distinguish between coexisting disabilities involving multiple developmental domains as revealed by formal functional assessment and the concept of risk discussed later.

Classification of Cerebral Palsy (CP)

Three crucial concepts underlie cerebral palsy (CP), a disorder of motion and posture resulting from insult or injury to the developing brain.[7,48,62] First, CP is nonprogressive. One of the essential tasks of the practitioner is to take a meticulous history and perform a clinical examination to establish the child's developmental rate and sequentiality. For instance, progressive loss of motor skills suggests a neurodegenerative disorder such as metachromatic leukodystrophy or active structural central nervous system (CNS) disease such as hydrocephalus. Second, peripheral manifestations may change. An individual may be hypotonic in early infancy. Choreoathetosis may then become prominent beginning in the second year of life. During the adolescent growth spurt, postural deformities may become more pronounced in individuals with spasticity. Third, other systems besides the motor may be involved. Persons with CP often have seizures, disorders of attention, perceptual problems, or communicative dysfunction.

In a London study of 527 children with CP aged 4 to 8 years born in an era of modern intensive care, Evans and colleagues found that 10% had hearing impairments, 26% had visual impairments, and 34% had cognitive impairments.[33] Shapiro and colleagues have offered an alternative definition of CP, which takes into account these associated deficits of cognitive and sensory processing. They define CP as

> a chronic neurological disorder of movement and posture due to a deficit or lesion of the immature brain. The motor disability serves as a neurodevelopmental marker indicative of associated cerebral dysfunctions such as mental retardation, learning disability, seizures, deafness, sensory loss and other dysfunctions.[83]

In addition to a basic definition of CP, a *physiological* (type of tone and movement disorder) and a *topographic* (pattern of limbs involvement) classification system is used.[25,43,92] Individuals are classified as predominantly *spastic, extrapyramidal/dyskinetic,* or *mixed* (both spastic and extrapyramidal). Tables 7-2 and 7-3 summarize the physiological and topographic classifications of CP.

TABLE 7-2 Physiological Classification of Cerebral Palsy

Extrapyramidal/Dyskinetic

Disordered movement, including athetosis, chorea, dystonia, and ballismus
Exaggerated and persistent primitive reflexes, including the Moro, ATNR,* STNR,** and †TLSR
Delayed postural development (equilibrium responses)
Variable muscle tone
Absence of clonus and Babinski's reflex, and a tendency to contracture. Tendon reflexes may be mildly hyperactive
Lead pipe, cog wheel, or candle wax quality to tone
Difficulty with oral, motor, and trunk control

Mixed

Combination of spastic cerebral palsy with a functionally significant movement disorder

Spastic

Increased muscle tone of clasp-knife quality
Increased deep tendon reflexes, including clonus; increased reflexogenic zone
Positive pathological reflexes, including Babinski's, Hoffmann's, and other upper motor neuron signs
Persistence of primitive reflexes, especially ATNR and positive support
Tendency to contracture
Spread and overflow of associated movements and difficulty with fine motor tasks
Signs are persistent, consistent, and continue even during sleep

* ATNR = asymmetric tonic neck reflex
** STNR = symmetric tonic neck reflex
† TLSR = tonic labyrinthine supine reflex

TABLE 7-3   Major Topographical Classifications of Cerebral Palsy

Monoplegia	One limb involvement; reflects incomplete hemiplegia, or incomplete diplegia
Hemiplegia	Unilateral involvement, with upper extremity involvement greater than lower extremity involvement.
Diplegia	Predominantly lower extremity involvement
Quadriplegia	Significant functional involvement of both arms and legs
Triplegia	Three limbs; reflects incomplete quadriplegia, or superimposed hemiplegia on a diplegia
Double hemiplegia	Spastic quadriplegia; arms are more involved than legs
Paraplegia	Refers to spinal cord conditions such as spina bifida or acquired spinal cord injury

(Adapted from Minear WL: A classification of cerebral palsy. Pediatrics 18:841–52, 1956; Denhoff E, Robinault IP: Cerebral Palsy and Related Disorders. New York, McGraw-Hill, 1960; Vining E, Accardo PJ, Rubenstein JE et al: Cerebral palsy: A pediatric developmentalist's overview. Am J Dis Child 130:643–49, 1976; Bax MC: Terminology and classification of cerebral palsy. Dev Med Clin Neurol 6:295–307, 1964; Hagberg B, Hagberg G, Olow I: The changing panorama of cerebral palsy in Sweden 1954–1970, I: Analysis of the general changes. Acta Paediatr Scand 65:403–408, 1976)

Some patients with CP present as pure *ataxia*. Usually these persons reflect a congenital cerebellar malformation. This type of presentation is rare but, because the signs of ataxia are not manifested readily prior to the first birthday, it is crucial to rule out acquired causes of ataxia such as central nervous system mass lesions or metabolic abnormalities. Some individuals present with motor delay and remain significantly hypotonic without weakness. This clinical picture is typical of Down's syndrome, Prader–Willi syndrome, and fragile-X. The hypotonia is believed to be a part of motor delays that accompany mental retardation. Other hypotonic persons eventually demonstrate spasticity or extrapyramidal signs. Their hypotonia evolves into CP. A third group, exhibiting hypotonia and weakness, often appear clinically the same as patients with a neuromuscular disorder such as myotonic dystrophy, congenital muscular dystrophy, congenital or metabolic myopathy, or spinal muscular atrophy. Thus, hypotonia should be viewed as a marker from which to distinguish either a central or a peripheral nervous system syndrome.

A third component of classification concerns divisions into etiological subgroups. Table 7-4 describes major etiological entities that cause CP and the corresponding time of insult. Another purpose of classification is to relate clinical findings to etiological and functional subgroups. For example, hyperbilirubinemia with kernicterus leaves as a sequela extrapyramidal CP, sensory neural hearing impairment, enamel hypoplasia, and difficulty with vertical gaze.[77] Prematurity resulting in intraventricular hemorrhage with periventricular leukomalacia causes damage to the pyramidal tracts and is evident as spastic diplegia.[95] Vascular events during pregnancy are associated often with later appearance of

TABLE 7-4   Etiological Classification of Cerebral Palsy

Prenatal

Developmental anomalies of the central nervous system, including agenesis of the corpus callosum, porencephaly, lissencephaly, and polymicrogyria. These disorders present as abnormal head growth, abnormal transillumination, developmental delay, and seizures

Fetal deprivation of supply: Maternal disorders involving toxemia, placental infarction, bleeding during pregnancy, multiple births, and small for gestational age infants.[39]

Inborn error of morphogenesis: Genetic malformation syndromes including chromosomal disorder

Teratogenetic exposure: Thalidomide, organic methylmercury (minimata syndrome), maternal hyperphenylalanemia (PKU), maternal alcoholism (fetal alcohol syndrome), and maternal diabetes

Viral teratogenesis: Toxoplasmosis, syphilis, rubella, cytomegalovirus, herpes simplex, and others

Perinatal

Prematurity
Asphyxia/hypoxia
Hypoglycemia
Hypocalcemia
Hyperbilirubinemia
Intraventricular hemorrhage
Neonatal meningitis
Inborn errors of metabolism (urea cycle, maple syrup urine disease, organic acid disorders)

Postnatal

Cyanotic congenital heart disease
Meningitis
Trauma (including child abuse)
Lead intoxication
Near drowning
Hypoxia

Mixed combination of the above

Infant with congenital rubella with a low apgar and both hypoglycemia and hypocalcemia (prenatal and postnatal etiologies for subsequent quadriplegia)

hemiplegia. For instance, the outcome of a twin pregnancy may be one live born infant and a macerated fetus. In such a situation, the live born infant may have porencephaly due to embolic migration from the macerated fetus to its twin. Despite these classic clinical pathologic examples, it is important for clinicians to realize that the majority of causes of cerebral palsy are unknown.[67]

The functional assessment classification of CP emphasizes the components of topography, physiology, movement disorder, and associated deficits. If an individual has not attained a level of gross motor skills appropriate to his age, it is imperative that primary care physicians ask five questions:

1. Is the inability to carry out a gross motor skill secondary to problems with spasticity?
2. Is the inability to carry out a motor skill secondary to a movement disorder that compromises balance and voluntary control?

3. Is there progressive deformity leading to mechanical instability, such as severe scissoring in diplegia or dislocated hips with scoliosis and quadriplegia?
4. What is the degree of maturation of individual motor responses, and has suppression of primitive reflexes been established?
5. Are there associated dysfunctions of cognition (*i.e.,* profound mental retardation) or sensory impairment (*e.g.,* blindness) interfering with independent ambulation?

A classification system should also include a functional rating system of the severity level of CP. Table 7-5 expands on the American Academy of Cerebral Palsy Classification of Functional Severity.[7,48,62,92]

TABLE 7-5   Functional Severity and Associated Deficits in Cerebral Palsy

Motor Function Capacity	Rehabilitation Therapeutic Intervention	Educational– Neurobehavioral Dysfunction	Ambulation Status
Class I Mild CP; no practical motor limitation	No treatment required. Walks at 2 yr	Risk of attention deficit disorder	Independent
Class II Moderate CP; slight to moderate motor limitation	Minimal bracing; habilitation. Walks by 3 yr	Risk of mild mental retardation or learning disabilities	Ambulation with supervision
Class III Severe CP; moderate to great motor limitation	Extensive bracing; assistive devices, targeted surgical intervention, multidisciplinary team required for long-term intervention. Walks by 7 yr	Communication disorder, mental retardation, seizure disorder; organic neurobehavioral disorders	Ambulation with assistance, household ambulator; may need wheelchair
Class IV Profound CP; no useful, purposeful motor activity	Completely dependent; highest risk for scoliosis, dislocated hips, positional and fixed contractures. Nonwalker	Oral motor dysfunction, communication disorder, sensory impairment, significant MR (IQ less than 50), seizure disorder, organic neurobehavioral disorders with stereotopy or self-injury	Wheelchair with assistance or wheelchair dependent. Transfers with assist or totally dependent

(Data taken from References 17, 18, 26, 62, and 92.)

Concept of Risk

Children who have potential developmental disabilities come to the attention of a primary care physician for three major reasons: (1) They have a medical diagnosis known to have a high incidence of handicaps, such as Down's syndrome; (2) they have medical disorders that carry a high risk of handicap, such as birth asphyxia, although their development to date may or may not be abnormal; or (3) they may have no previous medical diagnosis, but their parents suspect a primary developmental problem. The physician links his knowledge of the medical disorder or developmental concerns with knowledge of the spectrum of delayed development.

Children are at risk for disabilities if they have experienced any biomedical disturbance or serious environmental deficit which has been shown to be associated with an increased incidence of handicap. The list of risk factors has grown exponentially with advances in medical knowledge and treatment techniques. An exhaustive listing of conditions associated with increased risk for developmental disabilities is beyond the scope of this chapter. However, a list of general guidelines is given in Table 7-6. It is important for clinicians to realize that risk is a statistical concept and does not imply a one-to-one relationship. Infants with low birth weight are at risk for CP; however, 80% of infants who survive with birth weights below 800g do not have CP.[8] In the collaborative perinatal project, Nelson and Ellenberg found that 73% of cases of CP occurred in infants with a 5-minute apgar of 7 or higher.[66] The physician must use a combination of historical risk factors and functional neurodevelopmental assessment to detect developmental dysfunction. This is illustrated by the following case:

> *Case 1* Johnny was a 3-pound, 10-ounce product of a 36-week pregnancy to a 25-year-old primagravida. Pregnancy was uncomplicated. Labor was spontaneous. Apgars were 6 at 1 minute and 7 at 5 minutes. Initial physical exam revealed a small for gestational age, microcephalic infant. Diffuse petechiae were noted. Fundoscopic exam revealed a salt and pepper retinopathy. A cardiac murmur was thought to be consistent with peripheral pulmonic stenosis. Hepatosplenomegaly was present. The CT scan revealed extensive intracranial calcifications, and x-rays of long bones revealed a celerylike appearance. Cord immunoglobulin M (IGM) was elevated. Urine for cytomegalovirus (CMV) was obtained on the patient's second spontaneous void. The overall constellation of findings, consistent with congenital cytomegalovirus infection, was confirmed by viral urine culture.
>
> Initially the patient required gavage feeding. There were no complications of hypoglycemia or hypocalcemia. Mild jaundice responded to phototherapy. At 6 weeks of age, the child went home at a birth weight of 5 pounds. During the first 6 months of life, the child's growth parameters tracked parallel to, but less than, the third percentile. Head circumference, however, did not grow after 6 months. There were delays in attaining motor milestones. Rolling both ways did not occur until 9 months, and tripod sitting occurred at 12 months. Pulling to stand was just beginning at 18 months.
>
> Major parental concern at the 18-month visit was motor delay and the absence of language. Examination revealed a small, alert, interactive male in no apparent distress. Neurologic exam revealed hyperreflexia in the lower

TABLE 7-6   High-Risk Factors Predisposing to Developmental Disabilities

Children at Risk

Environmental Risk Factors

No prenatal care
Poor nutrition during pregnancy
Material substance use or abuse, especially alcohol and cocaine
Teenage mother
Mother over age 35
Low socioeconomic class
Parental school failures
Maternal psychoses

Biologic Risk Factors

Prenatal Factors
Twin pregnancy
Placental abnormalities (previa, abruptio)
Cord abnormalities
Preeclampsia, eclampsia
Prematurity
Small for gestational age
Congenital infection
Chromosome abnormality
Multiple congenital anomalies
Chemical teratogenesis (maternal diabetes, maternal PKU, maternal anticonvulsants, methylmercury)

Perinatal Factors
Inborn errors of metabolism (urea cycle and organic acid disorders; maple syrup urine disease)
Asphyxia
Metabolic abnormalities (hypoglycemia, hypocalcemia, hypernatremia, hyperbilirubinemia, hyperammonemia)
Hyperviscosity
Neonatal seizures, neonatal meningitis

Postnatal Factors
Trauma, including child abuse
Cyanotic congenital heart disease
Cerebral vascular accident
Hypoxia
Meningitis
Reye's syndrome
Recurrent seizures

extremities, tightness at the heelcords, and an obligatory positive support primitive reflex. (Table 7-14)

Problem-solving skills revealed mature pincer, easy release, and inability to make a pencil mark. The child was unable to stack blocks, imitate a stroke, or complete a pegboard. No spontaneous utterances were noted. The child did not respond to a one-step command and did not turn toward loud sounds. The initial impression was spastic diplegia with disproportionate language delay. Auditory evaluation revealed a severe neural sensory hearing loss.

The child was enrolled in a program for children with both language and motor handicaps. A total communication approach was used. At the age of 4 the child was able to walk. Perceptual skills and nonverbal language were assessed to be at a 2½-year level. The child had learned ten signs and had begun sign combinations.

This case reflects the complexity of developmental outcome in a small for gestational age infant. Based on the initial CT scan, the physician may have predicted major handicapping cerebral palsy and mental retardation. Overall, however, this child's major handicap was his deafness. By 4 years of age, he was a functional ambulator. His major developmental problem will be to function in the hearing world. Failure to recognize his hearing loss at 18 months would have led to an erroneous diagnosis of mental retardation. In the presence of motor and language delay, it is imperative that physicians assess the integrity of other neurologic and sensory systems.

History

Careful attention to parents' descriptions of developmental concerns and a functional developmental history are the key components in formulating a developmental diagnosis. Table 7-7 lists age of presentation and common parental descriptions of early developmental dysfunction. It is crucial that the primary care physician note these concerns are possible early markers of motor and cognitive handicaps. The following case illustrates the frustrations and distrust of parents when a systematic history is not accompanied by a complete functional assessment.

Case 2 Jane, a 7-pound, 11-ounce female, was a full-term product of an uncomplicated pregnancy. There were no problems with labor and delivery and no difficulties in feeding. Mother and infant went home from the hospital at 3 days. The mother became concerned about the child's development at 6 months because the child was not sitting up and had strabismus. The primary care physician reassured her that the child would outgrow the difficulties. He pointed out that the child was gaining weight appropriately, had no significant perinatal risk factors, and that the physical exam was within normal limits.

At the ninth-month visit, the mother expressed concern about a difficulty with diapering. Again, the physician reassured her that children often do not like to have their diapers changed. At the age of 12 months, the child was still not sitting and could not transfer. Her right hand was persistently fisted.

TABLE 7-7   Developmental Concerns of Parents and Their Functional Significance

Parental Concern	Functional Significance
0–3 Months	
Too good a baby	Lethargic baby with paucity of movement
Fussy	Organic irritability
Cannot see	No visual tracking
Cannot hear	Poor interpretation of environmental sound
Poor feeding/growth	Oral motor dysfunction, a
Recurrent aspiration/stridor	particular marker for extrapyramidal/dyskinetic cerebral palsy
Rolled early, especially from prone to supine	Exaggerated extensor posturing
3–9 Months	
Hard to diaper	Lower extremity spasticity
Persistent fisting	Upper extremity spasticity
Crossed eyes	Strabismus
Persistent hand regard after 5 mo	Delayed manipulative skills
Early handedness	Rule out hemiplegia on non-affected side

The mother brought her child to the United Cerebral Palsy Foundation, where a comprehensive multidisciplinary assessment was performed.

Neurodevelopmental examination was remarkable for alternating esotropia, increased tone of clasp-knife quality in the upper extremity, persistent fisting, and difficulty passively pronating and supinating the right upper extremity. There was limitation of motion at the hip, and clasp-knife quality on attempts at abduction. The heel cords were tight. In vertical suspension, there was scissoring and equinus posturing of the feet. Deep tendon reflexes were 3+ in the right upper extremity, and 4+ in both lower extremities. Pathologic reflexes included a bilateral plantar extensor response to the Babinski maneuver.

Functional assessment of fine motor skills revealed the absence of an extended reach and grasp. Language assessment revealed the inability to say "mama" or "dada," no response to a one-step command with gestures, and an inability to play gesture games. The history and exam revealed the absence of babbling. Razzing was present as the child could vibrate her tongue between the lips. Developmental diagnosis at this time was spastic triplegic cerebral palsy (spastic diplegia CP with a superimposed right hemiparesis) and mental retardation.

Early intervention and home-management techniques were developed. Over the following 2 years, motor skills progressed. Sitting occurred at 18 months, combat crawling at 3½ years. By 4 years Jane was learning to walk using parallel bars. Extended reaching and grasping developed at 2 years. Ability to pick up small objects was observed at 3 years, ability to remove clothes was observed at 4 years, and ability to feed herself occurred at 5 years. Language continued to be delayed. A communication board was introduced, and she rapidly learned functional signs for sleep, eat, drink, friend, and cookie. By 5 years of age she knew 5 body parts, nonsense commands, and color and coin identification. Her major handicaps were her cognitive deficits and communication disorder. Strategies to improve alternative communication continued to be employed.

The mother expressed appreciation that a multidisciplinary team effort had encouraged targeted developmental skills which enabled her daughter to conquer some developmental hurdles and to make significant gains during the first 5 years of life.

This case highlights the importance not only of listening to parents, but also of performing a functional developmental assessment so that appropriate therapeutic interventions can improve functional independence and facilitate parental management.

The key to the sequential elicitation of developmental milestones is that the primary care practitioner must use operational definitions and be systematic in his queries. Much confusion is embedded in such ambiguous terms as "rolling over," "sitting," and "walking," and therefore operational terms should be used. These appear in Table 7-8, which lists the sequential appearance of gross

TABLE 7-8   Gross Motor Milestones

Milestone	Month
Chin up in prone	1
Chest up in prone	2
On elbows in prone	
Head stable in vertical	3
On wrist in prone	
Rolls prone to supine	4
Rolls both ways consistently	5
Tripod sitting	6
Sits erect without using hand; 1 minute	7
Comes to sit with rail; quadriped crawl	8
Sits already without arm support for 10 minutes; pulls to stand	9
Cruises	10
Reciprocal crawl	11
Stands alone; walks hand held	12
Walks alone 2 steps	13
Walks short distance	14
Creeps up steps	15
Runs, climbs stairs (one hand held)	18

(Data taken from References 15, 26, 46, and 52.)

motor milestones and more explicit descriptions. For example, rolling prone to supine occurs on the average at 4 months. To elicit this information from the parent, the practitioner would phrase the question to a parent this way: "When did your child begin consistently to roll from his stomach to his back?" Often the term "sitting" is misinterpreted. A parent will think that sitting is the ability to remain in a seated position packed with pillows on both sides and held firm by a strap between the legs, such as in highchair sitting. It is necessary for the practitioner to ask the question this way: "When did your child demonstrate the ability to hold his head and trunk up when placed in a sitting position on a flat surface, such as on the floor?" Alternatively, the practitioner can ask: "When did your child not fall on his nose when placed in an upright position?" The milestone generally achieved at 6 months is tripod sitting. Specifically, the child is able to sit when placed on a flat surface and protect himself from falling forward with one hand.

There is also confusion about walking. Parents of infants with CP often describe their children as doing persistent automatic walking. Other parents confuse the ability to bear weight in the legs with the ability to take reciprocal steps. Taking reciprocal steps while holding onto something is called cruising and occurs at 10 months. The functional definition of cruising is the ability to hold onto a chair or table top and take steps around it. Independent walking, the ability to take steps without holding onto anyone or anything, occurs at 13 months. Thus, unless the milestone is asked in a functional way, the parent will provide descriptions either of weight bearing, pulling to stand, cruising, or walking.

The concept of the developmental quotient is another key to understanding milestones. Gesell and Armatruda define the developmental quotient as the ratio of normal to exhibited development present at any given age.[51,52] For example, if the average age of tripod sitting is 6 months, and a child is performing this activity on a regular and consistent basis at 6 months, the developmental quotient (DQ) is 100. On the other hand, if the child is only beginning tripod sitting consistently at 12 months, the DQ is 50 percent. The significance of the DQ is that it compares the child's current performance with age-specific norms. Children whose DQ is less than 70% are manifesting significant developmental delays. For instance, a child who still cannot get his chin up in prone at 3 months (DQ < 70%) cannot roll both ways at 8 months (DQ < 70%), or is not tripod sitting at 10 months (DQ = 60%) is manifesting significant motor delay.

Capute, Coplan, and their colleagues have developed a format for eliciting language milestones prior to the second birthday.[12,22,24] Table 7-9 lists a sequential series of developmental language skills reflecting understanding and expression. The importance of these scales is that primary care physicians can systematically assess language development even before a child talks in sentences.

Illingworth and Knobloch stressed the importance of fine motor and personal social milestones. (Tables 7-10 and 7-11) Fine motor skills form the basis of solving puzzles, drawing, and block construction tasks used in infant tests such as the Bayley and Cattell.[6,19] Personal social skills form the basis of adaptive scales such as the Vineland, Camelot, or the American Association of Mental Deficiency (AAMD) Adaptive Behavior Scale (ABS).[29,35,71]

Illingworth introduced the term *dissociation* to emphasize that development in one domain is sometimes out of step with development in other domains.[47] For

TABLE 7-9   Language Milestones

Receptive		Expressive	
1 Mo	Alerts to sound		
2 Mo	Social Smile		
		3 Mo	Coos
4 Mo	Orients to voice	*4 Mo*	Laughs
5 Mo	Localizes direction of bell	*5 Mo*	Ah goo, razz
		6 Mo	Babble
7 Mo	Orients to source and direction of bell in 2 stage manner, reacts to mirror		
		8 Mo	Mama, Dada, inappropriate
9 Mo	Orients to source and direction of bell in 1 stage manner		
10 Mo	Understands no	*10 Mo*	Imitates sound Mama, Dada, appropriate
		11 Mo	1 word
12 Mo	One step command with gesture	*12 Mo*	2 words
15 Mo	One step command without gesture	*15 Mo*	Immature jargoning 4–6 words
18 Mo	Points to one picture	*18 Mo*	Mature jargoning 7–10 vocabulary
21 Mo	Points to 2 pictures	*21 Mo*	Names 1 picture 20 word vocabulary 2 word phrases
24 Mo	2 step command, points to 5 pictures	*24 Mo*	50 word vocabulary Pronouns inappropriate Names 5 objects
30 Mo	Points to 7 pictures Points to objects by use	*30 Mo*	Names 5 pictures Pronouns, appropriate
36 Mo	2 prepositions, points to 12 pictures	*36 Mo*	Plurals; name, age, sex, names object by use

(Data taken from References 2, 12, 22, and 23.)

example, in a child with MR, motor development may be normal, but language and problem-solving behavior are delayed significantly. Accardo and Capute used the concept of dissociation as a key to formulating a developmental diagnosis.[2]

Table 7-12 illustrates the concept of dissociation in helping to decipher both the topography of cerebral palsy and its associated deficits such as mental retardation or communication disorder. In patients with spastic diplegia, the age of attaining gross motor skills such as sitting, cruising, and walking is delayed.

TABLE 7-10   Fine Motor Milestones

3 Mo	Predominantly unfisted
5 Mo	Extended reach and grasp
6 Mo	Transfer of objects
10 Mo	Mature pincer

(Data taken from References 46, 51, and 52.)

TABLE 7-11   Personal and Social Milestones

6 Mo	Chews
	Feeds self with biscuits
9–10 Mo	Helps dress (holds arm out for coat)
15 Mo	Feeds self fully using cup to drink, spoon to scoop
18 Mo	Begins to tell mother about wetting
2 yr	Mainly dry by day
3 yr	Mainly dry by night

(Data taken from References 46, 51, and 52.)

However, depending on upper extremity involvement, the ability to transfer and manipulate objects may be normal or may be delayed slightly. Overall, however, gross motor handicap exceeds upper extremity handicap. There may be some subtle delays in language, or language may be normal. In the personal–social sphere, sometimes the motor handicap may preclude the ready learning of such functions as toileting or dressing. In contrast, people with spastic hemiplegic cerebral palsy may be near-normal in onset of walking. In general, fine motor tasks are compromised, especially with respect to tasks involving bimanual dexterity. There may be difficulty with such personal–social tasks as dressing or holding a cup with one hand and pouring milk into the cup with the other. There are sometimes speech and language delays.

A person may be multiply handicapped with CP, MR, and a communication disorder, as illustrated in case 3 (Table 7-12)

Case 3 James, a 15-year-old boy with spasticity, upon neurological examination manifested delays in gross motor skills. He was unable to walk or to undress completely. Delays were apparent during the first 2 years of life and were nonprogressive. The combination of neurological signs of spasticity, in

TABLE 7-12   Use of Dissociation in Classification of Cerebral Palsy and Developmental Disabilities

Developmental Disability	Gross Motor	Fine Motor	Language	Problem Solving	Personal/ Social
CP—Spastic diplegia	Delay	Var*	Var	Var	Var
CP—Spastic quadriplegia	Delay	Delay	Var	Delay	Var
CP—Spastic hemiplegia	Var	Delay	Var	Var	Delay
CP—Extra-pyramidal	Delay	Delay	Var	Var	Var
Mental retardation	Normal–Delay	Normal–Delay	Delay	Delay	Delay
Communication disorder	Normal	Normal	Delay	Normal	Var

* Var = Variable

conjunction with nonprogressive upper and lower extremity dysfunction, established the diagnosis of spastic quadriplegic cerebral palsy.

Analysis of other functional domains revealed global delay in language, problem-solving, and personal–social skills. Language delays were severe and included absence of sentences and inconsistent responses to softly spoken requests. Problem-solving delay included inability to construct a staircase and copy letters of the alphabet. Personal–social delays included nocturnal enuresis. The disproportionate delay between language skills (less than 2-year-old level) and problem solving (less than 5-year-old level) were initially assessed as being due to a 40-decibel sensorineural hearing impairment. However, receptive language continued to be delayed despite a hearing prosthesis. This child had a mixed communication disorder with both peripheral and central auditory processing components. The global delays in language, problem-solving, and personal–social attainments indicated mental retardation. The disproportionate delays between language (DQ < 15) and problem-solving (DQ < 33), coupled with sensorineural hearing impairment, indicated a communication disorder. The combined delays in all streams of development revealed that James had profound cerebral palsy, severe communication disorder, and moderate mental retardation. Habilitation strategies were devised so that electric switches could be used to power a wheelchair and to facilitate access to visual information and leisure skills through use of a portable computer.

The developmental history should close with the practitioner's asking, "On the average, how old does your child act in each area of development?" Often the parents have already compared their child's current performance to what they have observed in a sibling. If a parent describes a child as significantly delayed with respect to performance as compared to that of a sibling at a comparable age, it is imperative that the physician conduct a functional assessment of that child. Coplan has documented that although parents may misinterpret the etiology of a child's developmental delay, their functional assessment of their child is usually highly accurate.[23]

Pedigree Analysis and Genetic Factors

A key component to the past medical history is the three-generation pedigree, concentrating on previous offspring of parents, history of miscarriages or involuntary infertility, stillbirths, unexplained infant death, and childhood epilepsy. In addition, phenotypical observation of other family members can be obtained by inspecting family photos. Especially with respect to the neurocutaneous syndromes, it is extremely important to examine other family members with a Wood's lamp. Whenever there is a possibility of a similarly affected sibling or other family member, medical records should be reviewed, and a comprehensive physical exam must be performed. Other factors to be included in pedigree analysis are maternal age (risk for autosomal trisomy), paternal age (risk for autosomal dominant disease), ethnicity and consanguinity (risk for autosomal recessive disease).

To establish pedigrees effectively requires open-ended and indirect questions. For example, "Has any family member had great difficulty in walking?" is a way to introduce concerns about CP. Another question would be, "Has any family member had any difficulty with talking or self-care?" This could indicate mental retardation. "Has any family member had difficulty learning to read?" could indicate learning disability or MR. Many of the neuropsychiatric disorders, which include depression, alcoholism, suicidal tendencies, and seizures are multifactoral. However, autosomal dominant disorders, such as Huntington's chorea and neurofibromatosis, should be kept in mind, as these disorders can present as familial tendencies to school failure, alcoholism, and suicide. The value of pedigrees is not only that they help determine genetic etiology, but also that they determine risks of recurrence. By excluding Mendelian patterns and by knowing the multifactorial inheritance of major syndromes, the practitioner can predict the risks of recurrence in subsequent pregnancies. Empirical data on risks of recurrence are available for hydrocephalus, spina bifida, cerebral palsy, and mental retardation.

The following case illustrates the importance of pedigree analysis and genetic factors in the etiology of CP (see Fig. 7-1).

Case 4 Joan, a 9-year-old white female, was followed for a complex seizure disorder. She was a 5-pound, 14-ounce product of a fullterm pregnancy to a 23-year-old primagravida. Pregnancy was complicated by maternal hypertension secondary to renal disease. As a teenager, the mother had been diagnosed with polycystic kidney disease, hypertension, and acne. Medica-

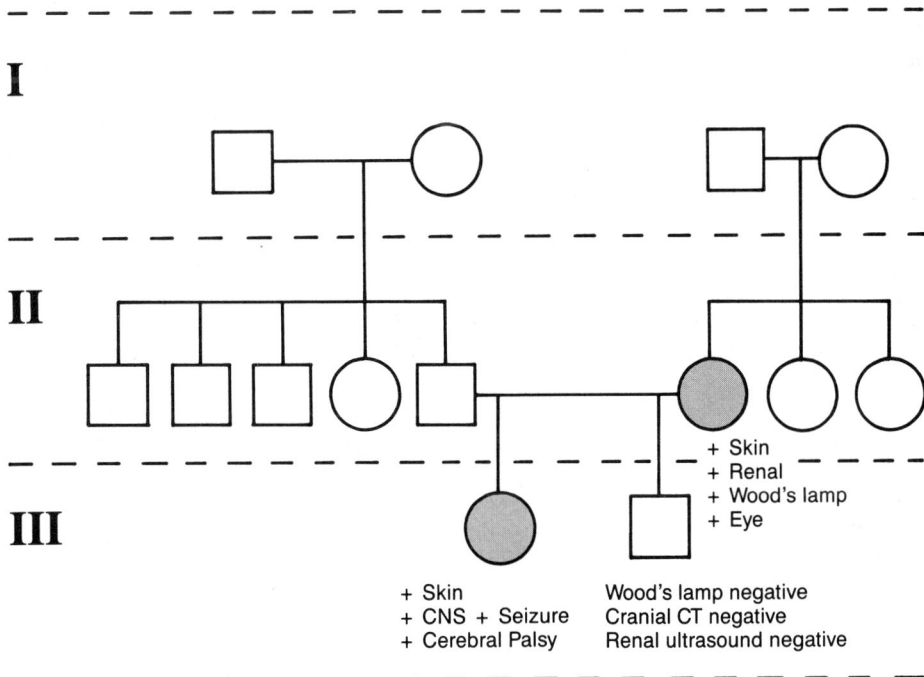

Figure 7-1. Pedigree of tuberous sclerosis, an autosomal dominant disorder.

tions controlled the hypertension. The perinatal period was without complications, but at the age of 6 weeks Joan developed salaam episodes (massive flexor spasms). At the age of 7 weeks, constant seizure activity was noted. At that time, Wood's lamp examination of the infant revealed depigmented macules. The dermatologic findings, in combination with the type of seizure and with calcifications found on cranial CT scan, confirmed a diagnosis of tuberous sclerosis. Anticonvulsants were initiated successfully.

Motor development was delayed. The child did not tripod sit until 21 months and did not cruise until 3 years. Examination at that time revealed increased reflexes in the lower extremity with unsustained clonus. Babinski's response was plantar extensor. Clasp knife hypertonicity was demonstrated on adducting the hips and on dorsiflexing the ankle. Observations of cruising revealed an obligatory positive support. Upper and lower extremity movement was ataxic. Over the next year, independent walking took place, but it was characterized by equinovarus posturing. This was corrected by lengthening the tendon achilles combined with intensive physiotherapy. Overall, the child was considered to have a seizure disorder and a mixed type of cerebral palsy with spasticity and ataxia.

Examination of the mother revealed cutaneous and renal aspects of tuberous sclerosis, but no seizure, developmental, or neurologic problems. Examination of the patient's brother revealed no evidence of dermatologic, renal, or neurologic aspects of the disease. This child's known syndrome, tuberous sclerosis, is the most common cause of a combination of infantile spasm-type seizure disorders and other developmental disabilities. The pattern of inheritance is autosomal dominant. Unfortunately, the mother's tuberous sclerosis aspects had not been detected during adolescence, when initial genetic counseling could have stressed that there was a 50% chance of a child being at risk for the spectrum of tuberous sclerosis. Despite being able to diagnose this condition, why the mother had a combination of dermatologic and renal findings, and the daughter had seizures and CP, can only be matters for speculation.

As more and more advances occur in genetic probes, cytogenetics, and classification of developmental disabilities, the primary care physician will become increasingly aware of the importance of evaluating pedigrees, prenatal concerns, and genetic contributions to etiology. A word of warning is necessary in this regard. Parental concerns discovered during prenatal, perinatal, or genetic counseling require a meticulous developmental and pedigree history matched by observations or documentation on the part of the physician. This includes evaluation of other affected family members with developmental disabilities and evaluation of past medical events and records. In the atmosphere of high anxiety and commotion in the delivery room suite, observers may perceive that all babies have a delayed cry or look blue. If a parent describes a child as blue, this observation must be weighed against more objective evidence such as apgars, seizures, feeding difficulty, lethargy in the newborn period, or other possible sequelae of significant asphyxia. Similarly, if a parent describes other mental disabilities, medical records, photographs, interviews with primary caretakers and, if possible, examination of affected and nonaffected family members, must take place.

Physical Examination

A focused approach to the physical examination of children is crucial. (Table 7-13). In the newborn period, it is imperative that all practitioners measure head circumference and graph length and weight on appropriate normative tables.[20,65,74] These simple physical examination techniques often reveal significant underlying problems. For example, in case 1 microcephaly and smallness for gestational age were markers for congenital intrauterine infection. An examination would thereby include assessment of the fundus to document salt and pepper retinopathy, which is found in congenital rubella or cytomegalovirus infection. Fundoscopy would also verify abnormal findings such as congenital toxoplasmosis. The presence of a cataract is often a preliminary indicator of a metabolic or congenital viral infection. Children with intrauterine growth retar-

TABLE 7-13   Key Items on Physical Examination of Children with Developmental Disabilities

Physical Parameter	Physical Findings
Growth	
Head circumference	Microcephaly
	Macrocephaly
Height	
Weight	
Growth chart monitoring	
Malformations and Organ System Assessment	
Dermatological (Wood's lamp)	Hypopigmentation
	Café au lait spots
Dysmorphic features	Epicanthal folds, malformed or posteriorally rotated ears; high, arched palate, scalp whorls; abnormalities of hands or feet
Skull	Shape, size of fontanelle; cranial bruits
Ocular	Optic atrophy, cherry red spots, colobomas (iris or retinal clefts)
Dental	Enamel hypoplasia, malocclusions, high, arched palate
Otolaryngological	Choanal atresia, cleft lip or palate; otic malformations, otitis media, stridor
Abdominal	Hepatosplenomegaly; protruberant abdomen
Genitourinary	Undescended testes; pubertal development
Musculoskeletal	Scoliosis, hip alignment, contractures

dation may have had chromosome teratogen exposure (alcohol or maternal phenylketonurea) or a genetic syndrome abnormality.[3]

Another component of the physical examination is the documentation of minor malformations. The physician should perform a systematic inventory of craniofacial and extremity dysmorphisms. These include such entities as epicanthal folds, low set or posteriorly rotated ears, alignment of the orbit, hypertelorism, shape of nasal bridge and philtrum, size of mandible, nuchal skin, ear pits, ear shape, syndactyly or polydactyly, nail dysplasia, webbed or wide toes, and unusual pigmentation. The presence of three or more minor malformations is associated with an increased statistical risk for other major malformations, such as congenital heart disease, spina bifida, renal malformations, and developmental disabilities.[60] In his textbook, *Recognizable Patterns of Human Malformation,* Smith describes a systematic approach to the measurement and description of dysmorphisms associated with inborn errors of morphogenesis.[88]

The purpose of the general physical exam is to detect signs of other organ dysfunction, such as dental caries, chronic obstructive upper airway disease, bronchospasm, heart murmur, organomegaly, genital urinary disorders, and unusual pigmentation. A focused musculoskeletal exam should include inspection of the entire spine from cervical area to sacrum and assessment for palpable vertebral defects, scoliosis, and dislocated hips. In addition, a description of developing contractures and classification as to whether or not they are flexible are vital. The classical neurologic exam should answer four questions: Is there cranial nerve dysfunction? Is there unusual tone? Is there a movement disorder? Is there a peripheral or cortical sensory defect?

The motor assessment of developmentally delayed individuals should focus on topography, physiological classification, and associated dysfunctions found in various syndromes of cerebral palsy. Also, it is important to perform a series of motor assessments based on chronological age.[11,30,70] In the newborn period, the exam combines primitive reflexes with the tradition of the French neurologists, which involves an assessment of tone in five cardinal positions: prone, supine, pull to sit, vertical, and horizontal suspension.[5] In addition, an assessment of asymmetries based on placing and automatic responses should be performed. Capute and colleagues systematically standardized a battery of primitive reflexes in early childhood.[13,14] The initial intent was to monitor maturation of motor status in a manner similar to the Apgar score, which is a measure of neonatal asphyxia. Table 7-14 describes primitive reflexes, their method of elicitation, and their functions.

Asymmetric, obligatory (examiner or therapist must break up reflex posture), and persistent primitive reflexes beyond the time that they should have disappeared are key indicators of motor dysfunction.[76] In addition to primitive reflexes, the primary care physician should have a systematic functional approach to the child with hypotonia. Dubowitz has stressed that a useful starting point is to distinguish children with hypotonia and significant weakness from those with significant hypotonia alone. Children with hypotonia and significant weakness may have diseases of the spinal cord or conditions affecting the neuromuscular junction.[31] Pediatricians and primary caretakers are most familiar with the assessment of hypotonia in the newborn,[31] which involves the Dubowitz neurological scale and includes such signs as the anterior scarf, popliteal angle, and foot to ear. Individuals with significant hypotonia continue to have these

TABLE 7-14   Primitive Reflexes

Reflex	Description	Functional Significance
Moro	Neck extension produces upper extremity abduction and extension, followed by adduction and flexion	Asymmetry indicates brachial plexus palsy, often absent in chromosome syndromes affecting CNS, such as TRISOMY 21, 18, 13
Asymmetric tonic neck reflex	Head rotation results in flexor posture on occiput side and extension on mandibular side	Prevents rolling. If obligatory, leads to hip subluxution and scoliosis
Tonic labyrinthine supine	Extension of head produces shoulder retraction and lower extremity extension	Prevents sitting with hips flexed; prevents midline hand use
Symmetric tonic neck reflex	When head is extended on midline, arms extend and legs flex. When head is flexed in midline, arms flex and legs extend	Exacerbates oral motor dysfunction; prevents crawling and standing with head up
Positive support	Bouncing child on balls of feet leads to leg extension and equinus position	If persists, tight achilles tendons and equinus deformity of foot result

(Capute AJ, Accardo PJ, Vining E et al: Primitive Reflex Profile. Baltimore, University Park Press, 1978)

findings. Other components of tone can be assessed by watching position with respect to these questions: Is there increased abduction at the hips? Does the infant get stuck on his face when in a prone position? Does the child slip through the axilla? Is there a posterior scarf? In the presence of hypotonia without weakness and of present deep tendon and primitive reflexes, hypotonia of central origin must be considered. The hypotonia serves as a marker for evolving motor and cognitive disabilities and includes such entities as Down's syndrome, fragile X syndrome, and evolving cerebral palsy.

A pediatric neurological examination includes also observation of postural and equilibrium responses (Table 7-15). Postural reactions are significant because they form the basis for mature motor skills. Their absence reflects very specific developmental disabilities. For example, the absence of an upper extremity parachute on one side is an indication of hemiplegia. Furthermore, postural reflexes have been used to develop prognosis with respect to walking. Specifically, Molnar has shown that the ability to have an anterior and lateral prop prior to age 2 is predictive of later walking.[63] After the age of 12 months, tone and movement disorders can be classified more formally. In addition, analysis of a child's ambulatory and movement skills can verify and supplement parental reports.

The primary care physician should have an ongoing mechanism available for visual screening.[28,89,90] In the newborn period, pupillary response, response to the opticokinetic drum, red reflex, fundoscopic exam, and time are the key

TABLE 7-15   Postural Responses

		Functional Significance
Head control	3 mo	Basis of head control
Landau	4 mo	Aligns body with trunk
Derotational righting (seg- mental rolling)	5 mo	Basis of voluntary rolling
Anterior prop	6 mo	Basis of tripod sitting
Lateral prop	7 mo	Basis of unsupported sitting
Posterior prop	11 mo	Basis of pivoting when sitting
Upper extremity parachute (prone extension of arms)	9 mo	Basis of crawling and functional use, both upper extremities

(Data taken from References 10, 15, and 46.)

hallmarks to detecting abnormalities of vision such as cataracts, coloboma, and congenital infections. The goal of visual screening for the primary care physician is to identify deficits in acuity, strabismus, and visual field. Early identification can lead to prompt correction and prevention of amblyopia and significant perceptual disabilities.

At 6 weeks of age the social smile and some visual tracking are present. The developmental pediatrician realizes that the defensive blink to threat does not appear until an infant reaches a mental age of 3 months. At 3 months an infant is able to follow 360 degrees, and at 4 months begins an extended reach and grasp.

At 6 months the infant can be tested for strabismus by the Hirshfield light reflex test. The examiner performs this test by shining a light in the patient's pupils. If the infant has strabismus, the light will be reflected back from a different part of the pupil and not in the center. Uncover test can be performed at this time. Sheridan has developed a series of graded balls ranging in size from ⅛ to 2½ inches in diameter.[85] Beginning at 6 months, the balls are presented in 3 different ways, which include rolling along the floor, for preferential looking, and mounted on sticks for fixed presentation in peripheral fields at 1½ feet. Sheridan developed a second set of miniature toys including a doll, chair, car, plane, knife, fork, and spoon, which can be used for children with a mental age of about 21 months to the age when letter cards can be employed.[87] Sheridan has developed also the Stycar panda letter test involving capital letters (A O U C H L T V X).[86] These letters are presented at 10 feet. Sheridan found that at the standard 20 feet it was often difficult to attract the infant's attention. The child points to a matching letter, rather than naming the letter, thus increasing the sensitivity of this test to visual discrimination rather than to both visual and auditory discrimination. Vision can also be tested by assessing competency in copying shapes and blocks (see Figs. 7-2 and 7-3). These tests simultaneously measure vision and perception and illustrate how simple items (12 blocks, paper, and pencil) can generate a wide range of developmental information.

The visual exam should also include an attempt to determine the visual fields. Prior to age 7, a child cannot cooperate in a formal test of peripheral vision. Screening for severe field defects of a child under 3 can be accomplished by bringing red rings from behind the child seated on the mother's lap. Beginning

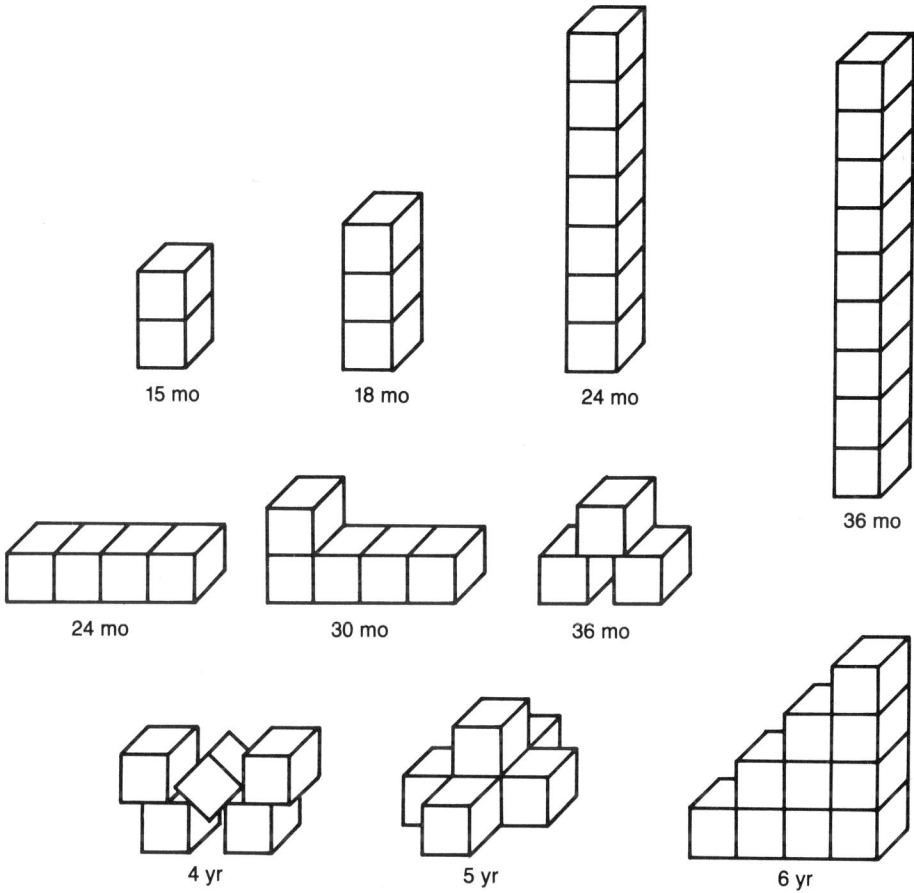

Figure 7-2. Visual perceptual assessment using cubes or blocks. (Data taken from References 14, 41, 46, and 51.)

at age 4, the practitioner can screen for severe visual field defects by direct confrontation. Once the child is enrolled in school, ongoing monitoring of vision includes Snellen charts, fundoscopy, extraocular movements, and visual fields by confrontation.[36,68,69]

A variety of definitions and confusing terms relate to visual impairments.[69] Total blindness is the inability to distinguish light from darkness. Legal blindness, a distant visual acuity of 20/200 or less in the better eye with correction, was unfortunately created for adults, not children. Partial vision has been defined as distant visual acuity better than 20/200, but worse than 20/70. There is a need for better functional screening and monitoring of severe visual impairment in the pediatric population, and primary care physicians can play crucial roles in achieving these goals.

Matkin, at Creighton University School of Medicine, developed a questionnaire that included three items related to auditory responsiveness and three

Spontaneous
scribble
(15 mo)

Imitate
stroke
(24 mo)

Imitate
horizontal
and
vertical strokes
(30 mo)

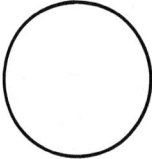

3 yr

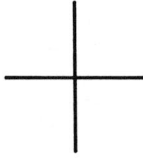

3½ yr

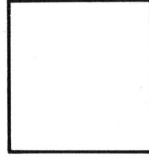

4 yr

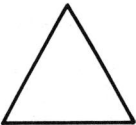

5 yr

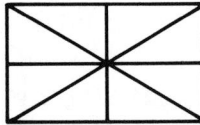

6 yr

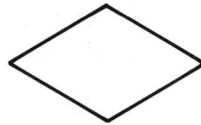

6 yr

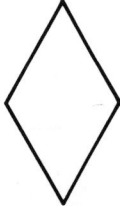

7 yr

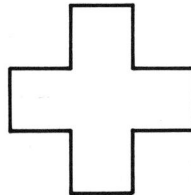

8 yr

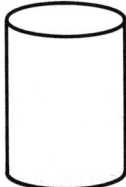

9 yr

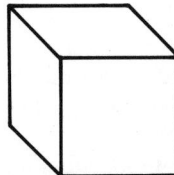

12 yr

Figure 7-3.   Visual perceptual assessment using drawing. (Data taken from References 1, 18, and 46.)

related to vocal output, in conjunction with one question related to social and motor development at ages 3 months, 6 months, and 9 months. (Table 7-16).[61] A referral for formal auditory screening is considered if one or more of the communication questions and one or more of the language milestones are answered no. A similar series of questions for children between 1 and 4 years of age serves for audiological assessment when speech is delayed.[61]

Beginning in the preschool period, teachers will often refer a child to the physician because of concern about speech and hearing. The primary care physician can use language milestones from Table 7-9 in conjunction with Matkin's auditory questionnaire. By utilizing family history, congenital infection, and anatomical malformations of the head and neck in conjunction with functional review of developmental aspects of language and hearing, primary care physicians can make a significant difference in the dismal statistic that over 50% of children with severe hearing impairment are not referred for audiometric assessment prior to their third birthday.[82]

Cortical sensory systems can be evaluated in children by having them identify such common objects as spoons, cups, and balls. Fur (a rabbits foot), cotton

TABLE 7-16   Auditory Function Screening

3 Months

Jumps to loud sound
Stirs from sleep when loud noise
Stops or decreases sucking when there is a sudden new sound

6 Months

Turns in general direction of loud sound
Stops crying when loud noise
Enjoys musical toys

9 Months

Responds to name, no, and bye-bye
Looks directly toward new sound
Knows if human's voice sounds friendly or angry
Enjoys ringing bell or rattle

12 Months—4 Years: Any Parental Concern About Hearing*

Turns to wrong direction when called
Fails to respond when spoken to in conversational voices and
    requires both gesture and verbal requests
Has difficulty understanding what others are saying in presence of
    background noise (TV, telephone)
Sits close to and adjusts TV to very loud levels
Cannot do several instructions combined in one long sentence
    without several gestures

* Any parental concern about hearing must result in audiological assessment for children of all ages. (Data taken from References 52, 61, 72, and 80.)

cloth, and a piece of sandpaper are also helpful. Beginning in first grade, graphesthesia can be assessed. Beginning at age 8, formal identification of American coins can take place.

Prognosis

Primary care physicians should acquaint themselves with methods of eliciting language, memory, perceptual, adaptive, behavioral, and educational function in school age children with motor impairments. Table 7-17 summarizes instruments

TABLE 7-17   Instruments for Monitoring Associated Deficits in School Age Children With Cerebral Palsy

Language

Single-word receptive vocabulary–Peabody picture vocabulary test
Single-word expressive vocabulary—Binet vocabulary cards
Serial commands
Action agents
Tests for auditory discrimination
Binet same/different discrimination
Binet vocabulary definitions
Binet cognitive situations

Memory

Binet digits forward
Binet digits reverse
Binet sentence memory
Visual memory
Object span—key, pencil, penny, blocks

Perceptual

Draw a person
Gessell figures
Bender-Gestalt figures

Educational and General Information

Oral reading paragraphs
Wide range achievement test (WRAT)
Includes subtest of single-word reading, spelling, and mathematics

Adaptive

Vineland social maturity
Barthel, PULSES, ESCROW
AAMD adaptive behavior

Behavioral

Checklists for hyperactivity and attention deficit disorders
Checklists for autism and organic neurobehavioral disorders

(Data taken from References 1, 29, 37, 39, 49, 53, 56, 57, 71, 80, and 91.)

TABLE 7-18   Laboratory Strategy for Genetic Causes of Cerebral Palsy and Developmental Disabilities

Onset	Physical Findings	Physical Techniques	Laboratory Tests
Prenatal	Multiple malformation Suspect central nervous system malformation or dysfunction	Measure and list anomalies Use reference texts of syndromes Use reference texts of teratogens	Chromosome studies Viral studies (Torch)* Targeted use radiographs and ultrasonography
Perinatal	Document pregnancy, labor, delivery records	Central nervous system Head circumference, transillumination, fundoscopy, Wood's lamp	If concern for seizures, electroencephalography; consider neuroimaging, audiometrics, viral studies
Postnatal	Recognize phenotypes for common treatable inborn errors of metabolism (see Table 7-20) Recognize Sanfilippo's syndrome, argininosuccinicaciduria, and biotinidase deficiency Recognize presentation of white matter disorders (spasticity, ataxia, optic atrophy) (see Table 7-22)	Vision and hearing screen, track head circumference	Fundoscopy using mydriatics, cranial sonogram; consider serial auditory tests
Mixed Perinatal and postnatal	Poor growth, recurrent symptoms	Rule out presence of storage disease: Corneal clouding, organ enlargement, dysostoses multiplex. Urea cycle, endocrine and organic acid disorders	Berry spot test on urine; fibroblast studies; urine thin layer chromotography. Thyroid function, ammonia, anion gap, plasma, amino acids, urine, and organic acids
Pre- and perinatal	Torch spectrum*	Pre- and perinatal chromosomal syndromes	Viral studies
Unknown	Recognize fragile x phenotype	Document macroorchidium, large forehead and jaw	Consider karyotype for fragile x, urine for metabolic screen

* Torch = Toxoplasmosis   Other, including syphylis   Rubella   CMV   Herpes

used at the Cerebral Palsy Clinic of Children's Hospital of Buffalo. This table illustrates that simple tools can be used to monitor a child's associated functional deficits in the office.

In an era of concern about the diagnostic utility of certain routine tests, the physician must have a specific approach to the use of the laboratory. We have found it most helpful to combine historic, malformation, and neurologic classifications so that appropriate use of the lab can follow. Our current approach

TABLE 7-19   Newborn Screening to Prevent Developmental Disabilities

Disorder	Incidence/Genetics	Untreated Phenotype	Diagnosis
PKU	1 : 12,500 AR*	Eczema MR† Gait abnormalities Behavior abnormalities, including autism	Plasma amino acids (increased phenylalanine)
Hypothyroid	1 : 4,000 Sporadic dysembryogenesis of thyroid gland	Short stature Large tongue Hirsute MR/CP‡ Umbilical hernia	Thyroid function test
Galactosemia	1 : 57,000 AR	Jaundice Neonatal sepsis Failure to thrive Vomiting irritability Cataract MR/CP Death	Urine reducing substance Enzyme analysis
Maple syrup urine disease	1 : 100,000 AR	Coma Opishtotonos MR/CP	Decreased glucose Increased ketones Plasma amino acids Enzyme analysis
Homocystinuria	1 : 100,000 AR	MR Hemiplegia Tall stature Dislocated lens Venous and arterial thrombosis	Plasma amino acids (increased methionine) Enzyme analysis
Biotinidase deficiency	1 : 50,000 AR	Intractable seizures Skin rash Failure to thrive	Urine organic acids Biotin
Argininosuccinic-acidurei	1 : 80,000 AR	Abnormal microscopic hair abnormality Failure to thrive Coma MR/CP	Urine amino acids Plasma amino acids Plasma ammonia

* AR = autosomal recessive
† MR = mental retardation
‡ CP = cerebral palsy

groups disorders by time of onset (Tables 7-18 to 7-21). Many of the tests used require as their basis a careful history and physical examination, plotting of growth, and functional developmental assessment. The way to work up a patient with cerebral palsy is not to ask how an individual child can get nuclear magnetic resonance scanning, CT scanning, and sophisticated electrophysiological investigations, but to ask if and how these tests contribute to better structural and functional classifications and etiological hypotheses.

We have found that the best procedure for management requires the targeted use of consultants and the ongoing involvement of the primary caregiver. Periodic monitoring by developmental physicians (pediatrician or physiatrist) and an orthopedic surgeon, in addition to the primary caregiver, is critical. Members of the rehabilitation team may include nurse, physical therapist, occupational therapist, speech pathologist, audiologist, psychologist, educational-vocational specialist, and social worker. A targeted use of these professionals is crucial so as not to overwhelm the child and family.

It is crucial to realize that no single technique of physical examination can substitute for a comprehensive, detailed neurodevelopmental and functional assessment. It is very important to examine children periodically in a comprehen-

TABLE 7-20   Treatment and Outcome of Developmental Disorders Detected in Newborn Metabolic Screening

Disorder	Treatment	Results	Unresolved Issues
PKU	Decreased dietary phenylalanine	Children treated before 3 mo are normal Improved behavior in older age	Offspring of maternal PKU
Hypothyroid	Thyroid supplement	No MR/CP if instituted prior to 6 wk	Subtle intrauterine damage
Galactosemia	Galactose-free diet	Prevents MR/CP, cataract, liver failure, death	Sepsis before action on results of screen
Maple syrup urine disease	Special diet Peritoneal dialysis Vitamin supplementation	Prevents MR/CP Promotes growth if started prior to 3 days	High degree of clinical suspicion has to initiate prompt treatment
Homocystinuria	Special diet Betaine Pyridoxine	Avoid complications of thromboembolism and dislocated lens	Betaine as new therapeutic strategy
Biotinidase deficiency	Pharmacological doses of biotin	Resolution of seizures Improved growth	Mass screening
Argininosuccinic-acidurei	Arginine supplementation	Resolution of coma	Prospective treatment before intrauterine toxicity of argininosuccinic acid

TABLE 7-21   Neurodegenerative Disorders That May Be Mistaken for Cerebral Palsy

Spasticity

Leukodystrophy	
Krabbe's	AR*
Metachromatic	AR
Adrenoleukodystrophy	X†
Zellweger's	AR
Cockayne's	AR

Small Molecule Disorders

Arginase deficiency	AR
Abetalipoproteinemia	AR

Movement Disorders

Wilson's disease	AR
Ataxia telangiectasia	AR
Lesh–Nyhan	X

* AR = autosomal
† X = linked

sive manner. Failure to do so ignores both the plasticity of children and the fact that minor central nervous system abnormalities often take their toll in cognitive processes such as language function or learning disabilities.

Motor Prognosis

Paine was the first to propose the continued presence of primitive reflexes and that increased intensity of primitive reflexes was highly predictive of motor delay.[75] Capute and associates compared four reflexes with the current ambulation status of 53 children with cerebral palsy.[13] Reflexes included asymmetric tonic neck reflex (ATNR), symmetric tonic neck reflex (STNR), tonic labyrinthine supine (TLS), and positive support (PS) (Table 7-14). The child's ambulatory status was graded as ambulation without assistance, ambulation requiring assistance, and nonambulation. This study found consistently higher primitive reflex scores in the nonambulators than in the ambulators.

Bleck found that if two of the following signs are present at 4 years, there is zero prognosis for ambulation: STNR, ATNR, absence of the parachute, positive supporting reaction, absence of foot placement reaction, absence of neck righting reflex, and Moro's reflex.[9] It is important for the primary care physician to realize that even though a child may not walk, ongoing developmental rehabilitation and orthopaedic monitoring is crucial. The goal for these nonambulating children is to have comfortable sitting and to avoid many severe secondary disabilities, such as acquired subluxation of the hip and progressive scoliosis.

Failure to monitor these secondary deformities in the severely involved child leads to additional difficulties with transportation, positioning, comfort, decubiti, and cardiopulmonary complications.

Molnar followed 359 children with cerebral palsy prospectively.[63,64] She found that all children sitting unsupported by age 2 years walked. In addition, all children who sat or walked by 2 years became community ambulators and did not require assistive devices. Molnar also found that 50% of children who sat by 3 years were independent community ambulators. The remaining 50% required crutches, braces, or had restrictions over community distances. No child who was not sitting by age 4 subsequently walked. Children who were not walking at age 7 were extremely unlikely to walk.

The prognosis for ambulation is related to type of cerebral palsy. Several series have shown that all hemiplegics walk.[25,64] Molnar followed 81 individuals with spastic diplegia.[63] She found that 65% walked independently, 20% required assistive devices, and 15% were nonambulators. Molnar also followed 144 spastic quadriplegics. She found that 33% were independent in walking, self-care, and activities of daily living (ADL). Thirty-three percent of the patients with spastic quadriplegia in this series walked with assistive devices, 25% were totally dependent in mobility and ADL, and 8% were nonambulatory but could perform some ADL tasks.

Kyllerman and colleagues studied 35 children with choreoathetoid extrapyramidal cerebral palsy and 81 children with dystonic extrapyramidal cerebral palsy.[54] Eighty percent of those with choreoathetoid extrapyramidal cerebral palsy (EPS) walked, whereas only 10% of those with dystonic extrapyramidal cerebral palsy walked.

In a study of 96 individuals with athetotic EPS cerebral palsy, Molnar found that 77% were ambulatory. Even in these 17 individuals there were considerable problems in oral motor control such as speech and swallowing, and upper extremity function such as feeding, dressing, and writing. Molnar also studied 38 mixed spastic and EPS individuals. Only 47% of these individuals were ambulatory. In summary, the prognosis for ambulation is best in hemiplegic and diplegic persons. Ambulation is less likely in individuals with spastic quad or extrapyramidal cerebral palsy.

Shapiro has pointed out, in a study of 152 profoundly mentally retarded, noninstitutionalized children (IQ < 25), that prognosis for walking is dependent upon absence of seizures, cerebral palsy, and sensory impairment.[83] Ninety-two percent of children with only profound mental retardation walked; however, only 53% of children with profound mental retardation and seizures, and only 11% of children with profound mental retardation and cerebral palsy and/or seizures, walked. In a separate study by Hreidarsson and Shapiro of seizures or sensory impairment in 185 home-placed children with MR only and not CP, 36% had mild MR, 23% had moderate MR, 21% had severe MR, and 20% had profound MR. All children with mild, moderate, and severe MR walked in each instance; and 35% of those with profound mental retardation walked. Seventy three percent of the patients with profound mental retardation who walked did so by age 2 years.[45]

In summary, the interaction among domains of development shapes a unique, yet dynamic, individual and that individual's functional capabilities.

Issues of Habilitation

The concept of habilitation covers a wide range of medical and nonmedical services. From the medical standpoint, diagnosis, evaluation, and therapeutic parameters address the management of oral motor problems in cerebral palsy, orthopaedic issues (including sitting, hips, and scoliosis), and visual and hearing impairments. Delivery of primary care and appropriate referral networks and provision of specialty clinics and preventive services can be utilized by the child with cerebral palsy. It is important, however, not to "overmedicalize" a child's care simply because of the existence of a disability. Disabled children may require a judicious use of special medical services and, at the same time, educational, social, recreational, and vocational services. Developmental goals based on children's ages are highlighted in Table 7-22.

The physician who manages the developmentally disabled or delayed child recognizes the strengths of the medical model in prioritizing known and treatable causes and in devising strategies for prevention. At the same time, he must recognize the limitations of the medical model, and the strength of a developmental–rehabilitation model for promoting functional independence, especially if information is incomplete. The physician must be aware of: (1) The untapped influence of parents, siblings, and peers in promoting self-esteem and coping behaviors; (2) the strengths of the interdisciplinary team, consisting of medical, habilitation, behavioral, and psychoeducational specialists, and (3) the legal

TABLE 7-22   Developmental Goals by Age Groups

0–3 yr	Establish diagnosis
	Attempt to determine etiology
	Monitor growth development and health status
	Screen for visual and hearing impairment
	Refer to infant stimulation
	Provide ongoing parental and sibling support
	Monitor progress in physiotherapy
3–6 yr	Assist with targeting goals and prioritization of needs for language, cognition, and behavior
	Surgery to prevent progressive deformity
	Strategies to enhance independence in activities of daily living
	Manage visual and auditory problems
7–11 yr	Monitor school progress
	Monitor peer and extracurricular experiences
	Avoid cycles of educational or therapeutic failure based on overoptimistic goals
	Prioritize areas of strength and work on success
12–18 yr	Target goals for early, middle, and late adolescence
	Enhance opportunities for independence
	Understanding of abilities and disabilities
	Hobby development
	Comprehensive sex education program
	Independent living
	Vocational/career counseling
	Manage acne, seizures, depression

mandate of special education to provide a full spectrum of services to all handicapped individuals.

Once a concern about the development of a child has been identified, the physician may recommend a stimulation program, such as Head Start or special services designed for the infant and toddler. Programs under the aegis of the Developmental Disabilities Act of 1967 now emphasize function rather than specific diagnoses. Thus, children eligible for these services must present with a ''substantial limitation in function'' in at least three of the following areas: self-care, receptive and expressive language, learning, mobility, self-direction, capacity for independent living, and economic self-sufficiency.

Medications for the child with cerebral palsy are usually needed for the control of seizures, spasticity and, at times, attention deficit disorder (Table 7-23). Medications have not been helpful in alleviating such significant movement disorders as choreoathetosis or dystonia. In using any medication on a child, the practitioner must ask such questions as: What are the indications? Is it helping? Can we use it at a lesser dose? Is it needed continually? A systematic approach to side-effects and cost benefits is necessary. For example, a child's spasticity at the ankles may be relieved by a medication such as Valium. However, if this leads to cognitive blunting, increased drooling, and truncal hypotonia, the child may not fully benefit from the original goal, which was ease in ambulation. Similarly, with respect to seizures, Vining and Mellits have shown that there are developmental and cognition effects of phenobarbital and phenytoin.[94] In addition, a person with developmental disabilities should not have to carry the burden of additional cosmetic stigmata such as gingival hypertrophy, hirsutism, or facial coarsening. Again, a targeted approach to seizure medications and the recognition that childhood seizures may not require lifelong chemotherapy are crucial to the approach of primary care physicians.[32] This is critically important for the primary care physician, as judicious tapering prior to adolescence can

TABLE 7-23   Medications in Cerebral Palsy

Children with seizure disorders	
Generalized tonic-clonic (grand mal)	Phenobarbital
	Phenytoin
Partial (focal)	Carbamazepine
Classical absence (petit mal)	Ethosuximide
Atypical absence (atonic, myoconic)	Benzodiazepine
	Valproic acid
	Ketogenic diet
	ACTH or prednisone
Children with spasticity	
Diazepam	
Dantrium	
Baclofen	
Children with attention deficit disorders	
Methylphenidate	
Dexedrine	
Magnesium pemoline	

avoid teratrogenicity of anticonvulsants to the fetus in women of childbearing age.

Public Policy

PL 94-142 established the constitutional right for handicapped children to receive educational services equal to those of their peers. The law states that social interaction is essential to effective high-quality educational services. The law requires that public schools provide to all handicapped children between the ages of 3 and 21 free and appropriate educational and related services and "due process" protections to parents. The law is a milestone in that it establishes equal rights of access for all children. Its implementation is problematic because of the definitions of handicapping conditions and the lack of definitive guidelines for the appropriate and utilitarian role of the physician. In addition, the meaning of "appropriate" educational services varies among professionals.

Wright outlined predominant issues that have an impact on the primary care provider's role. One problem is the inadequacy of guidelines that define learning disability and that can be a significant additional handicap among children with cerebral palsy. Criteria differ among states as well as among schools. On the other hand, many physicians have little exposure to the effect of chronic health-impairing conditions on learning and are often unfamiliar with the complexities of the educational system.

A second problem for a physician advocating for a child with a developmental disability is that appropriate educational placement and service is difficult, given the variability and heterogeneity of disabling conditions and individual response. Wright suggests that the ongoing involvement of the child's physician is crucial in order to ensure realistic and informed judgments about classroom type (*i.e.,* mainstreaming or self-contained), depth and frequency of related services (*i.e.,* speech, occupational, and physical therapies), and provision of primary health services in school, such as protocols for toileting, intermittent catheterization, and bowel management; special feeding techniques, ostomy care, nutritional services, and positioning, bracing, and timing of orthopaedic surgical interventions, policies on medication, school absence, and training of school staffs.

Funding problems and differing viewpoints on these issues often result in educational and medical professionals assuming adversarial relationships. One way of alleviating the problem is for physicians to be represented on committees for the handicapped. Such physicians should have had training and experience in *developmental disabilities* and primary care. Implementation of functional assessment and continuing evaluative followup of these children will also facilitate integration of the medical, social, and educational components of the service system for greater efficiency and effectiveness.

Adolescence

The adolescent with cerebral palsy is faced with increasingly complex challenges as he desires more independence. It is difficult for the young adult dependent upon others for physical and other assistance to achieve increased autonomy. The physician responsible for the management of the adolescent with cerebral palsy must take into account the patient's personal desires, as well as the changing needs of parents. Special needs of the adolescent include time with peers, time alone, activities that promote independence, leisure time, sexual counseling, and preparation for roles as a young adult.[79]

The following case illustrates the relationship between mild motor handicap, chronic health impairment, plateauing of school progress, adolescent issues, judicious use of ancillary tests, and a common environmental cause of attention and behavioral problems.

Case 5 Joe, a 13-year-old black male presented to the emergency room with diffuse abdominal pain. He had been premature and had weighed 1500 grams at birth. He had been followed since early childhood in hematology clinic for sickle cell anemia. At 2 years of age he toe walked, had tight heel cords, increased deep tendon reflexes, and positive Babinski. The diagnosis of mild spastic diplegia was made. Plastic anklefoot orthosis AFOs and active stretching resulted in plantigrade gait. There was a history of immaturity and attention problems attributed to recurrent hospitalization for complications of sickle cell anemia. He had made little educational progress since third grade. He was currently in the fifth grade and received resource help in language arts. During the preceding 3 months he had experienced increased difficulty in keeping up academically with peers. He complained of nausea after meals. His brother, who also had sickle cell anemia, had introduced him to the habit of chewing on magazine print in order to relieve him of his indigestion. Initial physical exam revealed a short, prepubertal black male with maloccluded teeth. There were no signs of acute abdomen. Initial diagnosis was sickle cell abdominal pain. Codeine was prescribed.

During the next 24 hours, the patient complained of headaches and diffuse bone pain. He refused solids. Clear liquids resulted in emesis. On return to the emergency room he was mildly dehydrated. During intravenous hydration, he became delirious. A grand mal seizure ensued. Anticonvulsants were administered. Revised diagnosis was central nervous system infarction.

Electroencephalogram revealed diffuse slowing, suggestive of a metabolic process. Cranial CT scan revealed no acute infarction. A lumbar puncture revealed no signs of infection or active bleeding. An exchange transfusion was performed to correct the anemia. On recovery from his seizures, the patient continued to complain of knee pain. There were no signs of injury or joint swelling. X-ray, however, revealed lead lines. Serum lead was 101 mcg, normal being less than 30. The diagnosis was lead encephalopathy. Chelation resulted in less irritability, decreased bone pain, and no recurrence of seizures. A review of the process of making printers' ink revealed that the ink was high in lead. After he recovered from coma, a neurodevelopmental assessment was performed. Memory and attentional and cognitive deficits were apparent. Strengths were in perceptual abilities. Full scale IQ was 75. There were difficulties with complex requests and abstract use of language. Reading and mathematics skills were at the second grade level.

Special education services were targeted to both cognitive deficits and generalized learning disability. Sugarfree gum was substituted for inkprint. A program of tutoring and ongoing pediatric support was initiated so that frequent absences would not lead to missed school days. Improved attendance resulted. Followup 1 year later revealed improved attention, concentration, and ability to handle complex language. He had made 1½ year of academic progress. His goals for his high school years included mastering functional academic skills so that he could pursue graphic arts.

This case illustrates the complexity of the management of an early adolescent with recurrent sickle crises. It also illustrates the consequence of not integrating medical, developmental, and behavioral approaches. This patient knew that narcotics made his abdominal pain worse. He felt that chewing on something gave him some relief, but he was concerned that chewing on gum would produce cavities. He was already worried about his maloccluded teeth. In addition, he kept his habit secret, as he was already embarrassed about his short stature, immaturity, and learning difficulties. In addition, this case illustrates that often mild spastic diplegia does not have major motor impairment as its long-term consequences, but can result in learning disability.

The role of primary care was to integrate medical, school, and counseling strategies so that cycles of absenteeism, chronic pain, and low self-esteem could be broken. A similar strategy can take place for other health impairments, including seizure disorders, diabetes, and asthma. By regarding the total child, medical, education, psychosocial, and environmental variables can be prioritized and addressed.

O'Reilly studied 336 adults with cerebral palsy over 20 years.[73] Twenty-six percent were working, 7% were in sheltered workshops, 39% were unemployed, and 11% were institutionalized. Seventeen percent had died. People with hemiplegia had the highest rate of employment (39%); people with total involvement (rigid quadriplegia) had the highest death rate (56%). No rigid quadriplegic was working or at a sheltered workshop. O'Reilly's study highlights the long-term difficulties that adults with cerebral palsy have in vocational adjustment.[73] Often the associated problems of learning disabilities, cognitive impairment, communication disorders, and seizures interfere more than the motor disability with being independent adults.

The role of the primary care physician has been well stated by the Ingram.[48] Job descriptions include relieving anxiety and stress on the handicap, seeking a way to circumvent the handicap, encouraging successes in areas least affected, and trying to produce a therapeutic program that includes the whole child and the child's need to be as independent as possible.

Integrating functional assessment into primary care will enhance the physician's role as coordinator of care, counselor, and advocate. By following and assisting children with developmental disabilities over time, the primary care physician can help integrate medical developmental, habilitative, and social services. This strategy promotes a child's independence no matter what level of handicap and makes a difference by restoring *caring* as a key therapeutic intervention for families.

References

1. Accardo PJ: A Neurodevelopmental Perspective on Specific Learning Disabilities. Baltimore, University Park Press, 1980

2. Accardo PJ, Capute AJ: The Pediatrician and the Developmentally Delayed Child: A Clinical Textbook on Mental Retardation. Baltimore, University Park Press, 1978
3. Allen M: Developmental outcome and follow-up of the small for gestational age infant. Semin Perinatd 8:123–156, 1984
4. Allen MC, Ichord RN: Developmental Outcome of Premature, Small for Gestational Age, and Asphyxiated Infants. Washington, DC, Instructional Course AACP DM Annual Meeting, 1984
5. Amiel-Tison C: A method for neurologic evaluation within the first year of life. Curr Probl Pediatr 7:1–50, 1976
6. Bayley N: Bayley Scales of Infant Development. New York, American Psychological Corp, 1969
7. Bax MC: Terminology and classification of cerebral palsy. Dev Med Child Neurol 6:295–307, 1964
8. Bennett FC, Robinson NM, Sells CJ: Growth and development of infants weighing less than 800 grams (28 ounces) at birth. Pediatrics 71:319–323, 1983
9. Bleck, EE: Locomotor prognosis in cerebral palsy. Dev Med Child Neurol 17:18, 1975
10. Bobath B: Abnormal Postural Reflex Activity Caused by Brain Lesions, 2nd ed. London, William Heinemann, 1971
11. Brazelton TB: Neonatal behavioral assessment scale. In Clinics in Developmental Medicine No. 88, 1984
12. Capute A, Accardo P: Linguistic and Auditory Milestones During the First Two Years of Life: A Language Inventory for the Practitioner. Clin Pediatr 17:847–853, 1978
13. Capute A, Accardo PJ, Vining E et al: Primitive reflex profile. A pilot study. Phys Ther 58:1061, 1978
14. Capute AJ, Accardo PJ, Vining E et al: Primitive Reflex Profile. Baltimore, University Park Press, 1978
15. Capute A, Biehl R. Functional developmental evaluation: Prerequisite to habilitation. Pediatr Clin North Am 20:3–26, 1973
16. Capute A, Palmer F: A pediatric overview of the spectrum of developmental disabilities. J Dev Behav Pediatr 1:66–69, 1980
17. Capute AJ, Palmer F, Shapiro B, Wachtel R: Expanded Classification of Cerebral Palsy. In Developmental Disabilities Fellowship Training Manual. Baltimore, John F Kennedy Institute, 1984
18. Capute AJ, Shapiro PK: The motor quotient: A method for the early detection of motor delay. Am J Dis Child 139:940–942, 1985
19. Cattell P: Measurement of Intelligence of Infants and Young Children, American Psychological Corporation 1940. New York, Harcourt Brace, 1980
20. Cole C (ed): Growth and development. In Harriet Lane Handbook, 10th ed, pp 318–330. National Center for Health Statistics, Courtesy of Ross Laboratories, 1985
21. Connolly KJ, Prechtl HFR (eds): Maturation and development: Biological and psychological perspective. In Clinics in Developmental Medicine, No. 77/78, 1981
22. Coplan J: ELM: The Early Language Milestone Scale. Tulsa, Modern Education Corp, 1983
23. Coplan J: Parental estimate of child's developmental level in a high-risk population. Am J Dis Child 136:101–104, 1982
24. Coplan J, Gleason JR, Ryan R et al: Validation of an early language milestone scale in a high-risk population. Pediatrics 70:677–83, 1982

25. Crothers B, Paine RS: The Natural History of Cerebral Palsy. Cambridge, MA, Harvard University Press, 1959
26. Denhoff E, Robinault IP: Cerebral Palsy and Related Disorders. New York, Mc-Graw-Hill, 1960
27. Desmond MW, Wilson GS, Voderman AL et al: The health and educational status of adolescents with congenital rubella syndrome. Dev Med Child Neurol 27:721–29, 1985
28. Diaz C, Fosarelli P, Groner J et al: Pediatric screening procedures: Vision screening. Adv Pediatr 29:418–33, 1982
29. Doll EA: Measurement of Social Competence: A Manual for the Vineland Social Maturity Scale. Circle Pines, MN, American Guidance Service, 1965
30. Dubowitz LT, Dubowitz V: Neurological assessment of the pre-term and full-term newborn infants. In Clinics in Developmental Medicine, No. 79, 1981
31. Dubowitz V: The Floppy Infant. In Clinics 2 in Developmental Medicine, 1980
32. Emerson R, Souza BJ, Vining EP: Stopping medication in children with epilepsy: Predictors of outcome. N Engl J Med, 304:1125–1129, 1981
33. Evans P, Elliott M, Alberman E, Evans S: Prevalence and disabilities in 4–8 year olds with cerebral palsy. Arch Dis Child 60:940–45, 1985
34. Ferry PC, Banner W, Wolf R: Seizure Disorders in Children. Philadelphia, JB Lippincott, 1986
35. Foster R: Camelot Behavior Checklist. Lawrence, KS, Camelot Behavioral Systems, 1977
36. Gammon JA: Visual systems screening in infants and young children. Pediatr in Review 4:71–73, 1982
37. Goodenough FL: Measurement of Intelligence by Drawing. New York, Harcourt Brace, 1926
38. Gortmaker SL, Sappenfield W: Chronic childhood disorders: Prevalence and impact. Pediat Clin North Am 31:3–18, 1984
39. Granger CV, Gresham GE (eds): Functional assessment in rehabilitation medicine. Baltimore, Williams & Wilkins, 1984
40. Hack M, Caron B, River A, Fanaroff A: The very low birth weight infant: The broader spectrum of morbidity during infancy and early childhood. J Dev Behav Pediatr 4:243–249, 1983
41. Hagberg B: The epidemiologic panorama of major neuropediatric handicaps in Sweden. In Clinics in Developmental Medicine, No. 67. Case of the Handicapped Child: A Festschrift for Ronald Mackeith, pp 111–124, 1978
42. Hagberg B, Hagberg G: Prenatal and perinatal risk factors in a survey of 681 Swedish cases. In Stanley F, Alberman E (eds): The Epidemiology of the Cerebral Palsies, pp 116–134. In Clinics in Developmental Medicine, No. 87, 1984
43. Hagberg B, Hagberg G, Olow I: The changing panorama of cerebral palsy in Sweden 1954–1970, I: Analysis of the general changes. Acta Paediatr Scand 64:187–192, 1975
44. Hagberg B, Hagberg G, Olow I: The changing panorama of cerebral palsy in Sweden 1954–70, III: The importance of fetal deprivation of supply. Acta Paediatr Scand 65:403–408, 1976
45. Hreidarsson SJ, Shapiro BK, Capute AJ: Age of Walking in the Cognitively Impaired. Dev Med Child Neurol 22:248–250, 1983
46. Illingworth RS: The Development of the Infant and Young Child: Normal and Abnormal, 8th ed. New York, Churchill Livingstone, 1983

47. Illingworth RS: Dissociation as a guide to developmental assessment. Arch Dis Child 33:118, 236–239, 1958
48. Ingram TTS: A Historical Review of the Dysfunction and Classification of the Cerebral Palsies. Clin Devel Med 87: 1–9, 1984
49. Jastak S, Wilkinson G: Wide Range Achievement Test Revised (WRAT-R). Administration Manual. Wilmington, Jastak Associates, 1984
50. Kiely T, Paneth N, Stein ZA et al: Cerebral palsy and newborn care, II: Mortality and neurologic handicap in low birth weight infants. Dev Med Child Neurol 23:650–59, 1981
51. Knobloch H, Pasamanick B: Gesell and Amatruda's Developmental Diagnosis: The Evaluation and Management of Normal and Abnormal Neuropsychologic Development in Infancy and Early Childhood, 3rd ed. Hagerstown, Harper & Row, 1974
52. Knobloch H, Stevens F, Malone A: Manual of Developmental Diagnosis. The Administration and Interpretation of the Revised Gesell and Amatruda's Developmental and Neurologic Examination. Hagerstown, Harper & Row, 1980
53. Koplitz EM: Bender–Gestalt Test for Young Children. New York, Grune & Stratton, 1963
54. Kyllerman M, Bager B, Bensch J et al: Dyskinetic cerebral palsy, I: Clinical categories, associated neurological abnormalities and incidences. Acta Paediatr Scand 71:53–550, 1982
55. Kyllermann M, Bager B, Bensch J et al: Dyskinetic cerebral palsy, II: Pathogenetic risk factors and intra-uterine growth. Acta Paediatr Scand 71:551–58, 1982
56. Levine M: Preschool child with learning disabilities. In Scheiner AP, Abroms IF (eds): The Practical Management of the Developmentally Delayed Child. St Louis, CV Mosby, 1980
57. Lloyd L, Dunn M, Dunn LM: Peabody Picture Vocabulary Test. Revised Form. Circle Pines, MN, American Guidance Services, 1981
58. McCarthy Scales of Children's Abilities. New York, The Psychological Corporation
59. Mahoney WJ, D'Souza BJ, Halber AJ et al: Long-term outcome of children with severe head injury and prolonged coma. Pediatrics 71:756–62, 1983
60. Marden PM, Smith DW, McDonald MJ: Congenital anomalies in the newborn infant including minor variations. J of Pediatr 64:357–71, 1964
61. Matkin ND: Early recognition and Referral of Hearing Impaired Children. Pediatr in Review 6:151–156, 1984
62. Minear WL: A classification of cerebral palsy. Pediatrics 18:841–52, 1956
63. Molnar GE: Cerebral palsy: Prognosis and how to judge it. Pediatric Ann 8:596–605, 1979
64. Molnar GE, Gordon SU: Cerebral palsy: Predictive value of selected clinical signs for early prognostication of motor function. Arch Phys Med Rehab 57:153, 1976
65. Nellhaus G: Head circumference from birth to 18 years: Practical composite international and interracial graphs. Pediatrics 41:106–114, 1968
66. Nelson K, Ellenberg J: Apgar scores as predictors of chronic neurologic disability. Pediatrics 68:36–44, 1981
67. Nelson KB, Ellenberg JH: Antecedents of cerebral palsy multivariate analysis of risk. N Engl J Med 315:81–6, 1986
68. Nelson LB: Pediatric Ophthalmology. Philadelphia, WB Saunders, 1984
69. Nelson LB: The visually handicapped child. Pediatr in Review 6:173–182, 1984

70. Prechtl H: Neurological examination of the full-term newborn infant, In Clinics in Developmental Med, No. 63, 1977

71. Nihira K, Foster R, Shellhaas M, Leland H: Adaptive Behavior Scale Manual: 1975 Review, p 14. Washington, DC, American Association on Mental Deficiency (AAMD), 1974

72. Northern JL, Downs MP: Hearing in Children. Baltimore, Williams & Wilkins, 1974

73. O'Reilly DE: Care of the cerebral palsied. Dev Med Child Neur 17:141–149, 1975

74. Ounsted M, Moar VA, Scott A: Head circumference Charts Updated. Arch Dis Child 60:936–39, 1985

75. Paine RS: Evolution of infantile postural reflexes in presence of chronic brain syndromes. Dev Med Child Neurol 6:354, 1964

76. Palmer FB, Shapiro BK, Wachtel RC, Capute, AJ: Primitive reflex profile. In Thompson GH, Rubin IC, Bilenher RM (eds): Comprehensive Management of Cerebral Palsy. New York, Grune & Stratton, 1983

77. Paneth N, Stark RI: Cerebral palsy and mental retardation in relation to indicators of perinatal asphyxia. Am J Obstet Gynecol 147:960–966, 1983

78. Perlstein MA: The late clinical syndrome of posticteric encephalopathy. Pediatr Clin North Am 7:665–687, 1960

79. Rubin IL, Bilenner RM (ed): Comprehensive Management of Cerebral Palsy, pp 171–179. New York, Grune & Stratton, 1983

80. Scheiner AP, Abrams IF (eds): The Practical Management of the Developmentally Delayed Child. St Louis, CV Mosby, 1980

81. Scheiner AP, Moomaw, M: Case of the visually handicapped child. Pediatr Rev 4:74–81, 1982

82. Shah CP, Chandler D, Dale R: Delay in referral of children with impaired hearing. Volta Rev 80:206–215, 1978

83. Shapiro BK, Accardo J, Capute A: Factors affecting walking in a profoundly retarded population. Dev Med Child Neurol 21:369–373, 1979

84. Shapiro BK, Palmer FB, Wachtel RC et al: Associated dysfunctions. In Thompson GH, Rubin K, Bilenner RM (eds): Comprehensive Management of Cerebral Palsy, pp 87–95. New York, Grune & Stratton, 1983

85. Sheridan MD: The STYCAR graded balls vision test. Dev Med Child Neurol 15:423, 1973

86. Sheridan MD: The STYCAR panda test for children with severe visual handicaps. Dev Med Child Neurol 15:728–35, 1973

87. Sheridan MD: Vision screening procedures for very young or handicapped children. In Gardiner P, MacKeith R, Smith V (eds): Aspects of Developmental and Pediatric Ophthalmology Clinics in Developmental Medicine, No. 32. New York, William Heinemann, 1969

88. Smith D: Recognizable Patterns of Human Malformations. Philadelphia, WB Saunders, 1982

89. Smith VH (ed): Visual disorders and cerebral palsy. Little Club Clinics in Developmental Med, No. 9. London, William Heinemnan, 1963

90. Smith VH, Keen J (eds): Visual handicap in children. In Clinics in Developmental Med, No. 73, 1979

91. Terman L, Merrell: Stanford Binet Intelligence Scale. Houghton Mifflin, Boston, 1972

92. Thurston JH, Thurston DL, Nixon BB et al: Prognognosis in childhood epliepsy. N Engl J Med 306:831, 1982

93. Vining E, Accardo PJ, Rubenstein JE et al: Cerebral palsy: A pediatric developmentalist's overview. Am J Dis Child 130:643–49, 1976
94. Vining E, Mellits ED, Cataldo M et al: Effects of phenobarbitol and sodium valproate on neuropsychological function and behavior. Ann Neurol Abstracts 10: 1983
95. Vohr B, Hack M: Developmental followup of low birth weight infants. Pediatr Clin North Am 29:1441, 1982
96. Volpe J: Neurology of the Newborn. Philadelphia, JB Lippincott, 1981

CHAPTER 8

Cardiopulmonary Rehabilitation

Richard A. Carleton

Cardiopulmonary diseases can be viewed as producing impairment primarily due to decreased stamina for physical tasks. Many heart or lung disorders can impair cardiopulmonary function. For clinical details of the manifestations of these disorders, the reader is referred to standard cardiology or pulmonary textbooks. To summarize briefly, the heart and lungs perform three fundamental functions: internalization of oxygen, removal of carbon dioxide with maintenance of acid-base balance, and delivery of sufficient oxygen and nutrients to all tissues of the body to maintain aerobic metabolism. The lungs must function at relatively low levels of work, with little effort of breathing, so the patient has energy for performing the activities of daily life. The heart must function with sufficiently low right and left ventricular preload levels to avoid systemic or pulmonary congestion. The major disabilities that are a consequence of cardiopulmonary disorders are dyspnea with exertion, angina pectoris, or disabling lassitude and fatigue.

People who are severely restricted by fatigue, dyspnea, or angina commonly experience physical deconditioning, a process by which performance is limited further by atrophy and loss of metabolic efficiency of muscles responsible for breathing, locomotion, and the tasks of daily living. Psychological depression typically aggravates the situation.

Rehabilitation of patients with cardiac or pulmonary disorders involves one or more of four approaches: surgery, pharmacologic therapy, lifestyle modification, and physical fitness training. Selected patients also may benefit from specialized physical therapy or emotional counseling. Fundamental to adapting to life with a cardiac or pulmonary disorder, as well as to the rehabilitative process,

168

is for the patient to thoroughly understand his or her condition(s), limitations, and capabilities. Development of a support system and inclusion of family and significant others in the counseling and educational process should not be overlooked.

Pulmonary Disorders

Disabling chronic pulmonary disorders can be restrictive, airway obstructive, and suppurative. Most chronic pulmonary disorders are combinations of two or three elements. Thus emphysema with its insidious destruction of alveolar walls is simultaneously restrictive, obstructive, and can be from time to time suppurative. Chronic bronchitis and bronchiectasis are also combinations of restrictive, obstructive, and suppurative disease. Certain pulmonary disorders (such as from asbestos exposure) primarily produce fibrosis and are restrictive. Specific rehabilitative interventions differ slightly from patient to patient, but general principles are applicable to all.

Surgical Therapy

Although surgery is seldom of value in treating chronic debilitating pulmonary disease, failure to consider surgery may limit rehabilitation. For example, selected patients with localized bronchiectasis may be spared the debilitating influences of hypoxia (due to a major ventilation/perfusion imbalance), as well as chronic suppuration and productive cough, by surgical lobectomy or segmental resection. Similarly, pleural stripping may rehabilitate the uncommon patient with restrictive disease related to marked pleural fibrosis. Pulmonary function may improve for some patients with severe bullous emphysema by resection of one or more giant bullae.

Pharmacologic Therapy

No curative pharmacologic therapy exists for true restrictive lung disease. Antibiotic and mucolytic therapy for severe chronic bronchitis or bronchiectasis often can produce temporary relief. Bronchodilator therapy, with steroids, frequently is useful in alleviating elements of reversible airway obstruction and may improve function dramatically. Low-flow oxygen (0.24 F_{IO_2}), including systems for ambulatory oxygen therapy, by providing relief from disabling hypoxia, may enhance mobility. Antibiotic therapy often helps in controlling bacterial infections that aggravate bronchial secretions and decrease air flow.

Lifestyle Modification

One key element in the rehabilitation of patients with pulmonary disorders is to prevent or retard progression of the disabling disorder. Cigarette smoking or sharing of smoke from others in the home or at work is a major factor in both the initiation and progressive exacerbation of many chronic pulmonary diseases.

Reduction of smoking or substitution of low-tar cigarettes is not an alternative. The increased puff profile that often follows a shift to low-tar cigarettes leads to further elevation of the levels of carboxyhemoglobin. With family support some persons who are motivated can stop smoking spontaneously. Others need a more formal program such as is offered by many health education centers, the American Lung Association, The American Cancer Society, and other agencies. Often the primary care physician's straightforward, unequivocal statement that smoking must stop can suffice.

Relaxation therapy can be effective for managing the stress that accompanies disabling illness. Progressive deep muscle relaxation according to the Jacobson technique[9] or primary relaxation response methods such as that proposed by Benson[1] are examples of relaxation therapy. Therapeutic benefits of relaxation for pulmonary disorders have not been demonstrated clearly.

Obesity markedly increases the amount of effort a patient with chronic pulmonary disease must expend to perform the physical requirements of work. The primary physician can counsel the patient to increase exercise and reduce calories, thereby achieving a more favorable caloric balance. A reduction of 3200 calories (1 pound) weekly can be achieved by a sustainable regimen of reducing high calorie foods (fats especially), as well as portion size, until the patient reaches his proper weight. An important element for the patient is positive feedback for each pound lost.

Physical Therapy

Breathing exercises designed to improve the mechanics of respiration are often helpful. Healthy people use the diaphragm for approximately 70% of the work of breathing. When greater expansion is needed, intercostal and accessory muscles of the neck and shoulders do the majority of the work of pulling the thorax upward and forward. The emphysematous chest is already expanded, however, and it is inefficient to move an already expanded thorax. Despite the limitations of the already flat diaphragm, diaphragmatic breathing exercises, having the patient push the abdomen outward during inspiration and inward during expiration, can sometimes improve the mechanics of ventilation even in the presence of severe emphysema. Have the patient place one hand on the abdomen and the other on the ribcage to illustrate whether the exercise is being performed correctly. The patient can observe diaphragmatic breathing most easily while supine or seated, but after learning it, he or she should apply it in the standing position, while walking, or while climbing stairs.

Pursed lip breathing and blowing exercises often help patients with airway obstruction. By pursing the lips during expiration, the patient delays reaching the critical closing pressure for small airways, thereby keeping the airways from collapsing. Other techniques for improving the mechanics of breathing include serial efforts to blow out a candle at gradually increasing distances from the pursed lips. Similarly, two bottles interconnected by rubber tubing, with a blow tube in each bottle, can be used to strengthen expiration by blowing water from one bottle to the other against the hydrostatic column of the water depth.

Postural drainage is useful in patients with suppurative lung disease. A spouse or other person may facilitate drainage of tenacious or purulent sputum

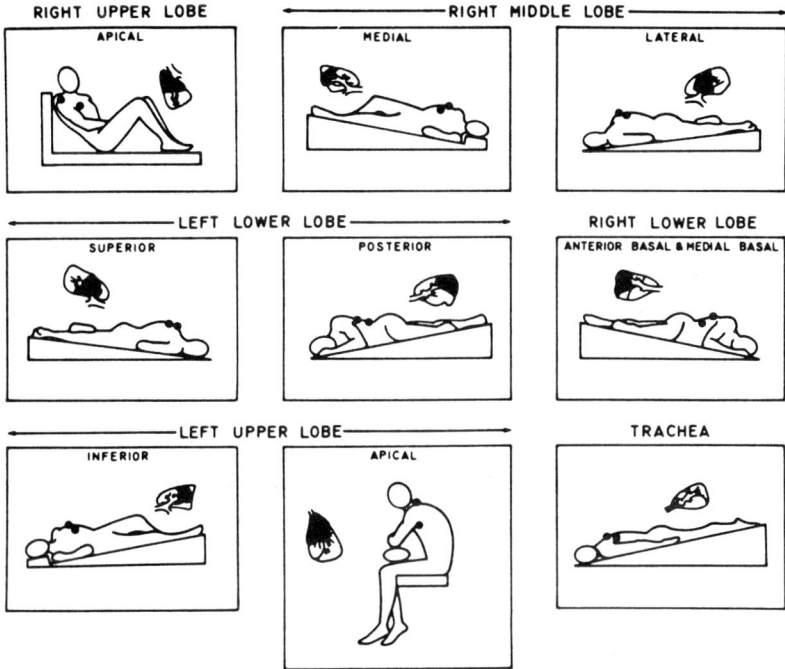

Figure 8-1. Basic postural drainage positions. Each position is used to drain the segment of the lung indicated by the *shaded areas*. ● indicates the points where percussion and vibration are to be applied. (Haas A et al: Pulmonary therapy and rehabilitation: Principles and practice, p 127. Baltimore, Williams & Wilkins, 1979)

from selected regions of the lungs by percussing the wall with cupped hands or by using an electric vibrator. To effect postural drainage, each segment of the lung requires a different position. The main positions for diverse lung segments are illustrated in Figure 8-1. The uppermost area of the chest in each position is then the appropriate location for rhythmic percussion.

Physical Fitness Training

The physiology of exercise includes a number of principles relevant to patients with pulmonary or cardiac disease. Whereas inactive skeletal muscles lose mass and strength and have increased oxygen demand per unit of work, repetitive use of muscles produces opposite effects. Although the effects have not been uniformly beneficial, patients with severely disabling pulmonary diseases have received cardiopulmonary endurance training. Many patients with pulmonary disease have coexistent heart disease with angina pectoris, atrial tachyarrhythmias, or right-sided heart failure from cor pulmonale. It is advisable, therefore, that patients with cardiopulmonary diseases who are about to start fitness training undergo monitored testing to determine safe levels of exercise.

Exercise testing by the Bruce[4] or Naughton[11] protocols provides valuable quantitative information about effort tolerance upon which to base a prescription for exercise therapy.

The general principles guiding exercise needed to produce a cardiopulmonary "training effect" are similar for healthy people and for people with heart or lung disease. Exercises should be isotonic rather than isometric. Isotonic exercises involve the development of relatively little force with rapid and repetitive movement of limbs. In addition, exercise should be aerobic, that is, at a less strenuous level than that which produces lactic acidosis and the attendent accentuation of respiratory drive.

In planning exercise programs, two general principles apply to all, whereas a third must be adapted for each patient. Exercise should be carried out at least 3, and preferably 5, times per week. Each exercise session should be at least 40 minutes long and should begin with 10 minutes of stretching, limbering calisthenics for arms, legs, and torso. A 5-minute "warm up" exercise phase should follow at a level of activity 25% less than the subsequent "training phase," consisting of at least 20 minutes of exercise at the prescribed level. A 5-minute "cool down" phase completes the program. With walking and jogging, the least expensive and most common form of isotonic exercise, as an example, the sequence would translate into calisthenics followed by a 5-minute slow walk for warming up, followed by a 20-minute brisk walk, walk/jog sequences, or jogging, followed by a 5-minute slow walk as a cool down phase.

Prescription of exercise is guided by several principles. In the absence of symptoms or of untoward effects, exercise can be prescribed in an amount that produces between 60% to 75% of the predicted maximal heart rate. The maximal heart rate can be predicted by subtracting the age of the person from 220 (e.g., for a 50-year-old person the predicted maximal heart rate is 170, and a 70% target rate equals 119). The exercise heart rate should be taken by counting the pulse (radial or, if necessary, carotid) for 10 seconds immediately after stopping the exercise and multiplying by 6. However, many patients with cardiac or pulmonary limitations cannot exercise strenuously enough to produce a heart rate in the desired range (including patients on beta blocking medications). For these patients, other guidelines must be used to recommend the appropriate amount of exercise. A rule of thumb is that an acceptable, safe level of exercise is attainable comfortably and while being able to converse in multiword sentences. Three to five exercise sessions carried out in 1 to 2 weeks are normally sufficient to achieve a training effect at the previous level of exercise and to permit increasing the exercise intensity. Each step in exercise intensity should increase by not more than 10%. The heart rate should be sustained in the previous range, as should comfort and ability to converse. Attainment of physical fitness is a slow process. Patients should not be discouraged if they progress only once every 2 or 3 weeks to steadily higher levels of exercise.

As the exercise program gradually increases, most patients find they can exercise more intensively while the symptoms remain at the same or a lower level than was possible in the beginning of the program. As physical fitness improves, patients find that general vigor increases and the exercise used in the program translates into increased endurance, permitting patients to perform many activities of daily living.

Finally, a diversity of exercises is feasible for a fitness training program for

TABLE 8-1   Supervised Walk-Jog Program

For the same patient as in the unsupervised walking program, train at 85% of 6 METS = 5.1 METS.

Walk ½ mile in 7.5 min, jog 50 paces, stop if angina is experienced. Wait until angina disappears, then resume walk at 4 mph. Repeat ½-mile walk in 7.5 min, then light jog for 50 paces (one pace = each time the left foot touches ground).

Day by day, as possible, extend jog out to 100 paces.

Try nitroglycerin or isosorbide dinitrate before exercise session to see if it eliminates angina response to jogging.

Try to extend walk to one mile in 15 min and jog to ½ mile in 5 min.

Warm-up—walk ¼ mile in 5 min.

Cool-down—walk ¼ mile in 7.5 min.

Alternatively, patients may be given a zone of target heart rates (70 to 85% of symptomatic threshold on the stress test) and advised to monitor their heart rate after 2-minute and 5-minute stints of exercise in any organized program of supervised exercise of the endurance-building type, such as walk/run, bicycle pedalling, calisthenics/jogging, swimming. If heart rates approach target zone and remain within it for the necessary training period (when monitored at 5-minute intervals), the supervised program probably is acceptable. However, the physical education instructor should be sufficiently familiar with exercise for cardiac patients to provide instruction in lessening the intensity of particular exercises by decreasing the cadence or the vigor with which the exercise is done. Jogging in the inner circle, for example, permits a cardiac patient to keep up with his peers who are exercising at higher heart rates and energy expenditures by jogging around the perimeter of a gymnasium.

(Reprinted with permission from The American Heart Association, The Committee on Exercise: Exercise Testing and Training of Individuals with Heart Disease or at High Risk for its Development: A Handbook for Physicians, 7320 Greenville Ave, Dallas, TX 75231.)

pulmonary patients. In general, one or at the most two exercises should be used primarily. Others can be used for recreational purposes and as supplements to the fitness training program. The most popular form of exercise for the training phase is walking or, as patients progress, walk/jog sequences, possibly culminating in a full jog. An example of a suitable fitness program using walk/jog sequences is presented in Table 8-1. Suitable alternative forms of exercise are stationary or mobile bicycling, swimming, jumping rope, aerobic dancing, and certain isotonic exercises.

A general guideline for adapting a new form of exercise for a patient who is already accustomed to a different one is to have the patient perform the new exercise at a low level for 3 minutes. The heart rate and the comfort level are then checked, and the exercise rate is adjusted up or down to a comparable level. Thereafter, the same schedule should be repeated, and the exercise rate should be increased by between 5% and 10% at 1- to 2-week intervals.

Emotional Counseling

Psychosocial factors have an important influence on the physiology of respiration. The respiratory system is very reactive. Anger or anxiety, for example, can increase ventilation and metabolism whereas depression or apathy can have opposite effects. Both conditions can affect an already precarious balance between the supply of and demand for oxygen, and both can lead to increased hypoxia or even hypercapnia.[7]

Pulmonary disorders, like cardiac disorders, represent a threat to life and can evoke marked anxiety. Patients with illnesses requiring prolonged artificial respiration can be expected to be very anxious in the anticipation of discontinuing respiratory assistance. Spakey and Davis[12] describe some of the physiologic and physical expressions of anxiety as they relate to the respiratory system. These include dysrhythmias, dyspnea, sighing, hyperventilation, labored "pant," suffocating or smothering sensations, substernal compression, chest pains, hiccups, diaphragmatic spasms, nasal reactions, allergic, bronchospastic, and other respiratory dysfunctions. They identify other distressing manifestations of anxiety including apprehension, uneasiness, helplessness, vulnerability, and loneliness. Anxiety also may cause disturbances of affection and cognition, concomitant with sensory and motor disturbances.

Patients with severe emphysema or unremitting bronchial asthma often are forced to restrict physical activities in order to avoid shortness of breath. Social contacts may diminish, interests may become increasingly focused on the disabling aspects of the disease, and depression and hopelessness may dominate. As activity and air flow diminish, sputum may not be moved adequately through the respiratory tract, and weakness and deconditioning may suppress adequate cough mechanisms. Insomnia, loss of appetite, confusion, marked irritability, and personality changes also may result from psychophysiologic reactions to pulmonary disorders. All of these conditions may accelerate or contribute to physical deterioration.

Management of Psychosocial Aspects

Management of the psychosocial aspects of pulmonary disease needs to be carried out in a series of steps. First, the patient and family need to be educated about the nature of the disease, its prognosis, its social and vocational implications, if any, and ways of decreasing risk factors associated with it (as described earlier in this chapter). The rationale for therapy regimens and treatment goals should be thoroughly discussed not only to help increase patient compliance, but also to help alleviate disabling fears or anxiety provoked by unknown aspects of the disease.

Second, the physician needs to identify the particular psychological and social situations that might perpetuate the patient's disability and dependence. Past and current family relationships, the physical set-up of the home, available transportation, friends and other support systems, the patient's attitudes toward disability, and his ability to accept or perpetuate dependency and a "sick role" may have an impact on disability and dependence. Depressed, anxious, and angry patients should have counseling available to them. The physician should explain that these emotions are both normal and appropriate; however, prolonged or severe reactions should be investigated and appropriate referrals should be made for psychological or psychopharmacological services. Referrals to community organizations for informational, social, financial, and vocational assistance also can be extremely valuable.

Third, the physician should help establish a supervised exercise program aimed at improving respiration, promoting the patient's satisfaction with life in general, and increasing the patient's activities and interaction with the environment. At the same time, exercising in a protected or supervised environment may help to decrease anxiety.

Finally, the primary care physician should be involved in coordinating treatment among physical therapists, social workers, home care providers, physiatrists, and so on. Patients should be followed initially at short intervals of 3 months or less; after 1 year of stabilization, office visits can be reduced to intervals of 3 to 6 months. During these visits, physicians should continue to evaluate the patient's adaption to his illness, coping mechanisms, and physical and emotional levels of disability. Continued reassurance, encouragement, and re-evaluation of needs are important in the successful rehabilitation of the patient with a pulmonary disorder.

Cardiac Disorders

Patients with cardiac disorders—especially that majority who have coronary artery disease—pose special challenges, but have better documented success rates from the rehabilitative process than patients with pulmonary disease. These patients deserve a systematic review to determine the type of therapy most likely to yield partial or complete rehabilitation.

Surgical Therapy

Unless they are relieved, limiting mechanical factors of many forms of cardiac disease make any rehabilitative process ineffective. The first step in the rehabilitation of a patient with congestive heart failure due to restrictive pericardial disease, disabling valvular disease, congenital lesions, or focal ventricular aneurysms is often full analysis by cardiac catheterization followed by appropriate cardiac surgery.

Patients disabled by angina pectoris should have an exercise tolerance test and electrocardiographic or radionuclide monitoring to determine whether they are at high risk for sudden death. If so, coronary bypass surgery should be considered as the primary means to their rehabilitation. Controversy persists concerning the indications for coronary surgery in patients with angina pectoris. In general, patients who continue to experience major disability despite good medical therapy should be evaluated for surgical intervention.

Pharmacologic Therapy

Pharmacologic therapy is the mainstay for most patients disabled by cardiac disease. Therapy enables them to increase their range of activities of daily living. Diuretics and often a digitalis glycoside, or afterload reduction, improve most patients with symptoms arising from systemic or pulmonary congestion. A digitalis preparation, beta blocker, or calcium channel blocking agent help patients disabled by rapid atrial tachyarrhythmias.

Patients disabled by angina pectoris can add to their range of somewhat taxing activities of daily living after therapy with a combination of nitrate vasodilators, beta blocking medication, or calcium channel blocking agents.

Lifestyle Modification

Several general principles concerning personal behavior apply to patients with cardiac disease. Patients with congestive heart failure usually benefit from a moderate restriction of sodium in the diet. All patients with cardiac disease who are overweight are able to improve performance if they can approach an ideal weight. A graduated program of weight loss of 1 pound per week is an appropriate target. This negative caloric balance can be achieved by a combination of curtailed nutritional intake and increased systematic exercise. Excess emotional tension is thought to hasten the development of coronary atherosclerosis; excessive time pressures and competitiveness may increase the likelihood of cardiac arrhythmias in susceptible patients. For these reasons, relaxation training by the Jacobson[9] or Benson[1,2] approaches are considered beneficial. Relaxation training has been proved to reduce participants' blood pressure and improve self-reported emotional states. The documentation of sustained benefits from relaxation training, however, remains controversial.

A process of careful patient education can improve compliance with antihypertensive regimens and other pharmacologic therapies. Developing a family support system for new lifestyles and compliance efforts is important. The cardiac patient who wants to improve virtually must stop smoking. With direct physician admonitions, a patient who understands and is motivated can be helped to cease smoking. If these measures are not successfully accomplished independently, then diverse agencies and organizations are available to provide programmatic assistance to stop smoking.

There is no proof that a sharp reduction in dietary fat and cholesterol will either retard the development of or decrease the size or number of atherosclerotic lesions in human coronary arteries. Yet, current understanding of the pathogenesis of atherosclerosis suggests that moderate reduction in fat intake to a level beneath 30% of total caloric intake is wise; a major proportion of fat should be polyunsaturated. Not only may this reduce excess weight but it may inhibit atherosclerosis.

Physical Therapy

Physical therapists have a role in the rehabilitation of cardiac patients by retraining them to perform many activities of daily living more efficiently by altering technique. Perhaps more important, physical therapists, occupational therapists, and vocational rehabilitation counselors can retrain the cardiac patient for less physically taxing employment. State Divisions of Vocational Rehabilitation often can provide invaluable assistance.

Physical Fitness Training

The physical fitness training program for patients with pulmonary disorders can be applied in an unsupervised setting to cardiac patients with valvular heart disease, mild congestive failure, or asymptomatic coronary disease. Because of the risk of arrhythmias and of sudden death in patients with active coronary artery disease—especially those with disabling angina pectoris and those soon after acute myocardial infarction—they should exercise in a medically supervised, electrocardiographically monitored setting, if at all possible. If medical supervision during exercise is not available, exercise within the previously described limits of heart rate, comfort and conversation ability is usually safe.

Most patients with cardiac disorders can safely perform exercise that is isotonic and aerobic 3 to 5 times weekly for 40 minutes or more per session. "Safe exercise" requires that the patient not exceed 75% of the predicted maximal heart rate while exercising. Such exercise also should be at a level just beneath that which produces symptoms such as angina pectoris and that permits conversation and is comfortable. These guidelines can be applied to many cardiac patients for whom supervised exercise is not possible.

Knowledge of the cardiac workload and metabolic requirements of specific activities is necessary to establish reasonable limits for their performance by cardiac patients. A customary way to establish the energy cost of an activity is to estimate the oxygen consumption required to perform it. A commonly used unit of measurement is the MET, which is equivalent to the amount of oxygen required for 1 minute by a person who is seated at rest, doing nothing with either arms or legs.[1] METS were described in chapter 2. A MET is approximately equal to consumption of 3.5 ml of oxygen per kilogram of body weight per minute. Various vocational tasks, recreational activities, and movements involved in activities of daily living have been classified in terms of the number of METS (multiples of the basic oxygen consumption) needed for their performance (as shown in Table 8-3). Cardiac patients can be placed on a program of gradually increasing activity based on these guidelines. Stress tests can be used to calculate heart rate during activity and to determine the MET levels the patient can safely perform.

Cardiac rehabilitation programs involving the MET measurement of task performance can begin as early as 1 to 2 days after a myocardial infarction. Even patients lying in bed are not at a continuous basal level of cardiac work; any movement by the patient (including changing position, reaching to the bedstand, or trying to sit up) increases oxygen consumption and cardiac work. Posture also affects these parameters.

> Sitting in an easy chair, fully relaxed, with support for the head, back, arms, thighs, and feet is a position of minimal cardiac requirement in which the cardiac output is only approximately 85% as great as when a person is lying in a supine position.[10]

During the acute stages of a myocardial infarction, activity is maintained at or below 1.5 METS. After the patient has stabilized, supervised calisthenic exercises of low MET value may be performed for short periods of time, followed by substantial rest periods. The intensity, number, and duration of these calisthenic exercises are increased progressively each day, assuming the patient shows no adverse effects. Eventually, walking, washing, and more strenuous tasks are allowed in addition to the exercise regimen. Prior to discharge from the hospital, the patient should be given an exercise program with the amount, duration, and MET equivalents carefully specified. (Tables 8-2 and 8-3 list the energy costs of common activities.)

TABLE 8-2   Energy Cost of Light Activities in Adults

Activity	Average Energy Cost (Kcal/min/70 kg)
Sleeping	0.9
Lying quietly	1.0
Lying quietly doing mental arithmetic	1.04
Sitting at ease	1.2 –1.6
Sitting, writing	1.9 –2.2
Sitting, playing cards	1.9 –2.1
Sitting, playing musical instrument	2.0 –3.2
Standing at ease	1.4 –2.0
Walking, 1 mph	2.3
Standing, washing and shaving	2.5 –2.6
Standing, dressing and undressing	2.3 –3.3
Light housework	1.7 –3.0
Heavy housework	3.0 –6.0
Office work	1.3 –2.5
Typing, mechanical typewriter	1.26–1.57
Typing, electric typewriter	1.13–1.39
Walking, 2 mph	3.1
Light industrial work	2.0 –5.0
Walking, 3 mph (average comfortable walking speed)	4.3

(Corcoran PJ: Energy expenditure during ambulation. In Downey JA, Darling RC (eds): Physiological Basis of Rehabilitation Medicine, p 187. Philadelphia, WB Saunders, 1971)

After 8 weeks, many patients are ready for formal cardiac rehabilitation programs to increase endurance and prevent deconditioning. Periodic exercise stress tests may be performed under a physician's supervision to establish exercise tolerance. It should be kept in mind, however, that MET equivalents are not absolute determinants of energy consumption; for example, temperature extremes, increased ambient carbon dioxide levels, inclines, and emotional stress at home or work may increase demands for cardiac work or reduce available oxygen.

Emotional Counseling

Coronary heart disease symptoms often have a sudden onset without any warning. In a matter of moments or hours, a person's functional capacity can be radically changed. If the person survives a myocardial infarction, he or she still is faced with the threat of future recurrence, disability, and possibly premature death. Psychological state of mind and lifestyle modifications that can increase survival odds are determining factors in surviving a myocardial infarction.

According to Follick and colleagues,[6] there are three phases of recovery from a myocardial infarction. The *acute* phase, which encompasses the first 24 to 72 hours after a heart attack, is typically a period of shock and disbelief. During this period the patient focuses mainly on the illness, is fearful of death, is restricted in mobility, and often feels a loss of personal independence and functioning. Anxiety and denial are characteristic reactions. The patient is likely to be

TABLE 8-3   Approximate Energy Cost of Common Vocational and Recreational Activities

Sitting: light tasks (1.5–4.5 METs)
Desk work, typing
Driving cars, trucks
Using hand tools, light assembly
Crane operation
Working levers
Playing cards, seated games
Machine sewing
Flying
Painting, recreational
Horseback riding, walk and trot
Golf cart, riding
Fishing from boat, seated
Riding mower

Standing moderate tasks (2.5–5.5 METs)
Standing quietly, working at own pace, light assembly or hand tools
Scrubbing, waxing, polishing
Assembly or repair of machine parts
Light welding, woodworking, interior carpentry
Power sanding
Stocking shelves
Light to medium assembly line work
Crank dollies, hitching trailers, operating large levers, jacks
Wiring house
Bricklaying, plastering, house painting, paperhanging
Hoeing, raking, weeding
Cleaning windows

Walking: light to moderate tasks (2.5–5.5 METs)
Gas station attendant
Carrying trays, dishes, etc.
Walking to 4 mi/h (6.44 km/h) on level
Billiards, bowling
Fishing, bait casting and fly with waders
Shuffleboard
Volleyball, noncompetitive
Archery
Sail small boat
Dancing
Gardening
Golf
Tennis, doubles
Calisthenics
Making beds
Mowing lawns, cast or power unit
Table tennis

Standing and/or walking: heavy tasks (Average or range of METs follows each task)

Pushing or moving heavy objects—75 lb (33.8 kg) or more, e.g., moving-van work	8.0
Cutting wood	
Power saw	2–4
Hand axe or saw	5–10
Digging, shoveling	4–8
Wheelbarrow	4–10
Plumbing	3–8
Snow shoveling	6–15
Lifting and carrying	
20–44 lb (9–19.8 kg)	4.5
45–64 lb (20.2–28.8 kg)	6.0
65–84 lb (29.3–37.8 kg)	7.5
85–100 lb (38.3–45 kg)	8.5
Pneumatic tool work	6.0
Skating, roller or ice	5–6
Badminton, competitive	5–7
Tennis, singles	6–9
Paddle ball, raquetball, squash, handball	7–15
Skiing	
Downhill	5–8
Crosscountry	6–12
Water	5–7
Hunting	
Small game	3–7
Big game	3–14
Swimming	4–8
Jogging, running	7–15
Basketball	5–12

(Brammell HL: Cardiovascular diseases. In Stolov WC, Clowers MR (eds): Handbook of Severe Disability, p 295. US Dept. of Education, Rehabilitation Services Administration, 1981)

unable to concentrate and may experience insomnia, tenseness, and an increased verbalization rate. Anxiety also may cause the patient to misinterpret information or medical procedures and, as a consequence, he or she may suffer from various misconceptions or exaggerated fears. Anxiety also may stimulate the autonomic nervous system, thereby threatening coronary stability.

Physicians and other health-care providers can help alleviate anxiety during this period by informing the patient accurately and completely of his condition, explaining routines or medical procedures in advance, and encouraging the patient to ask questions and participate in treatment. Relaxation training, used with caution, may help distract the patient from the noise of monitors or built-up tension. Denial during this stage is a normal reaction and helps the patient alleviate anxiety and cope more effectively. Physicians should not try to discourage denial at this time by forcing the patient to see the seriousness of the condition.

During the acute stages of a myocardial infarction, too often attention is paid only to the medical aspects of the experience. Consideration of the psychosocial aspects also is extremely important. Unresolved emotional upsets during the acute phase of an MI can result in an increased risk of mortality within 6 months following discharge. In a study by Garrity and Klein, 41% of patients who did not adjust within 6 months of discharge died, compared to 8% of patients who were considered to have adjusted well.[6]

The *second phase* of recovery from a myocardial infarction begins about 2 to 3 days after the acute attack. As the patient begins to stabilize, anxiety and denial subside as the medically critical period passes. After 3 to 4 days, however, depression is an almost universal phenomenon. According to Friedman,[7] a depressed mental state after a myocardial infarction is the largest psychological barrier to rehabilitation. During this phase of recovery, coronary patients begin to realize the impact the attack will have on work and family roles. They may focus on activities they always enjoyed prior to the attack, but now fear they will never do again. Hopelessness and helplessness are common feelings, and patients may experience crying spells, decreased appetite, insomnia, and a generally sad affect. Weakness and inactivity during this period contribute to the depressed state.

The second phase is very important to recovery. The way patients react to their disease during the first few days is an essential factor in the success of rehabilitation. Patients with *impulsive* reactions tend to minimize the disorder. These patients frequently pay no heed to recommendations that they modify their lifestyles. They resume activity quickly and may even be found in hospital corridors smoking cigarettes. Frequently they return to work ahead of the schedule recommended by the doctor. People who experience *regressive* reactions, on the other hand, tend to maximize the level of disability resulting from the myocardial infarction. These patients are frequently overwhelmed and confused. Fear prevents them from being motivated and participating in rehabilitation efforts. *Adaptive* reactions, the third alternative, represent constructive responses in which individuals take advice to reduce risk factors, face the disorder realistically, and follow rehabilitation routines.

Treatment during this second phase should focus on encouraging the patient to assume a responsible role in determining outcomes and modifying activity. Discussions with the patient should include prognosis, expected future problems, and available treatments. The physician or counselor should find out the kind of work the patient does, family roles and responsibilities, leisure activities, eating habits, vacation plans, and the amount and intensity of sexual activity, and offer concrete suggestions for modifying activities and lifestyle. Patients should be encouraged to talk about their feelings and fears, and all these issues should then be addressed. The common fear of never being able to have sex again, for example, can be assuaged by reassuring the patient that sexual activity is equivalent to climbing one flight of stairs and that most patients with uncomplicated myocardial infarctions can resume sexual activity within 6 to 8 weeks. Similarly, it is important to prepare the patient with an uncomplicated myocardial infarction for return to work, household, and social responsibilities.

Approximately 20% of all postcoronary patients with uncomplicated MI's do not return to work despite the fact that they are capable of doing so.[6]

Educating the patient about his or her condition, encouraging activity, and providing emotional support are all necessary to minimize fear and increase productivity. Family members should be included in discussions.

Phase 3 involves the posthospitalization period. During this time it is important for the physician to monitor the patient's progress and make attempts to modify his lifestyle. Of those surviving the heart attack initially, 15% to 20% will succumb during the first few weeks.[6] Many patients feel anxious, vulnerable, and unprotected outside the hospital confines due to the threat of death. Blue collar workers especially may worry about their ability to remain employed or to function effectively as a spouse or parent. Some men consider restrictions on drinking, smoking, and sex as synonymous with a loss of manhood. During hospitalization most patients' activity is limited; once home they may experience fatigue or even angina with increasing activity, causing them to become discouraged, resentful of their limitations, or even to feel hopeless.

Some posthospitalization anxiety can be relieved by offering the patient specific instructions and information about what to expect and how to cope with the disease. Physicians should refrain from vague instructions such as "take it easy," or "do it in moderation." Patients need to be given specific time and amount instructions for rest, work, exercise, recreational activities, personal care activities, sexual intercourse, and even travel. During periodic checkups, physicians should assess the patient's level of functioning in these areas and amend limitation of activity, if appropriate. Referral to a cardiac rehabilitation program is highly recommended because it may provide patients with the supervision and security needed to resume activities gradually. Group therapy and participation in heart clubs—at which individuals with coronary disease can share experiences, fears, and coping mechanisms—also are beneficial. Relaxation training may help some patients to deal constructively with their emotional stress and prevent recurrences of symptoms. Psychotherapy should be considered when post-MI depression is protracted and results in loss of libido, impotence, anorexia, insomnia or hypersomnia, or potentiates dependency in a sick role.[8]

Other types of cardiac patients can benefit equally from attention given to the emotional aspects of their disease. For example, physicians should be sensitive to the fact that reduction of anxiety can lead to the prevention of pre- and postprocedural complications of cardiac catheterizations and coronary bypass surgery. Studies have shown that the provision of accurate information about procedures, physical sensations, and expected postoperative feelings reduces complaints about pain, requests for medication, and length of hospitalization. Honest and informative discussions about the patient's cardiac state, prescription of realistic activity guidelines, and appropriate encouragement can help decrease patients' anxiety levels. This should enable the patient to cope better with his or her disabilities and thereby lead a more productive life. Indeed, psychological aspects must be incorporated into the comprehensive management of the cardiac patient.

Summary

Individuals with cardiopulmonary impairments frequently experience limitations due to fatigue, dyspnea, or angina. In addition to reduced stamina for activities, anxiety, fear, and mental depression may ensue, further restricting normal functioning and contributing to physical deconditioning.

Rehabilitation of the patient disabled by cardiac or pulmonary disorders is often possible by blending the principles of continuous primary care with active consideration of the options for surgery, appropriate pharmacologic therapy, lifestyle modification, specific physical therapy, exercise training, and emotional counseling. Adaption to these life-threatening disorders can be facilitated through patient education, encouragement, and strengthening the patient's social supports. Application of these principles by the primary care physician can be expected to improve the patient's quality of life and possibly increase longevity.

References

1. Benson H.: The Relaxation Response. New York, William Morrow & Co, 1975
2. Benson H et al.: Decreased systolic blood pressure through operant conditioning in patients with essential hypertension. Science 173:740, 1971
3. Brammel HL: Cardiovascular diseases. In Stolov WC, Clowers MR (eds): Handbook of Severe Disability. US Dept. of Education, Rehabilitation Services Administration, 1981
4. Bruce RA: Progress in exercise cardiology. In Yu PN, Goodwin JF (eds): Progress in Cardiology. Philadelphia, Lea & Feibiger, 1975
5. Dudley DL: Psychophysiology of Respiration in Health & Disease. New York, Appleton Century Crofts 1969
6. Follick MJ, Gottlieb BS, Fowler JL: Behavior therapy in coronary heart disease: lifestyle modification. In Sobel HJ (ed): Behavior Therapy in Terminal Care. Cambridge, MA, Ballinger, 1981
7. Friedman BH: Psychosocial factors in coronary risk and rehabilitation. In Stocksmeier U (ed): Psychological Approach to the Rehabilitation of Coronary Patients. Berlin, Germ, Springer–Verlag, 1976
8. Hackett TP, Cassem NH: Psychologic aspects of rehabilitation after myocardial infarction. In Wenger NK, Hellerstein HK (eds): Rehabilitation of the Coronary Patient. New York, John Wiley & Sons, 1978

9. Jacobson E: Progressive Relaxation. Chicago, University of Chicago Press, 1938
10. Kottke FJ: Common cardiovascular problems in rehabilitation. In Kottke FJ, Stillwell GK, Lehmann JF (eds): Krusen's Handbook of Physical Medicine and Rehabilitation, p 791. Philadelphia, WB Saunders, 1982
11. Naughton J: Refinements in methods of evaluation and physical conditioning before and after myocardial infarction. Am J Cardiol 14:837, 1964
12. Spakey PJ, Davis HL: Psychogenic dyspnea. In Bangar AL, Levine ER (eds): Dyspnea, Diagnosis & Treatment. Philadelphia, FA Davis, 1963

Additional Readings

1. Cohn P, Therapy of chronic angina pectoris. In Cohn P (ed): Diagnosis and Therapy of Coronary Artery Disease. Boston, Little, Brown & Co, 1979
2. Croog SH: Social aspects of rehabilitation after myocardial infarction: A selective review. In Wenger NK, Hellerstein HK (eds): Rehabilitation of the Coronary Patient. New York, John Wiley & Sons, 1978
3. Suinn RM, Bloom LJ: Anxiety management training for pattern a behavior. J Behav Med 1:25, 1978

CHAPTER 9

The Completed Stroke

As the proportion of the population over 65 years of age increases, vascular disease of the brain has become a major world public health problem and therefore one of the most pressing concerns for modern day medicine. Although there are a number of different definitions of stroke (the preferred term instead of "cerebrovascular accident"), the World Health Organization's (1971) definition is the most widely accepted. A stroke is characterized by

> rapidly developed signs of focal disturbance of cerebral function of presumed vascular origin and of more than 24 hours duration.[30]

According to this definition, a stroke includes most cases of cerebral infarction due to arterial thrombosis, stenosis or embolism, intracerebral hemorrhage, and subarachnoid hemorrhage. This definition of stroke does not include transient ischemic attacks and diffuse cerebrovascular disease of insidious onset.[30]

The primary care physician, rather than the neurological specialist, is most frequently responsible for the treatment of stroke, especially in elderly patients or those with a possible transient ischemic attack (TIA) precursor.[37] Comprehensive care of the stroke patient can be an extremely rewarding aspect of medical care since so much can be done for the patient. Stroke is a hospital-based problem only during the acute phase.[20] Comprehensive care of the stroke patient typically involves prevention of secondary complications such as decubitus ulcers, contractures, and urinary tract infections. Comprehensive care also is concerned with increasing patients' capabilities within their own homes through the use of physical and occupational therapy, adaptive aids, coordinated medical services, and local agency referrals for continued information and support.

The conventional wisdom is that the stroke patient will never be able to return to productive activity. In actuality, the prognosis for patients who survive the first 30 days following a stroke is variable. An estimated 10% will return to work, 40% will have residual mild disability, 40% will require some assistance with activities of daily living, and only 10% will need long-term institutional care. The goal of a comprehensive treatment program, therefore, should be to return the person with residual deficits to the mainstream by minimizing physical disability, by alleviating psychological and social maladjustment and, if possible, by reducing problems of vocational displacement.

This chapter is limited to the rehabilitation of stroke patients. Any health-care provider concerned with the stroke patient needs an appropriate background with respect to the epidemiology of stroke, mortality and morbidity of stroke, recurrence, classifications, types, outcomes, neurological involvement, risk factors and etiology, and methods of diagnosis. Information on these topics may be found in a variety of excellent sources. A list of titles we have found useful appears at the end of this chapter.

Management of the Stroke Patient:

A stroke is a catastrophic event both for the patient and his relatives. A previously normal, intelligent person may be suddenly rendered aphasic, paralyzed and incontinent. All too often nothing can be done, medically or surgically, to improve the situation in the acute phase. The quality of the remainder of the person's life will thereafter largely depend upon the degree of functional recovery which occurs. It is the aim of rehabilitation to help the patient make the best of his residual capabilities.[20]

Initially, management of the stroke patient focuses on attending to aspects of the acute situation. McHenry[31] lists five principal aims of managing the acute stroke: (1) maintenance of airway, (2) control of blood pressure, (3) stabilization of fluid, electrolyte, and metabolic balance, (4) bowel and bladder management, and (5) avoidance of pressure sores and postural contractures.

Once life-saving medical procedures have been applied, an accurate diagnosis has been made, and the patient has been stabilized, attention can be turned to assessing functional ability and to planning rehabilitative measures. The patient must be assessed with respect to self-care activities (including dressing, feeding, personal hygiene, and bladder and bowel management), mobility (including transferring to and from bed and chair and ambulation), communicative and cognitive abilities, psychosocial adjustment and family functioning, and household and vocational skills. The goals of the rehabilitation program for the stroke patient should be to (1) prevent avoidable problems that may limit performance and functioning, (2) increase capacity to perform and function, (3) modify the environment as needed so the patient can achieve his potential to perform and function.[34]

Improvement after a completed stroke involves both neurological and functional recovery. With the exception of some hemorrhagic strokes, after which recovery may continue at a slow rate over a long period of time, 90% of neurological recovery occurs within the first 3 months of onset.[2] Functional recovery, on the other hand, may not follow neurological recovery directly. Return of function is dependent upon the pattern and degree of specific deficits, as well as motivation and opportunities for retraining. Despite neurological limitations, functional recovery may continue after the patient is reintegrated into the life of the community because of his ability to adapt by using uninvolved limbs.[5]

For most patients with residual deficits from a stroke, rehabilitation is the most effective way of maximizing their functional recovery and narrowing the gap between disability in performance and potential capability. Studies of the effectiveness of rehabilitation on stroke patients have shown that whereas survival time may not be altered by rehabilitation, long-term goals that contribute to life satisfaction, such as greater independence in self-care and the ability to live outside the institution, are experienced more frequently by treated, as compared to untreated, patients.[8] Further, stroke rehabilitation has been shown to improve functional performance significantly even of patients who are elderly, medically ill, or have continuing neurological and functional deficits.[8]

Patients may enter the rehabilitation setting at many different levels, ranging from acute care in a general hospital to a specialized rehabilitation facility. Some persons enter the rehabilitation environment through less structured channels such as skilled nursing facilities, outpatient clinics, day care or day hospital programs, or stroke clubs.

To maximize functional return and help reduce the length of the hospital inpatient stay, rehabilitation should begin as soon as the patient is medically stable and able to tolerate a progressive activity program. In the past, stroke patients were confined to bed with the intention of limiting progression of the stroke. The efficacy of complete bedrest has not been established, and today the emphasis is on early mobilization to lessen complications that may stem from prolonged bedrest. Stroke patients are encouraged, at least, to begin sitting in a chair beside the bed as soon as the completed stroke has stabilized, usually within 48 hours of onset.[3] It is advisable that suitable patients be transferred to the rehabilitation unit if there is one. Studies have shown that patients treated in a specialized disability-oriented stroke unit within a hospital tend to ambulate sooner and are more likely to return home than those cared for in general wards within the same hospital. Patients in stroke units experience less morbidity and improved functional outcomes.[9] Although staff–patient ratios are generally similar to those on the general medical/surgical units, the success of the disability-oriented stroke units seems to be related to (1) better communication between the interdisciplinary team members, (2) a more consistent approach to problem solving, (3) the development of expertise in managing disability-related issues, and (4) greater patient interaction due to participation in group activities with others suffering from similar disabilities.[9]

The notion that the outlook for stroke patients is hopeless is both outdated and erroneous. Much can be done for the stroke patient. Not only physical limitations may occur following a stroke, but also shifts in personality, sexual patterns, position and role within the home, and degree of life satisfaction. Rehabilitation can help enhance independence, increase socialization, and reduce physical complaints, readmissions to the hospital, and psychological problems.

Peszczynski and colleagues[33] list nine goals in the rehabilitation of a stroke patient:

1. To prevent or minimize secondary complications such as contractures, infections (including those from skin breakdown), or effects of disuse which may interfere with natural recovery of function; the latter may be

motor (muscular weakness) or cardiovascular (inability to satisfy the energy requirements associated with standing, walking, or climbing stairs). Consequently, levels of performance demanded should be within the limits of current ability, and the patient should be protected from damage that may result from an abnormal or inadequate level of function.

2. To compensate for sensory loss which can result in a variety of deficits such as inability to walk effectively or judge whether the body is upright.
3. To encourage social participation and to provide the environmental stimulation needed for recovery.
4. To enable achievement of maximal psychological integration and stability.
5. To produce the high degree of motivation necessary for successful cooperation in a rehabilitation program; as each patient is different and has his own problems, individualized programs must be designed in order to achieve maximal motivation and results.
6. To substitute for a function either partially or totally lost once the level of recovery has been estimated or anticipated.
7. To enable independent home living or, if this is impossible, to attain sufficient improvement to permit future care with the least amount of assistance and supervision.
8. To achieve, in some cases, sufficient vocational rehabilitation to enable placement in competitive employment or in a sheltered workshop.
9. To provide a level of communicative skills adequate for establishing and maintaining interpersonal relationships.

Since neither age, sex, nor history of a medical problem currently under control tends to hamper functional return, and it is not possible to predict outcome on an individual patient basis, several authors conclude that all patients should be given a therapeutic trial unless they are too ill to participate.[1,10,25] Although almost every patient who survives the acute stroke may benefit from one or more rehabilitative services, not everyone requires an intensive, comprehensive program. The very severely affected stroke patient (*e.g.,* comatose or nearly so) will not benefit from a comprehensive program, and the mildly affected will not require it.[4] Ultimately, it is the severity of the disability which is of prime importance in determining improvement potential in all age groups. Using an interdisciplinary approach, pertinent rehabilitation services such as physical therapy, occupational therapy, speech therapy, and others are selected to achieve feasible goals.

In determining which patient is likely to benefit from care in an intensive and comprehensive inpatient setting, the physician must consider medical stability, survival potential, ability to participate in a progressive activity program, state of cognition and awareness, degree of neurologic impairment, and functional capacity.

Alternative Rehabilitation Settings

If a specialized rehabilitation unit is not available within a general hospital, it may be desirable to transfer the patient to a regional rehabilitation center. Such centers aim to move the stroke patient from a low level of functioning to a higher level within a short period of time. Other settings with rehabilitation services, such as long-term care in a chronic disease hospital or nursing home, tend to provide services to maintain functioning and prevent deterioration. Skilled nursing facilities, which provide therapeutic services such as physical therapy, social services, and occasionally occupational therapy, provide less intensive services than those available in a hospital or regional center, but more than is available in a custodial care nursing home.

Day hospital programs and day care centers are two other sources of rehabilitative services. Day hospitals provide intensive multidisciplinary rehabilitation and physician supervision on an ambulatory basis. Patients frequently go 2 to 3 or even 5 days per week. Daily programs may include the usual rehabilitative services, plus lunch and socialization activities, and some provide transportation services. Day care programs are less medically oriented than day hospital programs. They may have no formal therapy or medical services but focus on socialization activities such as arts and crafts, discussions, and entertainment. A meal may be included, and clients may attend from 1 to 5 days per week. Transportation often is provided. Finally, stroke clubs are comprised of persons who have had a stroke and their family members. As is true of other types of peer groups, their principal purpose is to provide information and to serve as catalysts for resocialization.

Functional Assessment of the Stroke Patient

Many different systems have been used to measure functional abilities of the stroke patient. These range from scales that rate according to gross level of disability (*e.g.*, no significant disability to severe disability) to complex delineations of specific tasks or movements. The activities of daily living (ADL), which include feeding, bathing, dressing, toileting, transferring, and ambulation, are a part of most scales. Other factors to be considered include use of the affected hand, mentation, and dependence upon others.[19] Periodic reassessments can be useful to describe the patient at different stages of rehabilitation and maintenance, for example, at hospital admission, hospital discharge and followup, and in other settings. If each assessment is consistently recorded and filed for reference, the functional status of the patient in the past can be compared with his current status.

Functional assessment will be helpful to most primary care physicians in assessing the stroke patient's status following stabilization of medical problems and prior to starting a rehabilitation program. The patient's functional status should be assessed at the conclusion of the rehabilitation program and during the outpatient period of followup care. However, physicians who see many stroke patients may wish to implement a long-range evaluation system (LRES), as described by Granger.[16,18,28] The LRES is a computerized data collection system on each patient with a disability, such as is characteristic of patients who have survived a stroke.

Data are collected and entered into the computer by means of precoded worksheets. The worksheets are completed by several health team members, *e.g.*, physician, nurse, therapist, or other allied health worker. The worksheets are designed to identify basic demographic data (*i.e.,* name, address, birth date, sex, marital status, household members, etc.). Also incorporated are functional data items such as motion of limbs, self-care, mobility, verbal, hearing and visual abilities, intellectual and emotional adaptability, financial ability, educational or vocational ability, and family and community supports.

The worksheets are used to collect data on-stream as a regular part of information entered into the patient's chart during the hospital stay, in any other facility, or as an outpatient. The worksheets are arranged as a series of checklists with mutually exclusive categories with regard to independent or dependent functional performance for each individual assessed.[28]

The Barthel Index, a 100-point scale, was modified by Granger (see Appendix 9-1) to assess 15 ADL tasks, including self-care, sphincter control, and mobility. A Barthel Index score is derived by accumulating points for accomplishing specific tasks in personal care. For example, a person who feeds himself and drinks independently is credited with ten points. If he is limited in some way that requires prior preparation of food such as cutting meat, five points are credited. If he needs actual assistance to eat or requires another form of help, three points are credited. He is credited with ten points for all forms of independent bladder management, five points if assistance is needed, and no points if he is frequently wet. A person who is continent, feeds himself, dresses himself, gets out of bed and gets up from a chair, bathes himself, walks at least one block and ascends and descends a flight of stairs would receive a score of 100 on the Barthel Index. A Barthel score of 100 does not mean that the person is able to live alone. He may not be able to cook, keep house, or meet the public, but is able to get along without personal attendant care. A score better than 80, but less than 100, indicates that the person probably requires assistance getting in and out of a tub or shower, climbing stairs, or walking 50 yards. A score of between 60 and 80 suggests that, in addition to the limitations described previously, the individual is likely to need assistance with dressing, bathing, and transfers to the bed or toilet. Sixty is a pivotal score on the Barthel. Those who score above 60 are likely to require fewer than 2 hours of assistance with personal care per day, whereas those who score 60 or below are likely to require 4 or more hours of assistance daily.

Both the admission and discharge Barthel Index scores were found to be related to outcome in a study of 269 patients admitted to an acute stroke unit of a general hospital.[28] Certain assumptions based on this study about rehabilitation potential can be made. An unfavorable outcome, that is, little likelihood of returning to community living, is predicted for acutely hospitalized patients with admission scores of 20 or less. Patients whose admission scores range between 21 and 40 had a better chance for a favorable outcome, patients whose admission scores were in the 41 to 60 range were ideal candidates, and those whose admission scores were above 60 were not likely to need a comprehensive rehabilitation program.

Either the self-administered form of the Barthel Index or the form completed by the physician or an assistant after interviewing the patient or a knowledgeable family member is useful as a case management tool in outpatient practice. Under certain circumstances, the clinician may observe the activities performed by the patient directly. This information on the patient's level of performance and the corresponding amount of assistance the patient requires can help family members set reasonable expectations for themselves and the patient. As a patient's functional performance changes, the index acts as an indicator, for example, of possible family stress if the patient needs additional assistance with personal care activities. Conversely, the index may reveal the patient's improvement, suggesting that family members need not offer as much help as they may have been giving. In either case the index can aid family-oriented case management of the patient who has long-term or severe functional limitations.

Fortinsky and coworkers described another use of the Barthel Index in the outpatient setting.[11] These authors used a modified Barthel Index to obtain information regarding a person's ability to perform ADLs in the home setting. The information obtained was then used to screen for eligible recipients and to direct home-care services efficiently. Further, these authors found a relationship between Barthel scores and psychological states. Lower Barthel scores were correlated with lessened ability to make decisions easily and an increased amount of depression, disorientation, and conceptual disorganization.

The PULSES profile is another functional assessment scale (see Appendix 9-2) consisting of six components that assess independence in life functioning.[15] The acronym stands for:

P   Physical condition (basic health/illness status)
U   Upper limb functions: self-care activities (feeding, dressing, washing, toileting)
L   Lower limb functions: mobility activities (transferring to chair/toilet/ tub or shower, walking, climbing stairs, propelling wheelchair)
S   Sensory components: sight, communications (verbal/hearing)
E   Excretory functions: control of sphincters (bladder/bowel)
S   Situational factors: psychological/emotional, family, social, financial supports

In general, the Barthel and PULSES scales measure similar changes in functioning; however, the Barthel Index measures more discrete functions (such as eating and ambulation), whereas the PULSES profile includes communication and aspects of psychosocial and means of support.[15]

In addition to predicting outcome and assisting in discharge planning from the short-term rehabilitation unit or hospital, the Barthel Index is helpful in providing organized, consistent feedback regarding a stroke patient's continued functional recovery once discharged home or to a long-term care facility (LTCF). Such periodic assessments are important in that they (1) help the patient to realize that improvement is continuing and is a basis for encouraging the patient to continue to strive toward functional goals, (2) help physicians to reassess the patient's progress and make appropriate referrals, (3) aid physicians in obtaining pertinent information regarding need for further services and supports, and (4) demonstrate problem areas that seem unlikely to improve and therefore suggest adaptations in the environment, modifications of family roles, or vocational plans that need to be discussed.

In addition to the very valuable role of functional assessment in guiding the primary care physician in monitoring stroke patients is the use of instruments such as the Barthel Index and PULSES profile in aggregating information about stroke patient populations. The data obtained from such efforts are useful in research, program planning, evaluation, and as a basis for triaging patients to facilities that most appropriately serve their needs. Statistical analysis and evaluation of the rehabilitation process is made possible by tracking the functional status of patient populations at different stages in the process of care. Functional assessment during hospitalization can serve to predict functional outcome and assist in discharge planning. For example, Granger and colleagues[17] used the Barthel Index to predict favorable rehabilitation outcomes, specifically, the patient's return to community living.

Problems Resulting from Stroke

Hemiplegia or Hemiparesis

Literally the term "hemiplegia" suggests a devastating loss—all voluntary movement on one entire half of the body—a sort of functional bisection. Fortunately, a permanent, complete hemiplegia is seldom encountered clinically and most patients with this common impairment, once the acute phase has passed, are left with varying degrees of less extensive motor deficit. Thus hemiplegia is usually "hemiparesis" actually and presents one of the most obvious rehabilitative and long-term care challenges. A number of important problems are associated with rehabilitating patients with hemiparesis. They are discussed briefly.

Skin Integrity

Some of the more common causes of skin breakdown in the stroke patient include:[32]

1. Paralysis that limits movement, rendering the patient increasingly susceptible to skin breakdown because of sustained areas of pressure and reduced circulation. In addition, disuse causes muscle atrophy and lessened muscle bulk causing increased pressure over bony prominences. The patient's position should be changed on a schedule. He should be turned at least every 2 hours from the supine to the side-lying position. The length of time the patient is on the affected side should be limited. Vulnerable bony prominences such as the heel and elbow should be covered with protectors. The sacral region should be examined each time the patient is turned for incipient decubiti. A footboard helps to prevent footdrop and the development of decubitus ulcers on the heel and lateral malleolus—two very vulnerable areas.
2. Continual excessive contact with moisture also may cause breakdown of the skin. Skin macerations may occur in the stroke patient as a result of urine or fecal incontinence, excessive perspiration, or drainage from wounds. Keeping the patient's room at a comfortable temperature and

changing wet clothes and wound dressings as soon as possible are good prophylactic measures.

If ulcerations occur despite preventive measures, efforts should be directed toward promoting healing and preventing concomitant complications. Greasy or sticky dressings should be avoided since they macerate the skin. Instead a protective film of tincture of benzoin on light gauze can be applied. Wet to dry saline dressings can be used for superficial debridement. In more serious cases, surgical debridement may be necessary.

3. Dry, cracked, or peeling skin, which allows bacteria to enter, increases susceptibility to infection. Lubricating lotions should be used to prevent dryness and soften skin.

Bladder and Bowel Function

A patient suddenly immobilized and partly obtunded by a stroke is likely to experience urinary or fecal incontinence, fecal impaction, or constipation. Bowel and bladder problems may be due to physical, neurological, or mental impairments, psychological reactions to lack of privacy, use of bedpan, or concomitant medical condition. It is very important to evaluate the basis for incontinence for purposes of both treatment and prognosis. Except for those with severe confusion or bladder dysfunction, most stroke patients have early and complete return of bowel and bladder sphincter control, a blessing of bilateral innervation.

Bladder

Early urinary incontinence may be due more to inattention to the patient's needs than to an organic neurologic deficit. The prognosis for a patient with a single hemispheric lesion for return of normal function may be excellent since (1) the reflex arc remains intact, (2) partial sensation of bladder filling remains, and (3) the patient maintains partial voluntary control over voiding.

Not all incontinence problems can be attributed to the stroke. Medical conditions especially in the age group affected, such as prostatic hypertrophy or other urinary tract disorder, may coexist. Before establishing a bladder rehabilitation program, therefore, the practitioner must assess the patient's voiding patterns prior to the stroke.

For male patients who are incontinent, an external condom catheter is preferable to an indwelling one, but it may be difficult to keep in place. If the male patient is relatively immobile, keeping a urinal in place is simpler and more effective than an external condom catheter. Internal catheterization or frequent straight catheterization may be necessary initially for men with urinary tract obstruction or retention problems (*e.g.,* prostatic hypertrophy) and for most incontinent women. Since indwelling catheters almost always result in bacteriuria within the first 3 weeks, clean, intermittent straight catheterization every 4 to 6 hours is preferred. By keeping the residual urine low, the risks of bacterial infection and stone formation are reduced. A bladder retraining program should be initiated as soon as the patient is alert. The purpose of the program is to establish a regular voiding pattern in order to avoid the need for an indwelling catheter and to protect against urinary retention or infection.

As soon as possible, a program of timed voiding should be initiated. Frequently this is all that is necessary to prevent incontinence. Usually every 2 to 4 hours the patient is provided with a bedpan, commode, or toilet privileges. Even patients unaware of a need to void can be maintained on a time patterned program without resorting to the use of indwelling catheters.[36] Several maneuvers can be tried with patients who have difficulty urinating due to neurogenic bladder dysfunction. Tapping the suprapubic area, stroking the medial thigh, or digital dilatation of the anus may help these patients. An anticholinergic drug may be beneficial in controlling the hyperactive neurogenic bladder.

Normal bladder control is frequently regained within 5 days, especially if the patient is able to use a bedside commode or toilet. The likelihood of success is guarded if more than 6 weeks of bladder retraining is required. Complicating disorders such as prostatic hypertrophy or infection must be treated before a bladder retraining program can be successful.[6]

Initial incontinence of the "dribbling, overflow" type may be experienced due to a flaccid, distended bladder. In the obtunded patient large amounts of urine may be retained without sensation, causing the patient to void in only small amounts. As mentioned previously, the resultant constant residual urine encourages infection and stone formation. Patients with a hemispheric stroke may experience frequency, urgency, and incontinence resulting from an inability to postpone the sense of urgency willfully. Bilateral lesions resulting from a brain stem stroke result in "a loss of all facilitation and inhibition of the micturition reflex."[36]

Bowel

Bowel incontinence also may occur after a stroke. Since peristalsis and fecal buildup continue automatically, the stroke patient who is unable to control the defecation urge or reflex may experience fecal incontinence. Most hemiplegic patients regain lost bowel control within a few days following the onset of stroke, especially once they are able to use a bedside commode or toilet. Failure to regain bowel continence within 3 to 4 weeks after a stroke generally indicates bilateral cortical injury or brain stem dysfunction.[36] As is true of bladder incontinence, bowel incontinence may be due to other medical conditions such as lower bowel and rectal abnormalities or diabetic neuropathy. Diarrhea precipitated by tube feedings, drugs, or fecal impaction may cause problems also.[32]

A major bowel problem for stroke patients is constipation associated with immobility, limited fluid intake, certain pharmaceuticals, and a weakened defecation reflex. Elimination can be helped by establishing effective intervals for offering the bedpan, commode, or toilet, supplemented with stool softeners and suppositories. Adequate fluid intake and diet sufficient in bulk and roughage is important. Foods and fluids which stimulate bowel activity (*e.g.,* prune juice, hot liquids, stewed fruit) should be encouraged. Enemas and harsh laxatives should be used only as a last resort. The most effective programs are those planned around the first meal, since defecation urges are strongest for about 10 minutes after that meal.[32] A bowel training program may include a stool softener given daily or every other day, prune juice or hot coffee in the morning, then a glycerin suppository and placement on a commode after breakfast. Defecation can also be stimulated by digital rectal stimulation. Because squatting rather than a supine position facilitates evacuation, bedpans should be avoided if possible. Periodic rectal examinations to identify and remove fecal impactions should also be a part of the rehabilitation routine.

Programs of bowel retraining like programs of bladder retraining must be individualized. The physician should have accurate information about the patient's elimination habits prior to the stroke. If he previously had bowel movements only every 2 to 3 days, caretakers should not be alarmed if the patient does not evacuate daily. The goal in bowel retraining is to return bowel habits to the situation that prevailed before the stroke.

Motor Function

Various forms of motor dysfunction may characterize the stroke patient, including incoordination, dyspraxia, and dystonia. The more common and important forms of motor dysfunction, however, are weakness (or paralysis) and muscle spasticity.

Weakness requires a careful and accurate evaluation of residual voluntary muscle contractility according to the muscle strength testing discussed under "examination" in Chapter 3. Evidence of residual active muscle function within 3 weeks of onset of the stroke indicates a good prognosis for functional restoration. This is particularly true of the distal segments of the limbs such as the hand and the ankle, since recovery usually proceeds from proximal to distal. Generally about half of the neurologic recovery destined to return is apparent at 3 months, and almost all is apparent at 6 months after onset. Physical and occupational therapy modalities are employed to re-educate lost or weak movements. There are numerous techniques for doing this, some of which employ neuromuscular facilitation methods and others of which use bracing and splinting. An important determinant for successful re-education of a weak or paralyzed muscle is the patient's proprioception and awareness of the position of the limb in space.

It is generally more cost-effective to incorporate re-education of specific muscles into retraining functionally useful movements, such as are required for feeding, grooming, dressing, and mobility, in order that the patient progress toward independence in personal care and independent living skills.

An important intermediate goal is permitting the patient to be independent or to be only minimally dependent in transferring to and from a toilet seat. This simple ability may make the difference between the patient's being successfully discharged or not. As many as 80% to 90% of patients able to benefit from an intensive rehabilitation program may be expected eventually to regain the ability to walk, even if some assistance from another person is required, or the use of a short leg brace or a walking aid such as a cane or walker is necessary. There are different types of short leg braces, and a physiatrist ought to be consulted as to the appropriate type for a given patient.

Spasticity is usually reciprocal with weakness: The more voluntary control the patient has the less likely spasticity will be a problem. Spasticity is involuntary and is due to a hyperactive reflex response so that muscles are actively contracting without being willed to do so. Spasticity is considered undesirable usually because it interferes with the patient's efforts to utilize modest voluntary ability; it may be associated with painfully stiff joints and it may predispose the patient to contractures that limit functional use. Such contractures commonly shorten the heel cord and thus limit standing and walking. They adduct the thigh so that scissoring either blocks walking or makes it precarious. Furthermore, contractures adduct the humerus, contributing to stiffness and pain in the shoulder, or they flex the wrist and fingers, rendering the hand awkward or useless. Spasticity is not always dysfunctional, however; it may help stabilize the knee for weight-bearing. Spasticity and its effects on the functions of the patient should be monitored constantly throughout the patient's life, as long as there is significant weakness, to assure that it does not insidiously rob the patient of some important function. The first maneuvers to control spasticity are passive range of motion and judicious stretching. In some cases cool applications over the affected muscle will facilitate the stretching. In other cases pharmacologic management is indicated using either diazepam, baclofen, or dantrolene sodium, usually in small doses or in combination.

Left-sided Brain Damage

Although the most obvious sign of cerebral damage is motor paralysis or sensory loss of the opposite side of the body, the stroke patient may experience other disturbing functional deficits. Right hemiparetics with left-sided brain damage behave differently from left hemiparetics with right-sided brain damage. Patients with left-sided brain damage frequently experience problems with language and speech. Patients with right-sided brain damage tend toward quickness and impulsiveness and may attempt to do things in an unsafe manner.[13] Caregivers should be cautioned that right hemiparetics may be interpreted erroneously as lacking intelligence, which can be psychologically devastating to the patient. Left hemiparetics may over-represent their capabilities verbally and should be carefully watched until the caregiver is sure of safe performance.

Communication Disorders

The right hemiparetic is likely to have a severely impaired ability to communicate. Cerebral dominance is related to "handedness." The higher nervous pathways for speech are located usually in the left hemisphere of the brain for righthanded persons, who account for 93% of the population; of the remaining 7% who are lefthanded, three fifths have speech centers in the left hemispheres and two fifths have them in the right hemisphere.[32] Inability to communicate is one of the most frustrating consequences of a stroke for many patients and their families. Communication may be affected by a language disorder, impairment of speech, or both. Inability to comprehend language or to interact verbally with others can be frightening and anger-provoking and may hinder some of the rehabilitative treatment approaches required for other manifestations of the stroke. In addition, because of the importance that society places on the ability to communicate verbally, a disability in either of these areas may be erroneously interpreted as lack of intelligence, which, as mentioned above, can be psychologically devastating to the affected individual.

Aphasia and *dysarthria* are the two primary speech disorders resulting from a stroke, and although frequently they occur concurrently, each has its distinct neuropathological mechanisms, symptoms, and management techniques.[27]

Aphasia

Aphasia is a general impairment of language function associated with localized cerebral pathology that is manifested by a reduced capacity for interpretation and formulation of symbols of communication. Aphasia is characterized by any one or a combination of the following impairments:

- Understanding
- Memory, sounds, or word finding
- Reading, spelling, or writing
- Gesturing
- Problem-solving ability
- Expression of thoughts using conventional sentence structure in a grammatical manner

Aphasia can result from strokes, head trauma, or any event causing oxygen deprivation to the brain that is not attributable to mental deterioration, confusion, memory loss, impaired senses or paralysis, although any of these deficits may be present concurrently.[36]

There are many terms that qualify aphasia and some are used inter-changeably. They may classify the disorder in terms either of the location of the cerebral insult that precipitated it or of the functional impairment that results. Localization of the lesion and identification of the underlying pathological and etiological conditions are essential to the physician who is responsible for establishing a diagnosis in instituting an appropriate plan of treatment for the patient with aphasia.[32]

One of the most universal descriptions of aphasia is *fluency.* In general, aphasia can be categorized as fluent, nonfluent, or global.

Fluent Aphasia The speech of patients with various forms of fluent aphasia is well articulated and involves normal intonational patterns. Although the patient is able to speak in long, grammatical sentences or phrases, the sentences convey little meaning.

The most common of the fluent aphasias, *Wernicke's aphasia,* also known as receptive or sensory aphasia, is usually the result of a lesion in the posterior part of the left superior temporal gyrus. Known as Wernicke's area, it is a storehouse for auditory association. Persons suffering from Wernicke's aphasia have impaired auditory comprehension and inability to monitor their own speech. They do not, however, have a hearing impairment.

Patients with Wernicke's aphasia produce words at a rate similar to or more rapid than that of normal speech. In fact, these patients often speak voluminously—seemingly unable to stop in spite of the many errors made in the use of words. Patients with Wernicke's aphasia transmit little information, and their speech frequently contains extraneous words and incorrect word substitutions. These incorrect words are called paraphasias and may be of three types: literal, verbal, and neologistic. O'Brien and Pallet[32] describe the differences: Literal paraphasias involve the insertion of incorrect sounds or syllables into words that would otherwise be correct. For example, "hence" may be substituted for "bench." Or completely unintelligible words are produced, such as "toofuf" for "toothbrush." Verbal paraphasia is the substitution of one word for another. For example, "chair" may be substituted for "bed." Although the substituted words may be related in some way, they are not necessarily related. Neologistic paraphasias are nonsensical substitutions, such as "ferbish" for "toothbrush."

Patients with Wernicke's aphasia are able neither to comprehend the examiner's words nor to repeat them.[32] Also, they may have difficulty naming objects. Since patients' written language is characterized by the same lack of content as spoken language, they cannot express their needs in writing. Because their auditory feedback system is damaged, patients with Wernicke's aphasia usually are not aware of their mistakes and therefore may be less disturbed than other aphasics by their disabilities. They appear to be at times even euphoric. If they express anger, it is usually aimed at others for not being able to understand them.

Anomic aphasia, another form of fluent aphasia, is associated with lesions in the area of the angular gyrus, located near the Wernicke's area, although localization of the lesion is not reliable. The person with anomic aphasia has fluent and rhythmic speech. The paraphasias typical of Wernicke's aphasia are not present. The essential finding with anomic aphasia is a problem recalling words, especially the names of objects and places. Frequently the individual uses circumlocution in place of the name he cannot recall. Since these patients have good auditory comprehension, they are aware of their errors and may become frustrated.

Conduction aphasia, a third type of fluent aphasia, is attributed to lesions in the arcuate fasciculus, which connects Broca's and Wernicke's areas. The damage is at the site of conduction, although language is properly interpreted at Wernicke's area. Comprehension and fluency are spared, but repetition and naming are difficult, even if the patient understands the words completely. The patient with conduction aphasia may produce many words, but little of his speech will be meaningful. Errors involving syntax and nonsense syllables may occur. Such patients cannot relate the sound of a word with the letters that form it. Although conductive aphasics cannot write from dictation, they can copy written words. Many patients with conductive aphasia cannot initiate speech themselves or repeat words spoken to them, although they are alert and able to comprehend everything they see and hear. They also have problems reading aloud.

Nonfluent Aphasia Also known as motor or expressive aphasia, *Broca's aphasia* is the most common of the nonfluent aphasias. It results from a lesion in the third frontal gyrus of the cerebral cortex, the portion of the brain located proximal to the motor association area that controls movement of the lips, jaw, tongue, soft palate, and vocal cords.[27] Broca's area apparently coordinates the muscles used to produce speech. Patients with Broca's aphasia have a disturbance in the ability to select, organize, and initiate the action of these muscles. The deficit may range from slight difficulty with articulation to complete inability to express spoken words.[32] Articulation for these patients requires tremendous effort and is often slow. Phrase length decreases to one or two words, and the patient usually speaks haltingly. In severe cases, patients may repeat a few words over and over, even though they are aware that the words are incorrect. Since Broca's aphasics may omit small words required for grammatically correct sentences and the ends of nouns and verbs, their speech is often referred to as "telegraphic speech." Patients with Broca's aphasia comprehend language normally. Although they usually understand what is being said by others, and they know what they want to say, they are unable to express themselves. They may be frustrated by their errors in speech, and for this reason may hesitate to speak.[27]

Global Aphasia The third type of aphasia results from a massive lesion in the left hemisphere affecting several language areas. Global aphasia is a combination of both Broca's (inability to transform sounds into words) and Wernicke's (impaired comprehension) aphasias. In severe cases the patient may not be able to communicate at all. Global aphasia usually occurs concomitantly with a severe hemiplegia.

> The patient with global aphasia has been likened to a visitor in a foreign land who does not recognize the local alphabet, cannot read or comprehend a single word he sees or hears, and although rational, able to retain the sum of his experiences, and in full possession of sound judgment, remains absolutely cut off from all communication with the world around him.[32]

Other Language Impairments

Dysarthria is a disorder of the motor component of verbal articulation caused by lesions in the cerebral hemispheres, basal ganglia, cerebellum, brainstem, or cranial nerves.[36] It is characterized by slowness, weakness, paralysis, incoordination or reduction in range of motion of the tongue, lips, jaw, and soft palate, resulting in slurred speech.

Not all language impairment is due to lesions in the specific language areas in the left hemisphere. Patients with right hemispheric lesions may have impairments of language (especially reading) due to visual–spatial and visual–motor deficits. A generalized reduction in cognitive function may affect language as well.

Functional Assessment of Speech Disorders

The primary care physician can make a simple bedside assessment of a speech disorder by noting the patient's spontaneous speech. Using a chart such as Table 3-7 (Chap. 3) as a guide, fluency concomitant with poor comprehension should alert the physician to the likelihood of Wernicke's aphasia. Nonfluency in the presence of good comprehension is suggestive of Broca's aphasia. Speech that appears less than normally intelligible, accompanied by oral–facial weakness in the presence of normal comprehension, suggests dysarthria.

More specific bedside evaluations, as discussed by Louis and Povse,[27] should cover the following areas:

1. Ability to comprehend spoken language—The patient should be asked a number of increasingly complex questions that require yes or no responses. The examiner then notes whether the patient answers the questions appropriately. If the patient is unable to speak, the examiner notes whether he responds correctly nonverbally (*e.g.,* nodding the head). Alternatively, the patient may be given simple one-step commands, such as "pick up the glass." If the patient responds appropriately, two- and three-step commands can be given to assess the level of functioning. The examiner must be careful to avoid giving clues or gesturing while giving directions.
2. Ability to speak—The patient should be assessed for production of any spontaneous speech. The examiner listens to hear if the speech is hesitant or telegraphic (indicative of Broca's) or fluent, or else melodic but lacking content (Wernicke's). Frequently the aphasic patient has a mixture of these two problems. If the patient fails to speak spontaneously, encouraging speech by asking openended questions such as, "Tell me about your family," should be attempted.
3. Ability to repeat spoken language—The patient should be instructed to repeat a sentence after the examiner says it. Initially the examiner speaks in short phrases or sentences, gradually advancing to longer ones.
4. Ability to comprehend written language—The patient should be given a series of simple commands printed in large handwriting and askcd to follow the written directions. Subsequently, two- and three-step commands can be given.
5. Ability to write—The patient should be asked to write his name or a short sentence. The physician should keep in mind in evaluating this ability that a paresis in the upper extremity may cause difficulty with writing.
6. Ability to name objects—The patient should be shown a series of pictures and commonly known objects and asked to name them. It is preferable to use pictures depicting only a few items to avoid confusing the patient. This test may identify even slight degrees of dysphasia.[32]

Although the physician can perform preliminary assessments at bedside to help pinpoint the anatomical area of deficit to determine residual function, referral to a speech–language pathologist is recommended. Speech pathologists have the knowledge and skills to determine the current level of mental status, language functioning, and perceptual and speech musculature deficits and can therefore provide assistance in diagnosis and prognosis. They also administer and evaluate standardized tests, such as the Wechsler Adult Intelligence Scales, the Minnesota Test for Differential Diagnosis of Aphasia, or the Boston Diagnostic Aphasia Examination, and interpret test results to the stroke rehabilitation team and family members. In addition to their evaluative abilities, they are also skilled in developing appropriate retraining programs and suggesting alternative communication modes.

Since only 20% to 30% of patients with severe aphasia recover completely, the realistic aim of speech and language rehabilitation is to help the patient communicate as effectively as possible within the limits imposed by motivation and brain damage. Therefore, the speech–language pathologist's approach may be to maintain or improve the patient's present language and auditory comprehension skills. If functional communication is not attainable, the speech–language pathologist may provide alternative communication modes. In either case, the family must be helped to understand and cope with the language deficit and its associated problems. Rehabilitation of the aphasic adult involves several different areas of intervention, including medical treatment, physical and occupational therapies, and psychological counseling.

Although the greatest amount of speech recovery occurs during the first 3 months poststroke, many patients continue to improve steadily for many more months. It is not unusual for improvement to continue at a very high level for 2 or more years after the onset of aphasia;[32] indeed, language recovery commonly extends over a longer period than physical recovery. For this reason, treatment should be planned over months and years rather than days and weeks. Younger patients usually recover to a greater degree than older patients. Global aphasics have a much poorer prognosis than other types of aphasics. The patient's premorbid level of intelligence, educational background, and personality traits, as well as general health and the site and extent of the lesion, all affect the prognosis. The patient's reaction to the illness and motivation to overcome the resultant disabilities affect language production and comprehension in important ways.[29,32] Language function can be very sensitive to fatigue or emotional upset.

> After a long day in therapy, or after an emotionally upsetting visit with family or friends, the patient may demonstrate a marked reduction in his or her ability to communicate.[27]

Speech pathology is the discipline best prepared to provide language retraining. However, the physician, the rehabilitation team, and the family can reinforce the learning process, assist the patient in achieving successful communication, and help reduce the patient's frustrations by applying some of the basic approaches used in speech therapy.

There are two main approaches to speech therapy for the patient with aphasia. The *programmed operant approach,* which concentrates on basic structural patterns of language, is based on the assumption that aphasia is a loss of language. The therapist employing this approach attempts to alter the patient's level of functioning by re-education using a stimulus–response approach. The view of aphasia as an interference and disorganization of language is the basis of the *stimulation–facilitation approach.* This model focuses on goal-directed stimulation related to the patient's needs and motivation and works optimally through repetitive sensory stimulation using real-life situations. The stimulation–facilitation approach does not employ re-education to convey new learning or a new vocabulary.[20,29]

Another approach that is gaining popularity is the *deblocking method* of Weigl.[21] The aim of this method is to evoke a language task that the patient is not performing by using a related task that the patient can still perform as a facilitative stimulus. Language rehabilitation therapy usually begins with the patient's repeating words, phrases, and sentences in unison with the therapist and writing from dictation. This approach's rationale is that it provides auditory stimulation, elicits feedback responses, and increases the patient's retention span. Complexity of material is increased as the patient progresses.[36] Automatic–reactive speech, including counting, reciting over-learned passages, and singing can be elicited early, even in severely affected patients, and may convince the patient that some speech is possible—thus encouraging feedback.[29] Since auditory processes are frequently impaired in aphasia, auditory stimuli in conjunction with visual stimuli may be helpful in improving language processing. Whatever the approach, the therapy must be individualized and based on a particular patient's situation and remaining capabilities.

Speech–language pathologists use a variety of techniques with aphasics. To increase attention span, stimulation is provided with a number of short words or phrases and progresses to longer words and sentences. Reading skills are exercised through the use of current newspapers and magazines or flash cards and pictures. Specific deficits also are treated. For the patient with dysarthria, exercises are taught including tongue protrusion, lateral rotation and elevation, whistling, blowing, and lip pursing. For patients with anomic aphasia, whose recall of even common objects is impaired, a therapist "shows a picture of an object to the patient, writes the word on a blackboard, pronounces it, and has the patient write and practice pronouncing it several times. The series of pictures is expanded to increase the number of words in the patient's vocabulary."[32] Patients with dysarthric speech or a tendency to produce paraphasias are helped by using a tape recorder to identify speech errors.

Although individual, clinician–patient therapy is the usual format for speech therapy, group therapy may be an important supplement. Participation in a group made up of people with communication problems alleviates feelings of isolation, provides an accepting environment, and enables patients to observe progress made by others.[29]

The primary care physician can play a pivotal role in reinforcing with families some of the concepts promoted by the speech–language pathologists. Some well-meaning families may try to force the aphasic patient to complete page after page of assignments in a published workbook. The patient may refuse to do the assignments because they are too boring or insufficiently challenging, or because they are too difficult and frustrating. Some patients may complete the assignments but fail to learn from them because they were merely copying rather than learning.[29]

During early stages of stroke recovery families should be encouraged to visit frequently with the patient, even if the patient seems unable to follow their conversation or does not acknowledge their presence.

Because a person cannot speak and be understood, or listen and understand does not mean that he is unable to communicate nor does this mean he cannot understand considerable language.[13]

Physicians must remember when working with the speech or language impaired hemiparetic patient that expressive difficulties do not always imply receptive ones.[18] On the other hand, physicians and family members must avoid overestimating an aphasic patient's understanding of speech because by doing so they can cause frustration, disappointment, and confusion. Overestimation may cause those working with the patient to label him as uncooperative, senile, or irrational if the therapist, physician, or family member believes the patient understands what is being said but acts as though he does not.

Some general guidelines for facilitating speech in the aphasic individual follow. The aphasic should always be addressed as an adult, and condescension should be avoided. All materials used should be geared toward an adult's interests. Family members should refrain from speaking too loudly or using a special childish voice. Language retraining of an adult stroke patient is not the same as teaching language to a child. Also comprehension difficulties may be exacerbated by poor attention span. It is therefore important to minimize visual and auditory distractions. Only one person should speak to the patient at a time and speech should be slow, allowing ample time for the patient to respond. Topics should be discussed in single words or short phrases, and words symbolizing concrete ideas should be used whenever possible. Nouns should be concentrated on first in language recovery, and verbs should be next; prepositions should be avoided if the individual has difficulty with them. Recall can be enhanced by repeating missing words, by suggesting that the person think of alternative words or phrases, or by asking the patient to fill in the word in a sentence that facilitates the association. It is preferable to stimulate spontaneous communication by discussing topics that are interesting and meaningful to the patient. A speech–language pathologist should be consulted for particular techniques to be used in facilitating speech.

> Many aphasic patients quickly develop effective communication without use of speech. They may develop an effective language by supplementing pantomine with gestures, groans, swear words or nonsense sounds.[12]

Sometimes the patient will substitute unusual words to express himself. Physicians and families must respond to the patient's language as it is; constant attempts to correct the patient or to insist that he use a language system that is confusing to the patient discourages attempts to communicate. As the patient improves, auditory feedback increases and he will be able to monitor his own speech, and many even indicate a desire for help in correcting errors. Initially techniques should be employed to increase auditory stimulation and communication. Pictures and objects familiar to a patient can be mounted on cards in a looseleaf binder that can be kept at the bedside. As the patient's language abilities increase, efforts should be made to encourage conversation, including asking the patient to talk about his family or describe a hospital routine.[27]

The speech–language pathologist and the physician can assist the patient and the family by constructive counseling efforts. It is important not only to provide factual information about aphasia, but to discuss its impact on their lives. The loss of functional communication can be psychologically overwhelming. Often the aphasic patient is dependent on others, unable to communicate needs or wants, or to comprehend what has happened or is occurring in the environment. Inability to express frustration or fear verbally may result in aggressive behaviors. Behavior may be inconsistent due to loss of ability to think in abstract terms or to evaluate situations as a whole. Memory may be affected and responses to stimuli may be delayed. Patients whose deficits are expressive only may be aware of their problems and concerned about improving behavior; those with receptive deficits may be less cognizant of their problems and more likely to exhibit unacceptable behavior in social situations.

A structured routine and secure environment is needed for patients with global aphasia. Since potential for language rehabilitation of these patients is almost nil, not every family will decide to take such a patient home and to deal with the complexity of problems that will ensue. Families that do attempt to care for a globally aphasic patient at home will need a great deal of support and encouragement. It is important for both physicians and family members to remember that most patients, whether severely aphasic or not, are aware of nonverbal positive and negative communication among hospital staff and relatives. Expressions of annoyance or impatience with aphasic patients are inappropriate.

Although the speech–language pathologist has the specialized skills to assist the patient with aphasia, the entire rehabilitation team, attending physician, and family can play important roles by providing opportunities for repetition and stimulation.

Right-Sided Brain Damage:

Patients with right-sided brain damage frequently have left-sided paralysis. As severe a deficit as paralysis is, damage to the nondominant parietal lobe, which is associated with one or more visual–spatial dysfunctions such as homonymous hemianopia, agnosia, or constructional apraxia, is also significant. Visual–spatial problems result in difficulty with perceptual tasks such as judging size, distance, rate of movement, position, form, and relationship of parts to the whole.[13] Intellectual functions such as a critical imagination and intuition also may be compromised. These deficits may present problems with activities such as dressing, because the patient is unable to distinguish top from bottom or may put on clothes inside-out. The patient with visual–spatial problems may have difficulty reading and writing. Letters and words involve shapes and designs. Such a patient may have difficulty following a straight line and may be unable to keep place reading a page of print. He may try to get through a doorway too narrow for the wheelchair or may walk or move toward the path of moving objects. Driving a car may become too complicated to manage safely.[13]

Homonymous hemianopia, the occlusion of the visual pathway posterior to the optic chiasm resulting in the loss of vision in the temporal field of one eye and the nasal field of the other eye, may occur in stroke patients with either right or left brain damage. Persons with right cerebral damage are more likely to have problems with visual field deficits and one-sided neglect (anosognosia).[12]

Unilateral neglect involves inability to integrate perception from the left side of the body or environment. The person may look at the involved arm while in bed and become angry "because someone else is in bed with him"[13] or may "neglect food on the left side of the tray, fail to shave the left side of the face, or not comb the hair on both sides of his head." He may slump to the left side of the chair or let the left arm dangle over the side of the chair near the spokes of the wheel, may fail to see others approaching from the left side, fail to read words from their beginning, and may mistake "men" for "women" in reading a sign to a public toilet.

The confrontation test is used to test a patient with unilateral neglect.[26]

When each field is tested separately, the patient with hemianopia will not see a finger or object as it is brought into view on the affected side, whereas the patient with unilateral neglect will. If the examiner simultaneously presents fingers or objects into both visual fields, however, the patient with visual neglect will not see the one presented from the left side, due to a phenomenon called extinction. Extinction to a touch stimulus can also be demonstrated if the examiner touches the patient's right and left limbs simultaneously.[26] During the acute phase of stroke, the reduced attention span and limited ability to communicate and cooperate may confuse the results. The visual fields therefore should be assessed more than once during acute and rehabilitative phases of treatment. Patients may have compounded deficits; left hemiparetics may have both homonymous hemianopia and spatial–perceptual deficits.

If visual–spatial dysfunctions are recognized early, measures can be taken to enhance functional recovery. Patients can be taught to encompass the right and left fields of vision by a technique known as "scanning." The patient is instructed to turn his head toward the side of the deficit and scan the area by sweeping the eyes horizontally and vertically. Visual scanning exercises can be carried out by using an $11\frac{1}{2}'' \times 8''$ magnetic alphabet board such as is found in most toy stores.

> Initially half the letters or numbers are placed within the patient's visual field and half on his hemianopic side. The patient is instructed to read the numbers and letters, beginning with those in his field of vision. He then turns his head to the hemianopic side to read the remaining letters. As he accomplishes this task, the letters on his hemianopic side are increased, expanding his visual field and reinforcing the scanning process.[23]

Since the verbal abilities of stroke patients with right brain damage are intact, frequent verbal cues and feedback for orientation can assist them as they attempt new tasks and as they complete each step. Patients should be reminded without nagging that they may have to be conscious of the neglected side since response on that side is no longer automatic. The patient with unilateral neglect may be helped to perform certain activities if some modifications are made in the environment. Rooms should be well lighted, simply decorated, and uncluttered to reduce distraction.

Other Rehabilitation Management Issues:

Sexual Functioning

Numerous physical impairments and organic disorders can affect sexuality, including damage to nervous system controls over the sexual response (arousal, orgasm), circulatory disorders, liver and kidney disease, pain, weakness, loss of stamina, and the side-effects of medication. Although physical disability "may necessitate a drastic change in sex technique, it need not preclude all options for sexual desire. . . ."[38]

The ability to function sexually has not been sufficiently researched. Although several articles have suggested that sexual activity or desire decreases after stroke, only the frequency of coitus has been assessed. Little attention has been paid to attitudinal or physiological factors related to the sexual activity of the recovering stroke patient.

One study of sexual functioning after stroke revealed that although the majority of survivors maintained their premorbid levels of sexual desire, most experienced sexual dysfunction including problems with erection, ejaculation, vaginal lubrication, amenorrhea, and reduced sensitivity.[4] Another study with similar results reported that although the degree of motor deficit did not change the frequency of sexual intercourse, impaired sensibility for touch reduced the frequency or caused the cessation of intercourse.[14]

Direct effects on sexual arousal of damage to different parts of the brain are still being investigated. There have been studies describing reduced libido and erectile ability in patients with temporal lobe and limbic tract lesions. Organic impairment of the brain also may affect levels of hormones involved in sexual arousal. Concurrent systemic disorders, such as diabetes mellitus, may affect libido and orgasmic response.[14] Nevertheless, there seems to be consensus that although physiological factors may account for the decline in sexual activity, other factors must also be considered if a patient experiences sexual dysfunction.

Thorton-Gray and Kern[38] discuss several issues associated with sexual dysfunction in both healthy and physically disabled persons. First they suggest that some health practitioners promote the notion that the physically disabled are physiologically unable to experience sexual response. Patients with hemiplegia, those who require indwelling catheters, or those who use wheelchairs may be discouraged from attempting sexual activity for unjustified reasons. Many practitioners mistakenly believe that if a patient is unable to achieve or maintain genital arousal and orgasm, he will have not sexual desire. This is rarely true. Physicians may reinforce the idea, already in the minds of their patients, that sexual activity will exacerbate an already established physical problem. Rather, sexual activity, as with other forms of physical activity, is to be encouraged as a means of giving pleasure, reducing stress, and strengthening muscles.

> Thus, the physically disabled patient has both the right to want to remain a sexual being and the physiological potential to express his or her sexuality behaviorally. Health practitioners can be among the first to help patients assert such rights or they can squelch this powerful source of gratification through active disapproval or through passive unwillingness to discuss sexual matters openly with patients.[38]

Lack of adequate information and unrealistic expectations about sexual performance related specifically to giving and receiving pleasure cause problems whether or not a person has had a stroke. Sometimes it is necessary to give patients accurate information to dispel their anxiety and disappointment. They may need to be assured that some of the problems they are experiencing, such as increased time to attain an erection, are normal physiological changes associated with aging rather than consequences of the stroke. Also patients should be aware that a variety of factors may affect their ability to function sexually. Physical fatigue or medications and drugs (*e.g.,* alcohol, CNS depressants and stimulants, narcotics, antihistamines, antidepressants, and antipsychotics) may influence sexual performance. Physical impairments such as hemiparesis or quadriplegia, cardiac and pulmonary conditions, and chronic pain may also change sexual performance. Age may cause diminished intensity of responses, but does not alone preclude sexual activity.

Problems in a couple's relationship may have predated the stroke. Newly acquired physical disability may be used as an excuse to avoid a partner who was unattractive prior to onset of the stroke. Thus, sexual dysfunction may reflect an unsuccessful coping process unrelated to the stroke.

Psychological factors can play a role. Anxiety, loss of self-esteem, conflict, anxiety, and depression, which are frequent sequelae of stroke, can affect a person's sexual self-image. An individual's basic feelings about sexuality (rightness/wrongness, pleasantness/unpleasantness, feelings about less familiar positions and methods of arousal, sexual preference, previous sexual experiences) may affect the ability and desire to adapt after the stroke.

Rehabilitation programs should address the sexual concerns of poststroke patients. To be effective the physician must obtain an accurate history to ascertain whether the patient was sexually dysfunctional premorbidly and his ability to cope with stress prior to disability. A thorough sexual history should enable the physician to assess (1) the individual's level of sexual knowledge regarding anatomy and physiological responses during the sexual experience, (2) the patient's previous sexual preferences, and (3) the patient's current attitudes toward acceptability of various sexual feelings and behaviors.

The physician can play a pivotal role by providing information and making specific suggestions, thus facilitating communication between partners. The physician can help also by giving permission through verbal and nonverbal cues that it is "OK" to want to continue to be sexual after disability, to ask questions about sex, and to learn about alternative means for sexual expression.[38] Practitioners can facilitate communication by setting up an atmosphere in which stroke patients feel that the physician regards their questions and problems as important and has the knowledge and skills to help them. Patients may not initiate questions about sexual matters, so it is important for the physician to provide subtle cues suggesting that it is acceptable to discuss sexual concerns. Nonetheless, some patients will be uncomfortable discussing sexual issues. When dealing with stroke patients, specific suggestions may include variations in sexual positions and alternative methods for sexual stimulation. Patients with catheters or patients who are incontinent may need instructions regarding preparation that should be made before attempting sexual intercourse. In some situations the patient may need to change from being the partner initiating sex to being somewhat passive. The physician should point out that sexual expression is not necessarily limited to coitus, but may include verbal, visual, tactile, and other forms of communication to express love and intimacy. It is important for the physician to discuss the patient's reactions to the need for significant change of sexual expression, and it is imperative that both partners be present to discuss these alternatives.

Sometimes permission for the disabled patient to be sexual, provision of adequate information, and suggestions for alternatives to traditional sexual expression may be all that is needed to alleviate sexual problems. If all of these approaches fail, referrals to specialists may be helpful. Physicians must be aware of the need to make appropriate referrals to a gynecologist, urologist, or sex therapist when disorders affecting arousal, orgasm, ejaculation, insufficient vaginal lubrication, or painful intercourse are reported. Since the origins of sexual dysfunction are frequently both physical and psychological, the practitioner working with stroke patients must be aware of both contributory possibilities.

Social Functioning

Functional recovery of stroke patients in terms of their muscle strength, mobility, and activities of daily living are well documented in the literature. The likelihood of resuming a premorbid level of social activities following stroke has received less attention. In the broad spectrum of rehabilitation, attention must be paid not only to maximum restoration of physical skills but to restoration of normal prestroke levels of social functioning. Research suggests that the attainment of physical independence is not necessarily correlated with participation in social activities.[7] According to several studies, social reintegration of stroke victims is the most difficult phase of rehabilitation.[24]

In a study of patients 6 months after onset of stroke, only 37% maintained two thirds or more of their previous activities; approximately 36% lost or reduced between one third to two thirds of their premorbid activities, and the remaining 27% lost or reduced more than two thirds of their previous activities. Activities assessed in this study included work or homemaking, hobbies or sports, pastimes, community activities, and socializing with family and friends. There was a significant correlation between depressed patients (those who described a loss of purpose, frequent crying, and trouble accepting illness) and the percentage of lost activities compared with premorbid activities.

It is not clear what causes the depression and poor psychological adaptation of stroke patients. Suggested reasons include reduced activities, loneliness, perceived loss of health, low self-esteem, and loss of transportation.[7] Labi and colleagues[24] found that women and those with more education had a more difficult time than men and the less educated in resuming activities. They proposed that this was probably due to a damaged sense of body image and fear of stigmatization. The temporary or permanent losses related to changes in functional capacity such as strength, appearance, control over body functions, mobility, cognitive abilities, and sensory acuity may attack the individual's sense of autonomy, body integrity, self-esteem, and "omnipotent fantasies of invulnerability."[35]

Depression after a stroke is not a static condition. One study[7] noted that some patients tended to have less depression 6 months after stroke than 2 months, whereas an almost equal number experienced new or increased depression during that same period. Physicians need to pay attention to this facet of stroke recovery, not only during the period following the acute attack, but for many months after the formal rehabilitative efforts have ceased.

The majority of stroke patients initially experience anxiety as much as depression. Later, almost all patients with physical limitations experience sadness and grief; at times they may appear apathetic, bitter, or angry. Denial is another common reaction and may involve an attempt to minimize the seriousness of the stroke and deny the need for help from others. In some instances stroke patients may project an appearance of being overly happy while inwardly they are feeling great despair. When interviewed 1 year poststroke, patients frequently are irritable, which might be expressed as aggressiveness and self-centeredness. Both of these behaviors may aggravate the difficulties of the caregiver's role.[22] Sometimes stroke patients are generally less energetic, less outgoing, and more worried than they were in the past. Such personality changes may be obvious to family members, but the stroke patient may be unaware of them. Less commonly, the stroke patient may develop a psychosis. If cognitive ability also is impaired, it may be difficult for the patient to regard his environment as other than hostile and threatening, and he might tend to become paranoid and withdrawn.[35]

Stroke patients need opportunities to mourn their losses, to deal with fears, and to evaluate current stresses. They may also need to ventilate about the circumstances surrounding the stroke onset and subsequent events in the hospital. They will need to vent feelings related to anger, guilt, and fear. Referral to a social worker or clinical psychologist may be of great benefit in helping patients to adjust. Family members must be included in the counseling. For patients of working age, discussions with the employer may be critical, and it also may be helpful to have a vocational counselor involved.

The social support system is the key to completion of the rehabilitation effort. Throughout the stroke recovery and rehabilitation periods, the family is under a great deal of stress. Initially, family members have to cope with a life-threatening event and the attendant fear of losing a loved one. When the medical condition stabilizes, the family has to come to terms with the long-term effects of permanent disability and the need for adaptations in work arrangements, living conditions, and lifestyle. Also they may have to cope with the patient's array of emotional reactions and possibly personality changes. Financial and emotional strains, in addition to physical fatigue, may further stress the family's coping mechanisms. The unpredictability of stroke recovery in terms of length and degree are additional concerns. Family members need to be active participants in the rehabilitation process. They need to be informed of goals and plans and of the patient's functional progress. Educating family members to focus on the patient's remaining and emerging abilities rather than on the inabilities can help them to provide needed support to the patient, revise expectations, and reduce unnecessary and unrealistic pressures on the patient.

There are many pamphlets and books available to help both the stroke patients and the family to adapt. *Up and Around: A Booklet to Aid the Stroke Patient in Activities of Daily Living,* by Mahoney and Barthel, is an example of many free materials for patient and family offered by the American Heart Association. This booklet, which diagrams methods for maneuvering in bed, transferring to a wheelchair, tub, chair, or toilet, and for climbing stairs, also suggests adaptive equipment for the bathroom and aids for dressing. *Clothes for Disabled People,* written by Maureen Goldsworth (BT Balsford, Ltd., London, 1981), discusses adapting clothing for the stroke patient's special needs as well as techniques for sewing, knitting, or crocheting suitable garments. *How to Create Interiors for the Disabled,* written by Jan Carey (Panther Books, New York), details ways to build or adapt fixed structures or furniture to maximize independent living. *A Stroke Family Guide and Resource,* by GP Bray and GS Clark (Charles C. Thomas, Springfield, IL, 1984), is another useful volume. Finally, informal support systems such as stroke clubs may enable patients and family members to share their burdens and joys, to develop new techniques for managing difficult problems, to socialize without stigmatization, and to weather stressful periods. The local chapter of the American Heart Association or the hospital social work department will help in locating such resources.

Summary

A stroke involves a disturbance of cerebral function of vascular origin. Nearly one half million Americans each year are afflicted. The factors implicated in the risk of having a stroke include advancing age, hypertension, diabetes mellitus, cardiac disease, oral contraceptives, cardiac surgery, increased blood lipids, high hematocrit, and cigarette smoking. Transient ischemic attacks are often prodromal warnings of a completed stroke.

The mechanisms of stroke include thrombosis, embolism, and hemorrhage. There are many variants in the site of lesion, type of onset, course, prognosis, probability of improvement, and rate of recurrence. It is important that the diagnostic workup be thorough enough to determine an accurate description of the type of stroke.

The goal of a comprehensive treatment plan after the patient has been stabilized medically is to minimize the physically disabling problems, consider pertinent psychosocial factors, and return the patient to as normal a life as possible. Some of the rehabilitation issues for the stroke patient are discussed such as noting the differences between involvement of the right and left cerebral hemispheres, communication disorders, perceptual problems, skin integrity, bowel and bladder retraining, sexual functioning, and social adaptations after stroke. Use of functional assessment to help manage the physically disabling problems of stroke is also discussed.

References

1. Adler MK, Brown CC, Acton P: Stroke rehabilitation: Is age a determinant? J Am Ger Soc 28(11):499, 1980
2. Anderson TP: Stroke and Cerebral Trauma: Medical Aspects. In Stolov WC, Clowers MR (eds): Handbook of Severe Disability. Washington, US Dept. Education, Rehabilitation Services Administration, 1981
3. Anderson TP: Rehabilitation of patients with completed stroke. In Kottke FJ, Stillwell GK, Lehmann JF (eds): Krusen's Handbook of Physical Medicine and Rehabilitation, 3rd ed. Philadelphia, WB Saunders, 1981
4. Bray GP, DeFrank RS, Wolfe TL: Sexual functioning in stroke survivors. Arch Phys Med Rehabil 62(5):187, 286, 1981
5. Buonanno F, Toole JF: Management of patients with established ("completed") cerebral infarction. Stroke 12(1):7, 1981
6. Chaudhuri G: Rehabilitation of the stroke patient. Geriatrics 35(10):45, 1980
7. Feibel JH, Springer CJ: Depression and failure to resume social activities after stroke. Arch Phys Med Rehabil 63(6):276, 1982
8. Feigenson JS: Stroke rehabilitation: Effectiveness, benefits and cost: Some practical considerations. Stroke 10(1):1, 1979

9. Feigenson JS, Gitlow HS, Greenberg DO: The disability oriented rehabilitation unit: A major factor influencing stroke. Stroke 10(1):5–7, 1979
10. Feigenson JS: Stroke rehabilitation: Outcome studies and guidelines for alternative levels of care. Stroke 12(3):372, 1981
11. Fortinsky RH, Granger CV, Seltzer GB: The use of functional assessment in understanding home care needs. Med Care 19(5):489, 1981
12. Fowler RS Jr: Stroke and cerebral trauma: Psychosocial and vocational aspects. In Stolov WC, Clowers MR (eds): Handbook of Severe Disability, p 6. Washington, US Dept. Education, Rehabilitation Services Administration, 1981
13. Fowler RS, Fordyce WE: Stroke: Why Do They Behave That Way? p 5. Washington State Heart Association, 1974
14. Fugl–Meyer AR, Joasko L: Post-stroke hemiplegia and sexual intercourse. Scan J Rehabil Med Supp 7:158, 1980
15. Granger CV, Albrecht GL, Hamilton BB: Outcome by comprehensive medical rehabilitation: Measurement by PULSES profile and the Barthel index. Arch Phys Med Rehabil 60(4):146, 1979
16. Granger CV: Health accounting: Functional assessment of the long-term patient. In Kottke FJ, Stillwell GK, Lehmann JF (eds): Krusen's Handbook of Physical Medicine and Rehabilitation, 3rd ed. Philadelphia, WB Saunders, 1982
17. Granger CV, Sherwood CC, Greer DS: Functional status measures in a comprehensive stroke care program, Arch Phys Med Rehabil 58:555, 1977
18. Gresham GE, Granger CV: Trends in stroke rehabilitation. Unpublished manuscript
19. Harrison MJG: The investigation of strokes. In Russel RWR (ed): Cerebral Arterial Disease. Edinburgh, Churchill Livingstone, 1976
20. Hewer RL: Stroke rehabilitation. In Russell RWR (ed): Cerebral Arterial Disease, p 262. Edinburgh, Churchill Livingstone, 1976
21. Hilton L, Kraetschmer K: International trends in aphasia rehabilitation. Arch Phys Med Rehabil 64(10):462, 1983
22. Jarman, CMB: Living with stroke. Postgrad Med J 58(684):58, 1982
23. Johnson JH, Cryan M: Homonymous hemianopsia: Assessment and nursing management. Am J Nurs 79(12):213, 1979
24. Labi MLC, Phillips TF, Gresham GE: Psychosocial disability in physically restored long-term stroke survivors. Arch Phys Med Rehabil 61:561, 1980
25. Lehmann JF, DeLateur BJ, Fowler RS Jr et al: Stroke rehabilitation: outcome and prediction. Arch Phys Med Rehabil 56:383, 1975
26. Louis MC: Visual field and perceptual deficits in the brain damaged patient. Crit Care Update, pp 32–34, April, 1981
27. Louis MC, Povse SM: Aphasia and endurance: Considerations in the assessment and care of the stroke patient. Nurs Clin North Am 15(2):265, 273, 1980
28. Lund BL, Healey ML: Evaluation of Functional Abilities: Workshop Manual, p 40. Medical Rehabilitation Research and Training Center, Boston, Tufts–New England Medical Center, 1977
29. Malone PE, Whitehead JM: Speech and language rehabilitation following stroke. In Meyer JS, Shaw T (eds): Diagnosis and Management of Stroke and TIA's. Reading, MA, Addison–Wesley, 1982
30. Marquesden J: Natural history and prognosis of cerebrovascular disease. In Russell RWR (ed): Cerebral Arterial Disease. Edinburgh, p 24. Churchill Livingstone, 1976
31. McHenry LC Jr: Cerebral Circulation and Strokes. St Louis, Warren H Green, 1978
32. O'Brien MT, Pallet PJ: Total Care of the Stroke Patient, p 117, 119, 127. Boston, Little, Brown & Co, 1978

33. Peszczynski et al: Stroke rehabilitation. In Sahs AL, Hartman EC (eds): Fundamentals of Stroke Care. Washington, US Dept. of HEW, 1976
34. Redford JB, Harris JD: Rehabilitation of the elderly stroke patient. Am Fam Physician. 22(3):153–160, 1980
35. Ripecky A, Lazarus LW: Family guide to the problems of the stroke patient. Geriatrics 35(10):47, 1980
36. Sahs AL, Hartman EC, Aronson SM: Stroke: Cause, Prevention, Treatment and Rehabilitation, p 263. London, Castle House Publishing, 1979
37. Starr LB, Robinson RG, Price TR: Reliability, validity, and clinical utility of the social functioning exam in the assessment of stroke patients. Exp Aging Res 9(2):101–106, Summer 1983
38. Thorn–Gray BE, Kern LH: Sexual dysfunction associated with physical disability: A treatment guide for the rehabilitation practitioner. Rehab Lit 44(5–6):138, 1983

Additional Readings

1. Barnett HJM: Progress towards stroke prevention: Robert Wartenberg lecture. Neurology 30(11):1212, 1980
2. Brocklehurst JC, Morris P, Andrews K, Richards B, Laycock P: Social effects of stroke. Soc Sci Med 15A(1):35, 1981
3. Dzau RE, Boehme AR: Stroke rehabilitation: A family–team educational program. Arch Phys Med Rehabil 59:236, 1978
4. Fisher CM: The anatomy and pathology of the cerebral vasculature. In Meyer JS (ed): Modern Concepts of Cerebrovascular Diseases. New York, Spectrum Publications, 1975
5. Gainott, G: Emotional behavior and hemispheric side of the lesion. Cortex 8(1):41–55, 1972
6. Garraway WM: The changing pattern of stroke. Practitioner 223:655, 1979
7. Gawler J: New diagnostic methods. Practitioner 223:805, 1979
8. Goldberg HI: CT scan and cerebral angiography in the diagnosis of cerebrovascular disorders. In Meyer JS, Shaw T (eds): Diagnosis and Management of Stroke and TIA's. Reading, MA, Addison–Wesley 1982
9. Goldberg RT, Bernad MS, Granger CV: Vocational status: Prediction by the Barthel index and PULSES profile. Arch Phys Med Rehabil 61:580, 1980
10. Grabois M: Rehabilitation of patients with completed stroke. In Meyer JS, Shaw T (eds): Diagnosis and Management of Stroke and TIA's. Reading, MA, Addison–Wesley Publishing Co., 1982
11. Granger CV: Stroke rehabilitation. In Reuben DB et al (eds): Handbook of Ambulatory Medicine. Littleton, MA, John Wright & Sons, 1983
12. Gresham GE, Phillips TF, Wolf PA et al: The Framingham study. Arch Phys Med Rehabil 60(11):487, 1979
13. Heinze EG: The differential diagnosis of stroke. Primary Care 6(4):699, 1979
14. Hutchinson EC, Acheson EJ: Strokes: Natural History, Pathology and Surgical Treatment. London, WB Saunders, 1975
15. Jancovic J: Differential diagnosis of stroke. In Meyer JS, Shaw T (eds): Diagnosis and Management of Stroke and TIA's. Menlo Park, CA, Addison–Wesley, 1982
16. Kannel WB, Wolf PA: Risk factors in atherothrombotic cerebrovascular disease. In Meyer JS (ed): Modern Concepts of Cardiovascular Disease. New York, Spectrum Publications, 1975

17. Kaplan J, Hier DB: Visuospatial deficits after right hemispheric stroke. Am J Occup Ther 36(5):314, 1982
18. Kinsella GJ, Duffy FD: Attitudes towards disability expressed by spouses of stroke patients. Scand J Rehabil Med 12:73, 1980
19. Lavy S: Medical risk factors in stroke. In Goldstein M et al (eds): Advances in Neurology, Vol. 25. New York, Raven Press, 1979
20. Marshall J: The natural history of cerebrovascular diseases. In Meyer JS (ed): Modern Concepts of Cardiovascular Disease. New York, Spectrum Publications, 1975
21. McCollum CH: Diagnosis and cardiovascular surgical treatment of extracranial occlusive disease. In Meyer JS, Shaw T (eds): Diagnosis and Management of Stroke and TIA's. Menlo Park, CA, Addison–Wesley, 1982
22. McDowell FH: Prevention of subsequent infarctions and TIA's. In Goldstein M (ed): Advances in Neurology, Vol. 25. New York, Raven Press, 1979
23. McDowell FH: Indications and selection of patients for extracranial artery surgery for stroke. In Goldstein M (ed): Advances in Neurology, Vol. 25. New York, Raven Press, 1979
24. Merritt JL, Lie MR, Opitz JL: Bladder retraining of paraplegic women. Arch Phys Med Rehabil 63(9):416, 1982
25. Meyer JS: Course and prognosis and medical management of patients with acute stroke. In Meyer JS, Shaw T (eds): Diagnosis and Management of Stroke and TIA's. Menlo Park, CA, Addison–Wesley, 1982
26. Miller HR: The place of computerized tomography and carotid doppler sonography in cerebrovascular episodes. In Goldstein M (ed): Advances in Neurology, Vol. 25. New York, Raven Press, 1979
27. Norman S: Diagnostic categories for the patients with a right hemispheric lesion. Am J Nurs 79(12):2126, 1979
28. Reinvang I: A plan for rehabilitation of aphasics. Scand J Rehabil Med Suppl 7:120, 1980
29. Robbins S: Stroke in the geriatric patient. In Reichel W (ed): The Geriatric Patient. New York, HP Publishers, 1978
30. Robson P: The study of stroke. J Roy Coll Phys London 14(4):241, 1980
31. Sacco RL, Wolf PA, Kannel WB, McNamara PM: Survival and recurrence following stroke: The Framingham study. Stroke 13(3)290, 1982
32. Shaw T, Meyer JS: Aging and cardiovascular disease. In Meyer JS, Shaw T (eds): Diagnosis and Management of Stroke and TIA's. Menlo Park, CA, Addison–Wesley, 1982
33. Toole JF, Grindal AP: Neurovascular diagnostic tests for stroke. In Meyer JS (ed): Modern Concepts of Cardiovascular Disease. New York, Spectrum Publications, 1975
34. Von Arbin M, Britton, M, DeFaire U et al: Accuracy of bedside diagnosis. Stroke, 12(3):288, 1981
35. Warren M: Relationship of constructional apraxia and body scheme disorders to dressing performance in adult CVA. Am J Occup Ther 35(7):434, 1981
36. Whisnant JP et al: Clinical prevention of stroke. In Sahs AL, Hartman EC (eds): Fundamentals of Stroke Care. Washington, US Dept. of HEW, 1976
37. Wolf PA, Kannel WB: Controllable risk factors for stroke: Prevention implications of trends in stroke mortality. In Meyer JS, Shaw T (eds): Diagnosis and Management of Stroke and TIA's. Menlo Park, CA, Addison–Wesley, 1982

APPENDIX 9-1   Barthel Index (Adapted Version)

	Can do by myself	Can do with help of someone else	Cannot do at all
Drinking and eating	10	3	3
Dressing upper body	5	3	0
Dressing lower body	5	2	0
Donning brace or prosthesis	0	−2	Not applicable
Grooming	5	0	0
Washing or bathing	4	0	0
Perineal care	4	0	0
Managing urination	10	5	0
Managing bowel movements	10	5	0
Getting in and out of a chair	15	7	0
Getting on/off a toilet	6	3	0
Getting in and out of a tub or shower	1	0	0
Walking 50 meters on the level	15	10	0
Going up/down one flight of stairs	10	5	0
IF NOT WALKING — Propelling or pushing a wheelchair 50 meters	5	0	Not applicable

Barthel Total: Best score is 100;   worst score is 3.

(Mahoney FI, Barthel DW: Functional evaluation: The Barthel Index. Md St Med J 14:61–65, 1965)

APPENDIX 9-2   PULSES Profile (Adapted Version)

P Physical condition: Includes diseases of the viscera (cardiovascular, gastrointestinal, urologic, and endocrine) and neurologic disorders:
   1. Medical problems sufficiently stable that medical or nursing monitoring is not needed more often than at 3-month intervals.
   2. Medical or nurse monitoring is needed more often than 3-month intervals, but not each week.
   3. Medical problems are sufficiently unstable to require regular medical or nursing attention at least weekly.
   4. Medical problems require intensive medical or nursing attention at least daily (excluding personal care assistance only).
U Upper limb function: Self-care activities (drink/eat, dress upper/lower, brace/prosthesis, groom, wash, perineal care) dependent mainly on upper limb function:
   1. Independent in self-care without impairment of upper limbs.
   2. Independent in self-care with some impairment of upper limbs.
   3. Dependent upon assistance or supervision in self-care with or without impairment of upper limbs.
   4. Dependent totally in self-care with marked impairment of upper limbs.
L Lower limb functions: Mobility (transfer chair/toilet/tub or shower, walk, stairs, wheelchair) dependent mainly upon lower limb function.
   1. Independent in mobility without impairment of lower limbs.

continued

APPENDIX 9-2   (*Continued*)

2. Independent in mobility with some impairment of lower limbs such as needing ambulatory aids, a brace, or prosthesis, or else fully independent in a wheelchair without significant architectural or environmental barriers.
3. Dependent upon assistance or supervision in mobility with or without impairment of lower limbs, or partly independent in a wheelchair, or there are significant architectural or environmental barriers.
4. Dependent totally in mobility with marked impairment of lower limbs.

S Sensory components: Relating to communication (speech and hearing) and vision:
1. Independent in communication and vision without impairment.
2. Independent in communication and vision with some impairment such as mild dysarthria, mild aphasia, or need for eyeglasses or hearing aid, or needing regular eye medication.
3. Dependent upon assistance, an interpreter, or supervision in communication or vision.
4. Dependent totally in communication or vision.

E Excretory functions (bladder and bowel):
1. Complete voluntary control of bladder and bowel sphincters.
2. Control of sphincters allows normal social activities despite urgency or need for catheter, appliance, suppositories, etc. Able to care for needs without assistance.
3. Dependent upon assistance in sphincter management, or has accidents occasionally.

S Situational factors: Consider intellectual and emotional adaptability, support from family unit, financial ability, and social interaction:
1. Able to fulfill usual roles and perform customary tasks.
2. Must make some modification in usual roles and performance of customary tasks.
3. Dependent upon assistance, supervision, encouragement, or assistance from a public or private agency due to any of the above considerations.
4. Dependent upon long-term institutional care (chronic hospitalization, nursing home, etc.) excluding time-limited hospital stay for specific evaluation, treatment, or active rehabilitation.

PULSES Total: Best Score is 6;   worst score is 24.

(Moskowitz E, McCann CB: Classification of disability in the chronically ill and aging. J Chronic Dis 5:342–346, 1957)

CHAPTER 10
Parkinson's Disease

Parkinson's disease, the most common degenerative disease affecting the basal ganglia, is a prominent cause of disability compared to other diseases. Parkinsonism affects both sexes equally and is found among all races and in all geographic areas. The onset of parkinsonism, also known as paralysis agitans, occurs most frequently between the ages of 50 and 65 years. A juvenile form is encountered on rare occasions. At present approximately 50,000 new cases of Parkinson's disease are reported each year in the United States.[13,27] An estimated 1% of the population over 50 years of age, and 3% of those over 65 years of age, either have or will develop Parkinson's disease.[14] These figures are significant to those involved in the treatment of the chronically ill, for the incidence of Parkinson's disease will increase in proportion to the increasing numbers of older people in the United States.

Parkinson's disease generally has an insidious onset and a variable course. Life expectancy is 20 to 25 years after onset and, as with other diseases, is not a direct result of Parkinson's but rather of complications arising from inactivity, poor nutrition, weakness, or infection. For the majority of patients, 10 to 20 years elapse before symptoms cause incapacitation, but in rare cases the disease progresses so rapidly that individuals become completely disabled within 3 to 5 years of onset.

Classification

Parkinson's disease is generally classified into three categories: (1) primary or idiopathic, (2) secondary, and (3) symptomatic.

215

Primary (Idiopathic) Parkinson's Disease

Primary Parkinson's, the prototypic form, is characterized by the appearance of three classical symptoms: tremor, rigidity, and bradykinesia. Pathologically, the disease involves a degenerative loss of pigmented (dopaminergic) neurons in the substantia nigra, the point of origin of the dopaminergic nigrostriatal pathway. On examination of the gross brain, this normally black structure appears pale. There may be additional neuronal loss in the caudate and putamen, and occasionally lesions can be seen elsewhere in the brainstem or cerebral cortex. For example, Kupersmith[15] reports finding dopamine in olfactory tubercles and in amacrine cells of the retina and suggests that Parkinson's disease may represent generalized disturbances of dopaminergic metabolism in the olfactory and visual systems, as well as in extrapyramidal tracts. Dopaminergic neuronal degeneration in the dorsal motor nucleus of the vagus and in the locus ceruleus is also a common finding. The cause of neuronal degeneration is unknown. Viral and genetic explanations, as well as a premature aging process in dopamine neurons, have been suggested. Reports of familial tendencies are variable. It is likely that a multifactorial explanation is responsible.

In addition to neuronal degeneration, idiopathic Parkinson's disease also involves a depletion of the neurotransmitter dopamine in the corpus striatum. The amount of depletion is directly proportional to the amount of neuronal degeneration in the substantia nigra. The lack of dopamine, which normally inhibits the excitatory neurotransmitter acetylcholine (Ach), is believed to cause an imbalance, resulting in the characteristic triad of Parkinson symptoms. Lewy bodies (laminated spherical or elongated inclusion bodies) are characteristically found in the cytoplasm of degenerated pigmented neurons. Occasionally neurofibrillary tangles and macrophages containing phagocytized melanin are also seen.

Secondary Parkinsonism

Secondary parkinsonism includes both of the basal ganglia structures and diffuse central nervous system involvement. "Postencephalitic Parkinson's" refers to a secondary parkinsonian disease resulting from an epidemic of encephalitis following World War I. The original disease was characterized by sleepiness, ocular and bulbar palsies, difficulty swallowing, and dramatic behavioral changes. The encephalitis (often referred to as von Economo's encephalitis or encephalitis lethargica) proved fatal to more than 50% of its victims and, in addition, severely crippled a large number of survivors. Although some of the survivors appeared completely cured, in the years after the epidemic neurological changes (including paralysis, tremor, rigidity, and mental dysfunction) appeared. The symptoms were similar to those of idiopathic Parkinson's, but in addition these patients had lateralization of neurological deficits, oculogyric crises (spells in which eye muscle spasms cause the eyes to look upward involuntarily for time periods lasting from minutes to hours), impaired pupillary reactions, dystonic postures, and bizarre tics. Pathologically, the negative loss of dopaminergic neurons and the neurofibrillary tangles were more prominent in the secondary than in the primary form, and there was an absence of Lewy bodies. Except for a few sporadic cases reported during the 1930s and 1940s, physicians rarely see patients with this disorder.

The arteriosclerotic form of secondary Parkinson's disease, referred to as "arteriosclerotic pseudoparkinsonism," is characterized by Parkinson-like signs and symptoms secondary to generalized cerebrovascular infarctions in the basal ganglia area. This form often follows a history of several minor strokes or a long history of hypertension. Unlike patients with primary parkinsonism, these patients do not have tremor, or it is insignificant. Secondary Parkinson's symptoms are: slowed movement; a short-stepping, shuffling gait; stooped posture; and difficulty speaking clearly. Other neurological signs, such as increased muscle tone, hyperreflexia, enhanced extensor–plantar reflexes, and cognitive difficulties, are present. According to Yahr,[28] symptoms of this form of parkinsonism tend to remain localized indefinitely, and major disability is restricted mainly to the lower limbs. A differential diagnosis between secondary and idiopathic Parkinson's disease is extremely important since arteriosclerotic pseudoparkinsonism patients respond poorly to antiparkinsonian drugs.

Another form of secondary parkinsonism is associated with normal pressure hydrocephalus. Patients with this disorder develop typical parkinsonian gait difficulties and rigidity. The rigidity of this form of secondary parkinsonism is different from the rigidity of the idiopathic form, however, in that resistance to passive movement is greater in general and more prominent in the lower limbs. Some patients develop a "magnetic gait," that is, resistance is so great that their feet appear to be held to the floor as if by magnets.[28] Normal pressure hydrocephalus patients frequently experience urinary incontinence and, if their condition is not surgically corrected, they may experience a rapid progressive dementia. A differential diagnosis is therefore extremely important. If normal pressure hydrocephalus is suspected, CT scans should be employed to aid in its early detection.

"Iatrogenic" or drug-induced parkinsonism is a secondary parkinsonian disorder found most commonly in psychiatric patients. Parkinson-like symptoms frequently occur in patients being treated with tranquilizers or medications for treatment of schizophrenia. Some of the drugs implicated include chlorpromazine (Thorazine), reserpine, and haloperidol (Haldol), which are believed to cause symptoms by blocking the actions of dopamine. Iatrogenic parkinsonian signs mimic those of idiopathic Parkinson's disease and, in addition, may include oculogyric crises and dystonic spasms. Unlike the primary form, drug-induced parkinsonism is reversible in most cases. Symptoms abate within days to weeks upon decreasing or halting the medication.

Symptomatic Parkinsonism

Symptomatic parkinsonian states are due to diseases, events, or toxic factors that damage the nigrostriatal fibers or injure the striatum directly. Secondary symptoms that are produced simulate those of parkinsonism but are not necessarily extrapyramidal in origin and do not normally respond favorably to antiparkinsonian drugs. For example, on rare occasions brain tumors, head injuries, and congenital malformations may involve the basal ganglia region. Carbon monoxide poisoning and manganese intoxication are two of the more common precipitating events. These are examples of symptomatic parkinsonian disorders. Striatonigral degeneration affects the basal ganglia rather than the substantia nigra and results in a greater degree of rigidity than is characteristic of the primary parkinsonian form. Progressive supranuclear palsy involves impaired

TABLE 10-1   Etiologic Classification of Parkinsonism

Idiopathic Parkinson's disease	Basal ganglia tumors
Secondary parkinsonism	Cerebral trauma
Postencephalitic	Syphilis
Arteriosclerotic	Behcet's disease
Normal pressure hydrocephalic	Striatonigral degeneration
Neuroleptic drug intoxication	Progressive supranuclear palsy
Symptomatic parkinsonism	Parkinson–dementia complex of Guam
Carbon monoxide poisoning	Shy–Drager syndrome
Manganese poisoning	(idiopathic orthostatic hypotension)
(possibly other heavy metals)	

(Adapted from Gelbart RO, Hamilton, DO: Parkinson's disease. Fam Phys 23(6):182, 1981)

eye movements and cognitive disturbances in addition to the classical features. The Shy–Drager syndrome features dysautonomic functions (*e.g.*, orthostatic hypotension, impotence, anhidrosis), neurogenic bladder, and cerebellar signs, in addition to the usual Parkinson features. The Parkinson–dementia syndrome of Guam is a rare, geographically specific disorder characterized by widespread, severe dementia in addition to parkinsonian symptoms. Senile dementia, "essential" or "familial" tremor, involutional depression, hysteria, and anxiety also may present with symptoms simulating those of Parkinson's disease. A differential diagnosis is extremely important when treating Parkinson-like symptoms, since drugs commonly used to treat dementia, cerebral ischemia, or essential tremor in the aged are contraindicated for Parkinson's patients. Table 10-1 summarizes the classification system for parkinsonism and some of the more commonly encountered Parkinson-related syndromes.

Diagnosis

The key to effective diagnosis of Parkinson's disease is dependent upon the clinical acumen of the physician. The observation of characteristic clinical signs and symptoms constitutes the main diagnostic source. The appearance of the classic triad of symptoms makes the clinical picture of advanced Parkinson's disease unmistakable. Earlier diagnosis, before all the characteristic features have appeared, may present difficulties. The patient may not notice early signs of parkinsonism or may attribute them to normal aging. Symptoms may be as benign as persistent tiredness, minor aches, or a vague sense of malaise. Table 10-2 lists some of the common premonitory symptoms. Because the symptoms usually are noted first by a spouse, friend, relative, or coworker, a family member or friends can provide useful information during history-taking.

Diagnostic Signs

Characteristic signs of Parkinson's disease are so obvious that there is only minimal need for confirmatory tests for diagnostic purposes, unless other concurrent disease processes are suspected.[28] Blood chemistry tests to rule out

**TABLE 10-2   Common
Premonitory Signs**

Marked slowing of bodily activity
Decreased facility of movement
Postural and equilibration disturbances
Immobilization of facial muscles ("masking")
Unblinking expression
Reactive depression

(Adapted from Yahr, MO: Early recognition of Parkinson's disease, Hosp Pract, 16(7):65, 1981)

thyroid and parathyroid dysfunction may be performed, but routine laboratory test results usually are within normal limits, with two exceptions. Normally there is decreased level of homovanillic acid (a metabolite of dopamine) in the patient's cerebrospinal fluid (CSF), and there is decreased urinary excretion of free dopamine. CT scans often show mild, diffuse superficial and deep cerebral atrophy, but there are no characteristic deficits. Initially, tremor, bradykinesia, or muscular rigidity may occur alone or in combination. As the disease progresses, varying degrees of all three symptoms frequently can be observed. A less common symptom may be falling without good explanation.

Tremor, often of several months' duration, is the initial complaint in 70% of patients.[12] The parkinsonian tremor often begins asymmetrically in the distal segments of the limbs. It is most frequently observed as a simple to and fro motion but may also involve supination or pronation of the forearm. Although eventually the tremor progresses in severity and spreads symmetrically, it may remain limited to the distal segments. Occasionally the tremor is seen in the lips, tongue, or jaw. The classic tremor occurs at rest (but not during sleep) with a frequency of 4 to 6 oscillations per second, producing a "pill rolling" movement of the fingers and thumb. The tremor may, however, occur with varying rhythms and severity in different parts of the body, or even in different fingers of the same hand.[5] This tremor, which disappears during sleep and increases in severity during periods of emotional stress, also is known to intensify with nervousness, pain, illness (*e.g.,* influenza, severe upper respiratory infections), trauma (*e.g.,* broken hip), anxiety, fatigue, and self-consciousness. Psychological trauma (especially the death of a loved one) frequently is reported to correlate with the onset of the tremor symptom. Movement supposedly abolishes the tremor, but a majority of patients continue to experience tremor to some degree even with intentional movement. In the early stages concentration or voluntary effort can frequently suppress the tremor for several seconds so that tasks requiring fine movements of brief duration can be performed. In later stages of the disease, however, tremors of 8 to 10 oscillations per second may occur even during planned movements and may become indistinguishable from ataxic tremor.

Although it is one of the most common and conspicuous symptoms of Parkinson's disease, the tremor is the least disabling. Patients may attempt to hide it, however, by avoiding social contacts, thus becoming reclusive. Because tremors are often perceived by patients as a loss of dignity, they are a source of humiliation both to the patients and to their families.

Rigidity, the second classical symptom, contributes to the abnormal postural reflexes, the dystonic deformities, the staring, the masked expression identifying many parkinsonian patients, the poverty of automatic movements, and the difficulties in balance and ambulation. Rigidity, which generally develops insidiously but is invariably progressive, may involve only the musculature of the extremities at first, but eventually the neck and trunk will be affected. Parkinsonian patients exhibit one of two types of rigidity. A "lead-pipe" type of rigidity is characterized by a plastic, hypertonic resistance to passive movement of a major joint. The resistance is relatively uniform throughout the arc of motion during both flexion and extension. The "cog-wheel" type of rigidity involves a stiff, passive resistance to movement and a superimposed ratchet-like mechanism of action. Cog-wheeling is perceived by the examiner as a series of interrupted jerks. Parkinsonian rigidity is clinically different from the hypertonus associated with spasticity, which is accompanied by increased tendon reflexes, clonus, and pathological plantar responses ordinarily not characteristic of rigidity.[5]

Although rigidity is only an objective sign, many patients have subjective complaints that are believed to be related to rigidity. These sensations include burning, tingling, numbness, persistent soreness or aching, cramps, fatigue, and weakness. The occurrence of foot cramps while walking is sometimes the initial symptom of parkinsonism. Headaches, low back pain, and chest pain (sometimes mistaken for angina pectoris) also may result from the tense, contracted muscles. Aspirin and other ordinary pain-relieving medication usually are not effective in relieving these discomforts; physical modalities such as hot baths, heating pads, and postural exercises often prove beneficial. Levodopa, a medication especially used to treat parkinsonism, may alleviate many of the painful or discomforting feelings. Rigidity also may be modified temporarily by passively changing postures.

One of the most disabling effects of rigidity is its effect on posture and the dystonic deformities that result from it. Flexor muscles become more hypertonic than extensors, resulting in the characteristic flexor posture of patients with advanced rigidity. Fingers and thumb may become flexed toward the palm, arms are adducted toward the body, head is bent forward, and hips and knees are flexed. Patients frequently walk or stand with their arms bent at the elbow. In the advanced stages of the disease, patients may assume a fetal position. As severity progresses, postural abnormalities shift the center of gravity, causing problems with equilibrium and gait. Patients fall frequently, because they are unable to move to correct the loss of balance. In severe cases patients remain lying on the ground for hours after a fall, awaiting aid from a passerby or family member. It is likely that abnormal vestibular and labyrinth responses contribute to these balance abnormalities.[5]

Bradykinesia, or akinesia, diminished volitional motor activity secondary to muscular rigidity, is the third classical Parkinson's symptom and includes a poverty of movements and difficulty initiating voluntary movements. Akinesia, the more severe form, is probably the most disabling feature of parkinsonism. Bradykinesia also involves the loss of automatic movements such as eye blinking, swallowing saliva, arm swings associated with walking movements, and expressive movements of the face. As a result, patients tend to have a staring, masked facial expression and dry, reddened eyes; they tend not to be able to control drooling saliva, and orientation and balancing reflexes also are likely to be impaired.

Bradykinesia is characterized by hesitation in initiating actions, slowness in performing movements and rapid fatigue, especially with repetitive movements. Patients may be able to initiate the activity, but slow down or stop abruptly before its completion. Patients have described the experience as a sensation of having their "batteries run down" or of being "restrained" while in movement.[9] In the middle of performing a routine task, a parkinsonian patient may suddenly find him/herself frozen and unable to complete the remaining sequence of actions needed to write, to feed, or to ambulate.

Parkinson's patients tend to perform better from a standing position than from a reclining one, and they complain frequently of difficulties performing finely controlled hand and arm movements. Common disabling problems include difficulty getting up from a chair, getting out of a car, turning over in bed, or putting on a jacket.

Another characteristic of bradykinesia is the inability to perform two activities simultaneously with ease, or to cease performing one activity to begin another. Frequently patients require so much concentration to perform each movement that they are overwhelmed by the effort, and they withdraw from social stimuli around them.

The changeability of bradykinesia, that is, its characteristic of varying from moment to moment and from one circumstance to another, is referred to as "paradoxical kinesia." Patients may be able to perform an activity at one time of day, but be completely unable to repeat that same activity at another time. For example, normally a patient may be unable to walk unassisted but suddenly ambulate to the bathroom independently. Family members or workers who witness such events and who are not familiar with this facet of the illness, often think the patient is faking dependency and is capable of doing more than he usually demonstrates. Families should be informed of this unusual aspect of bradykinesia.

Bradykinesia can be observed, although minimal bradykinesia may go unnoticed even by physicians. Family members may play an important role in reporting subtle changes in a patient's movements or facial expressions. The examiner's careful observation of a patient's gait patterns during physical examination may reveal this symptom. Parkinsonian patients may have difficulty initiating ambulation—that is, they may behave as if their feet are glued to the floor. After a delay they are likely to walk with a slow, shuffling gait. Steps may get progressively shorter, and walking may halt. Another useful diagnostic aid for bradykinesia is alternating hand slapping examination, as described in Chapter 4. Most patients are able to slap their hands alternately (although there may be a few initial hesitations), but after a few repetitive motions, speed and coordination deteriorate rapidly.

Early in the course of the disease, gait abnormalities may be barely perceptible. Usually the first sign of a disturbance is noted when the patient drags one lower limb during ambulation, due to the rigid musculature and failure of antagonistic muscles to fully stretch when the opposing muscles contract.[5] As a result, the patient walks with a shortened step of the affected limb, dragging that limb in an effort to stay even with the longer pace of the unaffected opposite limb. As the disease progresses and the opposite lower limb is involved, the chronic stiffness of the flexor muscles shortens the steps on both sides. The patient walks with tiny steps (marche à petits pas), the identifying characteristic of a Parkinson's patient in the early stage of bilateral rigidity.[5] Eventually, as the flexor posture increases, the bent trunk tends to precede the lower extremities during walking. The increased frequency of small steps, the *festinating gait*, is characteristic of advanced parkinsonism. Sometimes this symptom becomes so severe that the patient falls frequently. Some patients, either in addition to or in lieu of the propulsive festinating gait just described, have a tendency to initiate a short series of backward steps or to fall backward when backing out of a closet or opening a door inward. These symptoms, called retropulsion, are directly related to muscular rigidity.

Patients in earlier stages of the condition sometimes can break temporarily the pattern of festination by concentrating on lengthening their steps. Also, they often find it easier to walk upstairs than to walk on level terrain. As symptoms become increasingly severe, the patient may freeze during ambulation and be unable to initiate movement in the lower limb. The tendency to freeze becomes marked when the patient tries to turn, especially in a small space such as the corner of a room or a doorway, or when crossing the street. Loss of normal automatic movements, such as associated arm swings when walking, contribute to ambulation difficulties. Gait disturbances may increase in severity with anxiety, emotional stress, or fright. Fear of falling and of injuries, compounded by frustration and embarrassment, further inhibit attempts at ambulation and increase incapacity.

There are other symptoms and signs of parkinsonism, besides tremor, rigidity, and bradykinesia, that can help the physician confirm the diagnosis or prepare the patient for potential problems. In addition to generalized bradykinesia, bowel movements may slow, resulting in constipation. Slowing of the throat musculature frequently leads to slower eating patterns and difficulty in swallowing certain foods or medications. Poor eating habits further augment the constipation problem. Diminished swallowing, which may cause the saliva to pool in the mouth, may lead to uncontrolled drooling. A sluggish bladder may result in incomplete emptying and urinary frequency. Fortunately, bowel and bladder problems are usually not seriously disabling for Parkinson's patients. Autonomic dysfunction with hyperhidrosis and orthostatic hypotension sometimes occurs. Postural hypotension is further exaggerated by levodopa treatment. Two abnormal reflexes, the palmomental and glabellar, are frequent findings in parkinsonism. Bothersome conditions such as eczema and seborrhea also may occur.

Speech changes do not occur in all parkinsonian patients. When they do occur, however, patients characteristically tend to speak so softly (due to diminished chest movement) that it is difficult to hear them on the telephone, and they may speak in a rapid monotone. Soft, rapid, monotonous speech is an identifying symptom of parkinsonism. Occasionally there are pitch changes, and some patients speak slowly rather than rapidly. Speech usually improves with medication.

Microphagia is a characteristic symptom. Obtaining samples of patients' handwriting is a useful examination technique, especially if the samples can be compared with previous ones. Handwriting of patients with Parkinson's disease tends to get increasingly smaller, although letters remain well-formed. On careful examination (with a magnifying glass if necessary), squiggles may be apparent in each letter suggestive of a tremor. Usually drug treatment improves this symptom, but in some instances the problem will be overcorrected, and patients will write in large, bold letters.

Although acuity remains normal, visual problems may occur in patients who have Parkinson's disease of long duration. Patients may complain of difficulty reading because eye movements are poorly coordinated, necessitating the patient to work hard in order to read. Most Parkinson's patients are unaware of any visual impairments throughout the course of their disease.

Mental Alterations

Reports of psychological and behavioral disorders arising from Parkinson's disease are diverse. Mental changes frequently associated with the parkinsonian state vary from minor memory and cognitive impairment, or episodic confusional states, to chronic dementias. Certain Parkinson syndromes are typified by mental changes. Among these are the postencephalitic form, which frequently is accompanied by marked psychiatric disturbances; the arteriosclerotic form, in which cognitive and emotional impairments are common; and the parkinsonian syndrome of Guam, the rare familial form of amyotrophic lateral sclerosis, described previously, which is characterized by dementia and extrapyramidal involvement.

Typical reported psychic and behavioral changes include reduced alertness, spontaneity, and motivation, which may culminate in a paralysis of will or marked reduction in drive.[9] Mental changes may be as benign as drowsiness or excessive yawning, or as severe as hallucinations and paranoic states. Schizophrenic and psychotic behaviors are usually the result of medication intoxication. Mental changes may include impaired judgment and an inability to integrate multimodal stimulation. In a 1971 study significant differences were found between Parkinson patients and controls in problem-solving, sensory awareness, memory, general cognition, and abstraction abilities.[22] A recent study reports that 32% of Parkinson patients had moderate to marked dementia as compared with 10% of controls.[22] Parkinson patients are observed to be emotionally flat, corroborated by the masklike facial appearance, and depression and excessive dependence are frequently noted. Studies have found that the depression is not correlated with severity of handicap, age, or sex of the sufferer. Sometimes it may be difficult to differentiate functional disorders from the physical concomitants of Parkinson disease such as hypokinesia, facial masking, and withdrawal from the social environment in order to concentrate on movement.

There are several possible causes for the mental changes observed. Neuropathological changes may be due to disease etiologies such as encephalitis, vascular disease, or carbon monoxide or metallic poisoning. Second, psychic symptoms may result from a progressive, incapacitating disease, abetted by negative physician or family attitudes. Premorbid personality descriptions are crucial in evaluating this possibility. Third, medication may induce mental changes or aggravate those already present. Levodopa has been implicated in causing hallucinations,[22] for example. Fortunately drug-induced mental alterations usually are reversible within a few days to a few weeks by decreasing or halting medication. Fourth, Sroka and colleagues[23] report findings of increased cerebral atrophy in Parkinson's patients exhibiting organic mental syndromes. They suggest that whereas the demented population of Parkinson's patients may represent a subgroup of the usual parkinsonian population, prolonged disease does not suggest necessarily inevitable mental deterioration or cerebral atrophy.

Course of Illness

Duvoisin describes five stages in the clinical course of primary parkinsonism, as described below:[8]

Stage 1*. Mild, usually unilateral (hemiparkinsonism) disease*. The most common presenting symptom is tremor of one upper limb concomitant with a history of vague complaints of aches and pains and possible changes in posture, locomotion, facial expression, and speech. Patients may be unaware of any resulting disabilities. Clinical features presenting during this stage include:

- Postural changes: Slight lateral tilt of trunk away from side affected by tremor during standing or activity; flexion contracture at elbow
- Communication changes: Speech amplitude reduced; speech takes on deliberate quality; diminution of facial expression; possible micrographia
- Neurological changes: Mild rigidity; akinesia in affected (with tremor) upper limb; poverty of spontaneous movements; loss of unconscious associated movements (*e.g.,* diminished arm swing in affected limb while walking); impaired responses to rapidly alternating movements and finger dexterity tests; classic triad probably present in lower limb of affected side
- Other changes: Possible seborrhea of forehead; mild edema may be present

Stage 2*. Bilateral involvement, early postural changes*. Postural changes become more noticeable, and movement becomes more difficult. Slowness, fatigability, and limited range of motion may force patients to retire from their jobs or seek alternative employment. Patients may become socially isolated as they stay home more, withdraw from social activities, and abandon hobbies and interests. Reactive depression may develop. Physical disability still minimal; patient able to continue to perform activities of daily living (ADLs) independently.

- Postural changes: Patient assumes stooped posture when walking or standing; trunk inclined forward; flexion of knees, ankles, hips, and vertebrae continues to increase gradually; fingers adducted at rest; metacarpophalangeal and distal interphalangeal joints slightly flexed; proximal interphalangeal joints extended; wrist slightly dorsiflexed; foot in varus position
- Neurological changes: Gradual development of mild bradykinesia; poverty of spontaneous activity; development of slow, shuffling gait

Stage 3*. Pronounced gait disturbances and moderate generalized disability*. Gait disturbances and slowness in executing ADLs, especially dressing, cause increasing disability.

- Postural changes: Increased impairment of postural and righting reflexes
- Neurological changes: Progressive bradykinesia; onset of retropulsion and propulsion—progressive severity of these symptoms precipitates frequent falls; walking slows—involves hesitation and "freezing" phenomena

Stage 4. *Significant disability*. Increasing neurological symptoms limit patient's ability to live alone without constant supervision. Patients have difficulty dressing, turning in bed, rising from a chair, and preparing food; assistance required with ADLs

- Neurological changes: Tremors may be less marked; rigidity and bradykinesia increase in severity; slow, shuffling, festinating gait develops with subsequent falls; decreased finger dexterity; unsteady when standing

Stage 5. *Complete invalidism*. Patients who survive to this stage are complete invalids who cannot move without assistance and are confined to bed or chair; ambulation is impossible.

- Postural changes: Head flexed on trunk; arms adducted and flexed; wrists dorsiflexed; fingers deformed by dystonic posturing; legs slightly flexed at hips, adducted and held tightly together; knees partially flexed; feet plantar flexed
- Communication changes: Speech rapid and barely perceptible
- Neurological changes: Severe bradykinesia and rigidity; minimal tremor; little remaining voluntary motor function
- Other changes: Mouth constantly ajar; diminished swallowing causing constant drooling; face expressionless, with infrequent blinking and staring gaze; dehydration; often increased susceptibility to bronchopneumonia, urinary tract infections, bedsores, and other lethal infections

Treatment

Although there are no cures for Parkinson's disease, physical therapy, occupational therapy, speech therapy, and psychosocial therapies may be utilized to curtail the morbid effects of immobility, social isolation, and psychological withdrawal, all of which may contribute to increasing disability and eventual incapacitation or institutionalization.[25]

Parkinson's disease may strike at a time in life when a person is finishing up his career, looking forward to future leisure, and trying to add to retirement funds; or perhaps a spouse has died, the children have left home, and the patient is living alone. No matter what the circumstances, Parkinson's disease, because it alters physical and mental qualities, is likely to affect all aspects of its victim's life including vocational plans, family and social relationships, and emotional status. Treatment plans necessarily must deal with all of these aspects of life. The mainstay of treatment for Parkinson's disease is pharmacologic. Counseling, speech therapy, physical or occupational therapy, and adaptational techniques to help the patient perform activities of daily living may greatly assist the Parkinson's patient to cope with this incurable, progressively disabling illness.

Pharmacologic Intervention

The aim of pharmacologic intervention in Parkinson's disease is to maintain the delicate balance in the striatum between the neurotransmitters acetylcholine and dopamine. The degeneration of nigral dopaminergic cells and accompanying reduction in the dopamine previously produced by these now defunct neurons leads to an excess of acetylcholine, which is responsible for the activity underlying the major symptoms of the disease. Drugs to treat Parkinson's disease must be capable of crossing the blood–brain barrier and either reducing cholinergic activity or enhancing or replacing dopaminergic functioning in the remaining neurons. Enhancement can be accomplished by drugs that (1) increase the synthesis of dopamine (*e.g.,* levodopa), (2) delay the catabolism of dopamine (*e.g.,* monoamine oxidase inhibitor, MAO), (3) stimulate dopamine release or activity at receptor sites (*e.g.,* amphetamines), or (4) block the re-uptake of monoamines at the synaptic cleft (*e.g.,* anticholinergics).[27]

It is little wonder that no one drug is currently available to eradicate all adverse effects of the disease. Some symptoms, such as loss of finger dexterity, will not respond to any drug or combination of medications,[21] and even the most effective antiparkinson's medication frequently will exacerbate one or more symptoms or losses. In addition, the efficacy of medication varies from person to person and even from one time to another for the same individual. For this reason pharmaceutical management of the parkinsonian patient requires individualized treatment regimens, continuous monitoring of drug effectiveness, and regulation of dosages or use of adjunctive medications. The ultimate goal of treatment is to obtain optimal relief of disease symptoms with minimal adverse effects.

Pharmacologic intervention becomes necessary when symptoms begin to interfere with the patient's ability to function. It is generally better not to medicate during asymptomatic, nondisabling periods. The point at which any one symptom or group of symptoms becomes significant is variable and must be individually evaluated.

A slight tremor of the hand, for example, poses few functional problems to a retired patient whose manual activities are limited to dressing, cooking, cleaning, and other grossly manipulative tasks. But to a watchmaker or a barber, the same degree of tremor may constitute a catastrophic functional impairment. For the retiree, drug therapy would not be justified; for the watchmaker, it would be virtually mandatory.[28]

During the early stages of the disease, increased dopaminergic activity in undamaged nigral neurons can partially compensate for the dopamine deficiency caused by the destruction of nigral neurons. During this stage drug intervention focuses on the selection and use of agents that will enhance residual dopaminergic activity. In advanced stages the dopamine must be replaced or supplemented. Drugs for early parkinsonism include anticholinergics, antihistamines, and tricyclic antidepressants.

Anticholinergics are especially effective for treatment of mild to moderate tremors and may reduce rigidity to some degree. Although mainly used during the early stages of Parkinson's disease, anticholinergics frequently are taken in conjunction with levodopa—the principal medication used for more advanced stages—and often are prescribed for patients for whom levodopa or similar medications are contraindicated. Anticholinergics, especially beneficial in treating postencephalitic parkinsonism, in contrast to levodopa, can reverse the iatrogenic parkinsonism induced by certain tranquilizer drugs.

Examples of anticholinergic drugs are trihexyphenidyl (Artane, Tremin), procyclidine (Kemadrin), cycrimine (Pagitane), and biperiden (Akineton). The usual dose of trihexyphenidyl is 2 mg 3 times a day; if well tolerated, this can be increased up to 15 mg per day in divided doses. More than 15 mg per day rarely provides any additional benefit, and some patients may not tolerate this amount.[27] Benztropine mesylate (Congentin) is a more potent drug than trihexyphenidyl.

As is true with all current antiparkinsonian medications, anticholinergics have frequent side-effects, including dry mouth or throat, blurred vision, anhidrosis (in severe cases, warm weather may precipitate a fever or even coma), constipation, and urinary symptoms, especially urinary retention. Other side-effects include flushing, elevated body temperature, lightheadedness, and rash. Anticholinergics may exacerbate narrow-angle glaucoma. Toxic manifestations may include ataxia, dysarthria, hypertension, tachycardia, heart block, or other cardiac abnormalities. It is advisable for cardiac patients to obtain an ECG before initiating treatment. Mental changes such as recent memory loss, mild confusion, hallucinations, and depression also may occur. Adverse symptoms are usually alleviated by lowering the dosage. Elderly patients particularly may have adverse reactions to these medications.

In addition to anti-allergic actions, antihistamines are helpful to parkinsonian patients because they contain mild CNS anticholinergic and sedative properties. Two examples of antihistamines specifically used in Parkinson's treatment are chlorphenoxamine (Phenoxene) and orphenadrine hydrochloride (Disipal); a third, diphenhydramine, has also been used with some success.[9] Because these drugs are far less potent than primary anticholinergic substances such as trihexyphenidyl, they must be used in larger dosages. Although they are only minimally effective in alleviating parkinsonian symptoms, frequently they are invaluable as adjunctive drugs. Aside from the anticholinergic side-effects previously mentioned, antihistamines may cause dizziness, sedation, and hypotension in elderly subjects.

Amantadine, another therapeutic drug, was accidently found to have antiparkinsonism effects in the treatment of mild symptoms. The exact mechanism of its action is unknown. Although amantadine has a fairly rapid response (within days), its actions are short-lived and it loses its effectiveness within 3 to 6 months. According to Duvoisin,[9] however, the drug regains its effectiveness if the patient stops it for a period of time and then begins it again.

Like the anticholinergic medications, amantadine has some disturbing side-effects such as peripheral edema, insomnia, confusion, and psychotic symptoms (*e.g.,* hallucinations). Also a condition characterized by the legs assuming a purplish appearance, livedo reticularis, may occur. This condition reportedly is harmless and usually disappears within 1 to 2 months after stopping the drug. In rare cases amantadine has been reported to induce heart failure or cause reversible central vision failure.[12] It is contraindicated in patients with impaired renal functioning.

As Parkinson's disease progresses, increasing the dopamine activity in the remaining neurons can no longer compensate for the dopamine depletion from continuing nigral neuronal degeneration. At some point in this continuum, pharmacologic intervention must focus on replenishing dopamine reserves. Dopamine cannot be directly administered since it does not cross the blood–brain barrier. Instead a precursor, L-dopa (also known as levodopa or 3,4-dihydroxyphenylalanine), is employed. L-dopa is transformed into dopamine by a decarboxylation reaction. Unfortunately, because dopa decarboxylase, the catabolizing enzyme, is present both in the central and peripheral nervous systems, only 1% of L-dopa is able to enter the brain and be converted for therapeutic purposes. The other 99% is catabolized extracerebrally,[24] resulting both in a tremendous waste of medication and in active metabolites forming from the breakdown of dopamine in the periphery. Even so, L-dopa remains the most effective and least toxic antiparkinson's medication to date.

Levodopa, the only pharmacological agent to alter the clinical signs and symptoms of Parkinson's disease[12] significantly, is effective in reducing rigidity, improving gait and postural abnormalities, diminishing excessive seborrhea and oiliness, ameliorating drooling, and relieving pain, numbness, and associated aches. Levodopa greatly reduces or even abolishes tremor in most patients and normally abolishes bradykinesia or akinesia in mild to moderate cases. The most distressing, persisting problem for the majority of parkinsonians,[9] bradykinesia, may be only partially alleviated by levodopa.

Initially L-dopa is administered orally in daily dosages of 250 mg 3 times a day,[27] and then slowly increased about 500 mg every 4 to 7 days until an optimal limit is reached.[24] Normally most of the therapeutic effects begin at a dosage of about 2 to 3 g. The average optimal dose is 5 to 6 g but in rare cases as much as 8 g daily may be needed for desired symptom control. No single dose should exceed 1.5 to 2 g, so multiple doses are necessary. Since L-dopa does not "cure" Parkinson's disease, eventually a time will come when a previously effective dose fails to control the adverse symptoms, or dyskinesias begin to occur. A sign that optimal dosage has been reached is apparent when dyskinesia increases as the dose of L-dopa is increased. In general the object of management of parkinsonian symptoms by pharmacologic means is not to eradicate symptoms completely, because high doses almost always lead to severe side-effects, but to maintain a balance between adequate symptom control and minimal adverse medication effects.

The patient on L-dopa must be carefully monitored, and dosage and use of adjunctive drugs must be adjusted to individual requirements. Although effective in primary parkinsonism, levodopa is not helpful in treating iatrogenic parkinsonism. Certain agents should not be used in combination with L-dopa. Pyridoxine for example, frequently found in vitamin supplements, is a cofactor in the catabolism of L-dopa and may reduce its effectiveness by stimulating extracerebral decarboxylase activity. Monoamine oxidase inhibitors should not be given concomitantly with levadopa, as serious life-threatening effects, such as palpitations, shortness of breath, severe headaches, convulsions, and coma can result. Anticholinergics, used prior to administration of L-dopa therapy, should be continued probably as long as 6 months, to help maintain symptom control until optimal L-dopa responses have been obtained. Then the dosage of anticholinergics can be gradually reduced and L-dopa can be adjusted accordingly.

Long-term responsiveness to L-dopa varies from patient to patient. Although some patients continue to enjoy good symptom control with L-dopa for more than 10 years, numerous recent studies have reported that effectiveness diminishes for the majority of patients after 4 to 7 years. One group of investigators reports that, with some exceptions, 1 to 2 years after the commencement of treatment effectiveness declines steadily.[2] The "on–off" effect is one of the complications that occurs with continued use of L-dopa. This can be of two types: (1) The "wearing off" course, whereby effectiveness begins to wane at the end of the dose period and potentially adverse mid-dose effects appear, and (2) the "yo-yoing" course, whereby symptoms seem to improve, then worsen, then improve again, or the reverse. Increasing the dosage only intensifies the oscillations of clinical responsiveness, which may last from hours to days. Although the mechanism of this see-saw response is unknown, smaller, more frequent doses seem to improve the on–off phenomenon. Another indication that the effectiveness of L-dopa therapy is beginning to fail is "start–hesitation," a patient's inability to begin a movement such as walking. The patient's feet reportedly feel as if they are "frozen to the ground." Sometimes this effect is dose-dependent, but lowering the amount of L-dopa does not necessarily relieve the symptom. Evidence of levodopa toxicity may be akinesia, dyskinesia, or psychiatric symptoms. Some patients become totally unresponsive to L-dopa after 7 to 10 years. A recent study by Bauer and colleagues[2] found that 47% of the patients in their study were at the pretreatment level of disability after 10 years. However, these investigators stress that the interim improvement afforded to these individuals while the L-dopa was therapeutically beneficial affirms its effectiveness as an important antiparkinsonism medication. Because of the apparent reduction in its effectiveness after long-term use, L-dopa should be postponed until more effective treatment than can be achieved by use of anticholinergics or amantadine alone is needed.

Although controversial, a "drug holiday" is sometimes given to the patient exhibiting symptoms of long-term levadopa use. A full drug holiday involves the total cessation of levodopa for a period of 3 to 21 days, whereas the partial drug holiday involves the dramatic reduction of the levodopa dosage to a minimal level for a specified period of time. Another alternative drug holiday is the intermittent form, which involves a withdrawal of the dopaminergic medication for 2 consecutive days each week. Patients unable to tolerate withdrawal of medication according to this regimen are quickly identified by an increase in tremor or bradykinesia.[7]

Drug holidays have a dual advantage. First, although slow manipulation of dosage on an outpatient basis by a titration approach is most desirable, the range between an effective therapeutic dose of medication and a dose that produces excessive dopaminergic reactions is very narrow in patients prone to levodopa toxicity. The delicate process of drug titration is difficult to sustain on an outpatient basis and may prove stressful to families of Parkinson's patients. A one-time withdrawal of medication while the patient is hospitalized may be easier to manage and more efficient. Second, some studies have indicated that a drug holiday increases motor responsiveness and decreases levodopa-induced side-effects for as long as 9 months.[1] In some instances, titration of medication following either a full or partial holiday period required only half of the initial daily dose for improved motor function.[2] The lower doses required after the holiday also resulted in a lessening of dyskinesias[3] and a marked improvement in patients with psychiatric complications.[5] A decrease in side-effects during the two-day cessation of dopamine medication has been reported for patients participating in the weekly drug holiday. Although some patients claim a decrease of side-effects throughout the week,[6] results from this form of holiday may not manifest for 6 months.

Although the immediate results of drug holiday as a pharmacological manipulation are demonstrable, the long-term benefits are still questionable. The maneuver is repeatable, but the specific benefits derived from periodically lowering the doses of dopaminergic preparations seem to diminish with time. Depending upon the severity of the patient's condition when beginning the drug holiday, the physical and psychological risks are considerable. Although the temporary withdrawal of doapminergic preparations is expected to produce only transient results, the potential for complete immobilization of the patient during the process may prove life-threatening. Furthermore, unmasking of the actual extent to which the parkinsonian state has progressed may prove traumatic both to patient and family and may require intense emotional support.

The patient also requires acute medical support and supervision during the various stages of the drug holiday. Constant assessment, evaluation, and support is necessary to prevent systemic side-effects secondary to inertia. The patient therefore should be hospitalized during the entire holiday period, and a multidisciplinary team should manage the consequential problems.

In summary, lack of control of symptoms in response to increased dopaminergic medication or the presence of dyskinesias may be early indications that a drug holiday may be necessary. A drug holiday is a dramatic intervention, however, and it should never be undertaken without consulting a neurologist and without carefully evaluating the risks versus the potential benefits. Also a drug holiday should not be attempted without informing both the patient and the family of the ramifications of withdrawing pharmacologic support and without the availability of intensive nursing, medical, and psychological support for the patient before, during, and after the holiday.

Physicians should be aware of the many side-effects of levodopa. Nausea, vomiting, and anorexia, which are common symptoms due to the effect of dopamine on the central emetic center, are almost universal during the initial treatment period. However, many patients develop a tolerance to the drug as therapy proceeds. Involuntary adventitious movements such as head nodding, facial grimaces, tongue protrusion, exaggerated gestures and arm swings, and other chorealike movements are present in 80% of patients receiving L-dopa treatment. These movements diminish if the dosage of L-dopa is reduced, but some patients are never free of them. If the movements are mild, treatment should continue at full dosage. If they become excessive, however, medication should be decreased. Other side-effects of L-dopa include cardiac irregularities or palpitations, the most frequent of which is sinus tachycardia. Precautions must be taken in administering dopaminergic medication to patients who have a history of cardiovascular or pulmonary disease, and the drug is usually contraindicated for patients with recent myocardial infarction. Although orthostatic hypotension is another common side-effect of levodopa treatment, when severe orthostatic hypotension coexists with parkinsonian symptoms a diagnosis of Shy–Drager syndrome should be considered. Constipation is a distressing, but very common, consequence of L-dopa therapy. Patients should be advised to maintain healthy diets and drink plenty of fluids; in more severe cases laxatives may be used. Patients who may notice discolorations in urine and sweat and, at times, stains on the sheet at night or darkened urine may fear blood loss. These discolorations, however, are usually due to metabolic breakdown products of L-dopa.

Although L-dopa has proved to be an effective antiparkinsonism drug, its large required daily dose, delayed onset of therapeutic benefits, and frequent side-effects are a source of disappointment. Improved results have been achieved through the simultaneous administration of L-dopa and a dopa decarboxylase inhibitor, carbidopa. The addition of carbidopa to L-dopa increases from 1% to 3%[24] the proportion of L-dopa that enters the brain and reduces the required dosage by up to 80%.[17] Fewer peripheral side-effects are reported, and a faster onset of response (days instead of weeks or months) occurs if carbidopa is combined with L-dopa. The combined drug has similar therapeutic effects, but provides slightly better control than an L-dopa preparation alone. Furthermore, the combined drug accounts for a significant reduction in gastrointestinal disturbances and may prevent L-dopa-induced cardiac arrhythmias.

At present, the combined drug is obtainable in a single pill in combinations of 10 : 100 mg, 25 : 250 mg (the average dose), or 25 : 100 mg carbidopa to levodopa. Since approximately 75 mg of carbidopa are needed to inhibit peripheral dopa decarboxylase, the pills are usually taken 3 or 4 times a day. Unfortunately the combined pill makes it difficult to regulate individual amounts of carbidopa or levodopa, and 20% of patients remain totally unresponsive to the combined therapy.[7] Side-effects of the combined drug are similar to those of L-dopa alone.

Research continues for new antiparkinsonian drugs. For example, bromocriptine, an analog of dopamine, is now being studied extensively. Early reports are conflicting. Generally it is agreed that bromocriptine improves functional abilities in parkinsonians, but other authors report that it is not as effective as L-dopa and is much more costly. Other agents, such as monoamine oxidase beta inhibitors, may reduce the on–off effect of L-dopa and slow the catabolism of dopamine, but are also costly and have adverse side-effects. The future holds promise for better pharmacologic management of Parkinson's patients.

Supportive Counseling

The success of rehabilitative efforts depends upon a patient's outlook and motivation, especially for Parkinson's patients who commonly react with progressive disinterest and withdrawal from social situations, increased dependency, and depression. The health-care team must provide encouragement and support and should assure parkinsonian patients that the gradual onset and slow progressive nature of the disease makes them good rehabilitation candidates. Both patients and their families should be told the nature of the disease and that patients can lead active lives and enjoy minimal disability for long periods after the initial symptoms begin. Patients should be prepared for some of the classical symptoms, and health-care providers should counsel them about ways to overcome some of their disabling consequences. Related issues such as sexual functioning should also be addressed. Although sexual functioning normally remains intact in parkinsonian patients, activity may be limited by severe rigidity and tremors.[2] Fortunately L-dopa effectively alleviates most of these problems.

Vocational issues also should be discussed. Most patients have to readjust vocational plans to some degree. Blue collar workers are affected especially, as lifting, carrying, and climbing will become increasingly difficult for the Parkinson patient. Muscle stiffness may also cause parkinsonians to fatigue easily and may limit their ability to perform heavy physical labor. The loss of fine rapid movements of the hands may disrupt careers requiring manual dexterity. Jobs dependent upon positive social interaction, such as salespersons, may be compromised due to drooling, lack of facial expression and characteristic monotone voice, qualities that Parkinson's patients develop. Jobs involving stress or temperature extremes also should be avoided. Cold temperatures tend to increase stiffness, whereas hot climates accentuate hyperhydrosis symptoms. Stressful jobs exacerbate tremor symptoms; sedentary, low-pressure jobs requiring light workloads are preferable, although patients must avoid prolonged sitting, which threatens to increase stiffness and contractures. Jobs with flexible time limits also are desirable. Patients will need to allow for increased time for dressing and eating to avoid being late for work, or they may need additional time for lunch hours. Transportation is another important consideration when choosing a job. The typical swaying motion of public transportation may present a problem for patients whose balance is already precarious. Finally, many parkinsonians have difficulty ambulating in crowded places and therefore should plan lifestyles that avoid this barrier.

Although patients must learn to adjust activities to their present level of ability, they should strive to keep physically active. Part of the adjustment process includes allowing adequate time to complete tasks. It is essential that unemployed Parkinson's patients remain physically and mentally active. Health-care providers can spur motivation by encouraging patients to make lists of daily activities they wish to accomplish.

Both patients and families find it difficult to cope with progressively debilitating illnesses such as parkinsonism. Physicians should discuss family situations with the patient and significant others during checkup examinations. Together, they should identify problem areas. Depression, for instance, is a common feeling in Parkinson patients and may be associated with feelings of helplessness and hopelessness. When necessary, patients should be referred for formal counseling.

Communication and Speech Therapy

Improving communication skills is an important aspect of rehabilitation. Patients should be urged to exaggerate face, eye, and lip movements (smiling, frowning, grimacing, puckering, and so on) in a mirror. This may keep facial muscles toned and prevent the characteristic masked face of Parkinson's patients. Reading aloud, especially rhythmic poems and numbers, may help the patient to improve the characteristic soft, monotone speech or to slow rapid speech. Since breath control is important in speaking, breathing exercises should be practiced regularly. Routine movement of the chest during exercise may also help deter contractures in this musculature.

Patients should be encouraged to overcome feelings of embarrassment and to communicate rather than withdraw from social interactions. Speech may be adversely affected by tremors, bradykinesia, and diminished gestures. Speech impairments that may threaten job security and interpersonal relationships contribute to already elevated levels of anxiety and frustration. A speech therapist may help by evaluating disabling speech consequences of the disease and by suggesting methods to improve communication. The speech therapist also can help if the patient is experiencing chewing and swallowing difficulties by evaluating the underlying mechanisms and teaching the patient and family compensatory techniques.

Physical Therapy and Exercise

Physical therapy is an important form of adjuctive therapy for parkinsonism. Physical modalities including heat can alleviate the rigidity that can cause stiffness, muscle cramping and contractures, and resulting muscle aches, headaches, and low-back pain. Therapists can carry out exercise and conditioning programs to increase muscle strength, improve coordination, maintain range of motion in the joints, and assist in transfer and ambulation skills. Although exercise will not alter the disease course, it may help to maintain function, reduce disuse atrophy, prevent unnecessary complications such as contractures, and relieve discomforts. Physical therapists can also help patients with gait training and postural training. With occupational therapists patients can be helped to improve coordination, to develop adaptive skills for the performance of ADLs, and to increase motivation. Therapists can help patients develop exercises that they can do within their own homes. Patients can be encouraged to develop a walking program, for example, or to practice walking and turning for 15 minutes each day. Therapists also can teach them the proper way to rise from a chair and can help them to perform other transfer maneuvers with greater ease. Practical tips such as techniques for getting up from the floor after a fall or modified dressing skills also can be discussed. Active participation by the patient in a physical fitness program can encourage a sense of well-being and increase motivation and independence.

Surgery

Before the discovery of levodopa, surgical procedures were performed commonly in the treatment of Parkinson's disease. Stereotactic thalamotomies, for example, were performed to interrupt one or more of the neural pathways that produce parkinsonian symptoms, but sparing normal sensory and motor pathways. This procedure had several drawbacks, however. Often unilateral surgeries were only temporarily successful; as the disease progressed, symptoms reappeared on the contralateral side. Bilateral surgery often resulted in disturbances of speech and residual muscle weakness. Surgery rarely relieved bradykinesia, gait disturbances, postural abnormalities, or voice problems. Its main benefit was the eradication of tremor or mild rigidity in an upper limb and was therefore applicable only to patients in the early stages of the disease. Today, due to the success of L-dopa, surgical procedures are almost obsolete; those still performed are limited to patients with a unilateral tremor unresponsive to medication.

Activities of Daily Living Aids

Dressing becomes increasingly difficult for parkinsonian patients. Tremors, contractures, and dystonic posturing produce deformities and reduce dexterity. Bradykinesia further complicates the picture by increasing the amount of time required for the patient to dress. To simplify dressing routines, the patient's clothes should have velcro closures or zippers; or overhead shirts instead of buttoned garments should be worn. Large buttons can replace less manageable ones, and elastic shoe laces (which do not have to be tied and untied) and slip-on shoes make dressing easier and reduce dressing time.

Difficulties in eating and food preparation are a frequent cause of malnutrition and associated bowel problems. Patients should be urged to eat a well-balanced diet. High protein meals reduce the absorption of levodopa and may require dosage adjustments. Salt pills may be required by parkinsonians with hypotension. Fluids and roughage should be encouraged to reduce constipation, which is exacerbated by levodopa, and fruit juices, such as cranberry juice, may be beneficial in acidifying the urine to ward off urinary tract infections—especially important in older, more disabled patients. Vitamins may be taken to supplement regular meals, but vitamin B6 excesses are discouraged, as pyridoxine has been shown to interfere with the action of levodopa. This precaution is not necessary with Sinemet. Kitchen utensils should have large, comfortable handles. Foam rubber wrapped around knives and forks makes them easier to hold. Suction devices on the bottoms of cups, plates, or bowls, and lid-covered cups will help prevent spillage—a common problem due to tremors. Warming trays can be used to keep food warm for the slow eater. Patients who have difficulty swallowing should be told to eat slowly and take small amounts of food in each mouthful.

Ambulation can be improved in a number of ways. First, patients with shuffling gaits should be urged not to wear rubber-soled shoes, as they tend to stick to the ground and cause falls. Leather or hard-soled shoes should be worn instead. Patients with retropulsion problems may benefit from wearing heeled shoes; slippers, sandals, or other flat-soled footwear actually may encourage retropulsion. Weighted walkers or three-legged canes may prevent backward falling but are of most benefit for patients with weakness, balancing disturbances, or forward propulsion problems. Carrying a weighted bag such as a shopping bag while walking may help counteract the tendency to list to one side (lateropulsion).

Concentrating on walking patterns also helps to improve ambulation. With each step patients should practice lifting their toes and placing the heel of the foot down on the floor first as they walk. Concentrating on keeping their feet wide apart (12 to 15 inches) as they walk or turn also helps. Patients who freeze during ambulation should be encouraged to relax and try dorsiflexing their toes or shifting their weight to the opposite foot. Another trick to counteract freezing is to step backward first and then forward. Patients can practice many simple ambulation improvement techniques in their homes. One such technique is to place several sticks equidistant from each other on the floor. Patients should practice stepping over each one, trying to lift each foot high as they do. Other gait training and balancing exercises can be provided by a physiatrist or a physical therapist.

Bathrooms should be equipped with grab rails. A raised toilet seat will help the patient to stand more easily. As a safety precaution, stairways should be equipped with double handrails, when feasible. Since rising from a sitting position is difficult for many parkinsonians, patients should be advised against sitting in low, upholstered chairs; instead, straight-back wooden chairs should be used. Raising rear chair legs or shortening front legs 2 to 4 inches can help patients get out of a chair. In the bedroom, a firm mattress will enable the patient to turn more easily in bed and facilitate getting off the bed. A knotted rope tied to the foot of the bed can be used to pull the patient to a sitting position. Many books are available now suggesting home aids for the disabled. Local librarians or hospital occupational therapy departments can help patients in selection of appropriate literature.

Parkinson's Disease Organizations

In the current trend toward providing psychosocial support to patients with a variety of diseases, groups concerned with Parkinson's disease patients are well represented. Membership in support groups is comprised of patients, family members, and health practitioners who have an interest in or are concerned with research, education, financial support, and treatment interventions for patients with Parkinson's disease.

There are several national organizations that support these various aspects of Parkinson's disease. The Parkinson's Disease Foundation, 640 West 168th Street, New York, NY 10032, maintains a registry of Parkinson's patients and sponsors research on the cause, cure, and prevention of Parkinson's disease. The United Parkinson's Foundation, 220 South State Street, Chicago, IL 60604, a membership organization comprised of 10,000 patients, families, and medical practitioners, assists patients and families through medical referrals and education. The National Parkinson's Foundation, 1501 Ninth Avenue, Miami, FL 33136, provides diagnosis, treatment, rehabilitation, and educational programs for physicians, nurses, and patients and engages in research on Parkinson's disease. The American Parkinson's Disease Association, 116 John Street, New York, NY 10038, sponsors information and referral centers at leading university and hospital-affiliated centers. The latter organization also annually presents the Dr. George C. Cotzias Memorial Research Fellowship for research in Parkinson's disease.

Local support groups, branches of these national organizations, play a pivotal role by helping affected patients socialize with other persons with Parkinson's disease and by providing educational materials and forums on specific aspects of the disorder and ways to cope with them. Each group publishes a newsletter and can provide numerous references for information on symptoms, treatment, medication, rehabilitation modalities, and aids for daily living. Local support groups also contribute to efforts to sensitize the general public and health practitioners to needs and issues concerning Parkinson's disease patients and their families. These groups also strive to help families develop increased confidence and sensitivity and to play a more active role in the treatment of Parkinson's patients.

Summary

Parkinson's disease is a degenerative disorder affecting the basal ganglia and resulting in a chemical neurotransmitter imbalance. Clinical symptoms usually initiate between the ages of 50 and 65 years, primarily causing a disturbance of motor abilities and significant disability. Life expectancy is 20 to 25 years after onset of symptoms, however, and frequently many years elapse before patients experience serious incapacitation.

Parkinson's disease is generally classified into three categories: primary (the prototypic form), secondary (disorders involving diffuse central nervous system [CNS] involvement in addition to basal ganglia structures), and symptomatic (disorders that produce secondary symptoms simulating those of parkinsonism but not necessarily extrapyramidal in origin). A differential diagnosis is important when parkinsonian symptoms are observed, as drugs used to treat primary parkinson's disease may be ineffective or even contraindicated for other forms. Several other pathological states, including functional disorders, may have similar features and must be distinguished from actual Parkinson's disease.

Diagnosis of Parkinson's disease is dependent upon observation of a triad of characteristic signs which include resting tremor, bradykinesia, and rigidity. Although the combination of all three symptoms provides an almost unmistakable diagnosis of Parkinson's, occasionally one or two of the symptoms never develop. There are no laboratory tests to confirm the diagnosis, but a decreased level of homovanillic acid in a patient's cerebrospinal fluid and a decreased urinary excretion of free dopamine may support clinical evidence. Additional symptoms include urinary retention, constipation, autonomic dysfunctions, facial masking, micrographia, and postural and gait abnormalities. Parkinsonians develop a stooped posture, dystonic deformities, and a festinating gait, frequently accompanied by start hesitations. Primary parkinsonism follows a progressive course of disability, beginning with unilateral disturbances (usually tremor of an upper extremity) and terminating in complete invalidism.

There are no cures for Parkinson's disease. Treatment is based on providing maximal control of adverse symptoms and maintaining physical and mental functioning. The mainstay of therapy is pharmacological intervention. In early stages, anticholinergics, antihistamines and amantadine are the drugs of choice; as the disease becomes progressively disabling, L-dopa usually is prescribed to replenish the dopamine deficiency caused by an excessive degeneration of striatal dopaminergic neurons. L-dopa relieves all three cardinal symptoms to some degree and helps alleviate other physical and sensory complaints. In addition to drug therapy, counseling, physical therapy, speech and occupational therapy are employed. Many adaptive aids for the home and personal care can help the parkinsonian patient compensate for functional losses. Physicians play an important role in educating patients about the disease and encouraging them to continue to pursue active and meaningful lives.

References

1. Barbeau A, Roy M, Gonce M, Labreque R. Newer therapeutic approaches in Parkinson's disease. In Poirer LJ, Sourkes TL, Bedard PJ (eds): The Extrapyramidal System and Its Disorders. Advances In Neurology, Vol. 24. New York, Raven Press, 1979

2. Bauer RB, Stevens C, Reveno WS, Rosenbaum H: L-dopa treatment of Parkinson's disease: A ten year follow-up study. J Am Geriatr Soc 30 (5):322, 1982

3. Birkmayer W, Riederer P, Rausch WD: Neuropharmacological principles and problems of combined L-dopa treatment in Parkinson's disease. In Pirier LJ, Sourkes TL, Bedard PJ (eds): The Extrapyramidal System and Its Disorders. Advances in Neurology, Vol. 24. New York, Raven Press, 1979

4. Cailliet R: Rehabilitation in Parkinsonism. In Licht S (ed): Rehabilitation and Medicine. New Haven, Elizabeth Licht, 1968

5. Cooper IS: Involuntary Movement Disorders. New York, Harper & Row, 1969.

6. Corcoran PJ: Neuromuscular diseases. In Stolov WC, Clowers MR (eds): Handbook of Severe Disability. Washington, US Dept. of Education, Rehabilitation Services Administration, 1981

7. Dasmasio AR, Caldas AC: Neuropsychiatric aspects. In Stern G (ed): The Clinical Uses of Levodopa. Baltimore, University Park Press, 1975

8. Duvoisin R: Parkinsonism. "Parkinsonism." Clinical Symposia 28(1), New York, CIBA, 1976

9. Duvoisin R: Parkinson's Disease: A Guide for Patient and Family. New York, Raven Press, 1978

10. Erb E: Improving Speech in Parkinson's Disease. Am J Nurs 73:1910, 1973

11. Escourolle R, Poirier J: Manual of Basic Neuropathology. Philadelphia, WB Saunders, 1978

12. Gelbart AD, Hamilton, WJ: Parkinson's disease. Family Phys 23(6):182, 1981

13. Gersten JW: Rehabilitation for degenerative diseases of the central nervous system. In Kottke FJ, Stillwell GK, Lehmann JF (eds): Krusen's Handbook of Physical Medicine and Rehabilitation. Philadelphia, WB Saunders, 1982

14. Goldenson RM: Parkinson's disease. In Goldenson RM, Dunham JR, Dunham CS (eds): Disability and Rehabilitation Handbook. New York, McGraw–Hill, 1978

15. Kupersmith MJ, Shakin E, Siegel IM, Lieberman A: Visual system abnormalities in patients with Parkinson's disease. Arch Neurol 39(5):284, 1982

16. Lieberman AN et al: Bromocriptine and lergotrile: Comparative efficacy in Parkinson's disease. In Poirer LJ, Sourkes TL, Bedard PJ (eds): The Extrapyramidal System and its Disorders. Advances in Neurology, Vol. 24. New York, Raven Press, 1979

17. Marsden CD: Combined treatment with selective decarboxylase inhibitors. In Stern G (ed): The Clinical Uses of Levodopa. Baltimore, University Park Press, 1975

18. O'Connor AB: Nursing in Neurological Disorders. New York, American Journal of Nursing, 1976

19. Riley TL, Massey EW: Managing the patient with Parkinson's disease. Postgrad Med 68(3):85, 1980
20. Rusk HA: Rehabilitation Medicine. St Louis, CV Mosby, 1977
21. Schwab RS: Parkinson's disease: Symptoms and drug therapy. In Barbeau A, Doshay LJ, Spiegel EA (eds): Parkinson's Disease: Trends in Research and Treatment. New York, Grune & Stratton, 1965
22. Serby M: Psychiatric issues in Parkinson's disease. Compr Psych 21(4):317, 1980
23. Sroka C et al. Organic mental syndromes and confusional states in Parkinson's disease. Arch Neurol 38(6):339, 1981
24. Stewart RM: Parkinson's disease: New treatments. Compr Ther 7(4):38, 1981
25. Szekely BC, Kosanovich NN, Sheppard W: Adjunctive treatment in Parkinson's disease: Physical therapy and comprehension group therapy. Rehab Lit 43(3–4):72, 1982
26. Taylor JW, Ballenger S: Neurological Dysfunctions and Nursing Intervention. New York, McGraw–Hill, 1980
27. Yahr MD: The Parkinsonian syndrome. In Beeson PB, McDermott W (eds): Textbook of Medicine. Philadelphia, WB Saunders, 1975
28. Yahr MD: Early recognition of Parkinson's disease. Hosp Pract 16(17):65, 77, 1981

CHAPTER 11
Multiple Sclerosis (MS)

One of the gravest dangers facing the MS patient is ignorance concerning the nature of the disease, the complications that may arise and what can be done to combat them.[2]

The cause of multiple sclerosis (MS) is elusive, the course is unpredictable, and the cure is unknown. The most common disease affecting the central nervous system of young adults in the United States (several hundred thousand Americans have MS and closely related disorders), MS is characterized by disturbances of motor, sensory, and excretory functions. Clinical symptoms usually appear between the second and fourth decades of life; onset is rare before 15 years of age or after age 50. The ratio of women to men with multiple sclerosis is 3 to 2. Prevalence is highest in temperate zones with areas of high sanitation standards.

Although there are many theories about the cause of MS, none explains its etiology. MS is not an inherited disease but does tend to evidence familial occurrence. There is a 12- to 15-fold increased incidence of MS among first degree relatives of individuals with MS compared to the incidence in the population not related to an MS patient.[55] There is also a slightly elevated prevalence among monozygotic twins.[32] The unusual worldwide geographic pattern of MS (Fig. 11-1) may be due to genetic factors but is more likely indicative of an acquired exogenous disease resulting from exposure to an environmental factor during late childhood or adolescence.[11] Fischman[14] discusses the possibility that onset of the pathology in MS is dependent upon passing through puberty; this would explain why few cases are found under 15 years of age, and why females have an earlier age of onset than males. Many researchers believe that the disease is acquired before clinical onset of symptoms and that there is a long latency period. Current research suggests that MS is a disease of the immunological

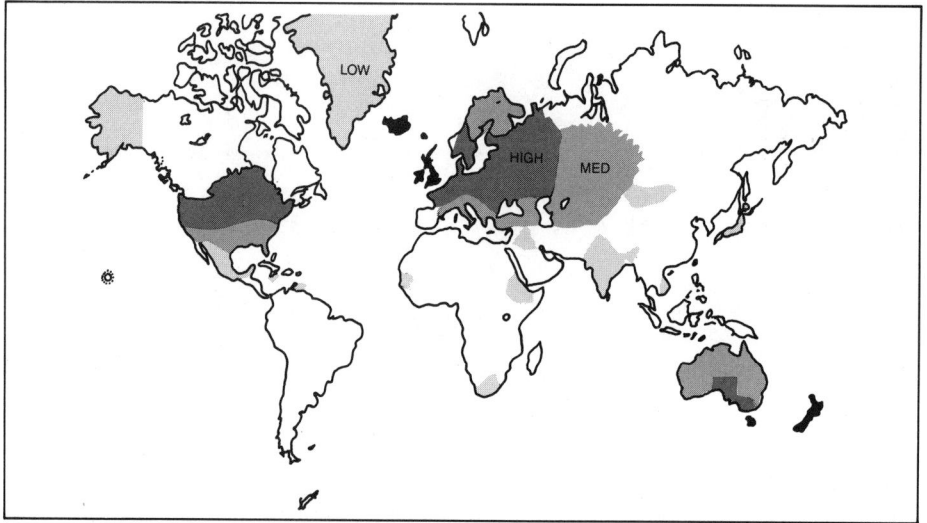

Figure 11-1. Worldwide distribution of MS according to high- (solid), medium- (dotted), and low- (diagonal dashed) risk areas as of 1974. The high-risk area of Europe may reach the head of the Adriatic Sea in the Balkans. (Kurtzke JF. Multiple sclerosis: An overview. In Rose FG (ed): Clinical Neuroepidemiology. London, Pitman Medical Publishers, 1980)

system and that the cause is either an infectious agent such as a virus or an autoimmune reaction, most likely involving myelin or its constituents.

Although the cause is unknown, the presenting pathology of MS has been well established. Multiple sclerosis is a demyelinating disease, characterized by circumscribed regions of myelin loss scattered throughout the white matter. The myelin is replaced by greyish translucent areas called "plaques," which eventually harden and form sclerotic tissue. The regions in which the plaque forms fail to maintain normal nerve conduction so that messages are distorted and blocked. Acute phases also normally involve inflammation around the blood vessels and swelling of the tissues.

Multiple sclerosis may affect any area of the central nervous system including the cortex, cerebellum, brain stem, or spinal cord; peripheral nerves, however, are spared. Clinical symptoms vary from individual to individual, depending on the area of the central nervous system affected by the plaques. Clinical deterioration is believed to be due either to the expansion of old lesions or to the formation of new ones. Functional deficits necessarily will be dependent upon the location and size of the areas of demyelination, as well as how critical these anatomical regions are for normal physical or mental functioning.

For example, a plaque as small as a few millimeters in the optic nerve may lead to a significant blind spot or scotoma, whereas a plaque several centimeters in diameter at the margin of one of the lateral ventricles in the brain may not cause a deficit detectable either by the individual or observers, including physicians.[42]

Course and Prognosis

The natural course of MS varies greatly from one patient to another, and even for any one patient at different times. Characteristic clinical courses that typify patients' experiences are acute (malignant), benign, progressive, and relapsing MS (Table 11-1).

Acute MS is a rare form, characterized by a rapid, progressive development of signs and symptoms, which can lead to death within months. Death is rarely a direct result of MS but rather the consequence of secondary complications, such as urinary tract infections or infected skin ulcers from pressure.

Benign MS, affecting approximately one third of MS patients, involves occasional acute phases followed by complete or nearly complete remissions. Persons with the benign form, although not necessarily symptom-free, are generally not restricted in their ADLs or employment performance and enjoy long periods of stability.

Progressive MS begins as a chronically progressive disease in 10% to 15% of cases. Patients become gradually more dysfunctional and remissions and relapses are no longer clear-cut. Steady progression from onset is more common among those acquiring MS after age 25 than among younger persons and is especially common in persons for whom onset occurred after age 40.[42] This form of MS very commonly evolves from a relapsing form, which is described below. The progressive form usually results in early severe disability within 2 to 10 years from onset.[25] Occasionally the progression is very slow, enabling the patient to retain a high level of functioning for many years.

The *relapsing* form, characterized by periods of acute exacerbations and remissions, is the most frequent course of MS. Characterized by sudden onset of neurological symptoms, which remit either partially or completely over a period of several days to several weeks, there is wide variation in the duration of acute bouts. Relapses occur an average of every 2 to 3 years but decrease in frequency as the disease increases in duration. Approximately 80% to 90% of patients follow the exacerbation–remission course during the first 10 to 20 years of illness; thereafter the course of the disease, for almost 60% is slowly progressive.[7]

According to Brown and colleagues,[7] prognosis for improvement following an acute exacerbation is related to the duration of the phase up to the time the patient is seen. Eighty-five percent of patients whose exacerbations last for 1 week or less are expected to improve; 50% of patients whose exacerbations continue for 1 month experience spontaneous improvement. Only 7% of patients whose functional deficits continue for 1 to 2 years are expected to show improve-

TABLE 11-1   Clinical Course of Multiple Sclerosis

Severe relapses, increasing disability, and early death
Many short attacks, tending to increase in duration and severity
Slow progression from onset, superimposed relapses, and increasing disability
Slow progression from onset without relapses
Abrupt onset with good remission followed by long latent phase.
Relapses of diminishing frequency and severity; slight residual disability only
Abrupt onset; few if any relapses after first year; no residual disability

(McAlpine D, Lumsden CE, Acheson EP: Multiple Sclerosis: A Reappraisal. Baltimore, Williams & Wilkins, 1972)

ment; no improvement is expected for patients who have had no remission for more than 2 years. Schneitzer[48] claims that the longer the interval between the initial attack and the first relapse, the better the prognosis. Monosymptomatic attacks, he adds, have a better prognosis than polysymptomatic ones. In addition, cranial nerve, visual, and sensory symptoms offer a better hope for remission or a benign course than motor or cerebellar symptoms. An acute onset of symptoms generally is associated with a better prognosis, less future disability, and a lower mortality rate[25] than an insidious onset. Kraft[25] points out that 3 to 5 years after diagnosis, when the disease course is established, patients at minimal or low disability levels tend to remain at those levels (with the exception of periods of acute exacerbations), whereas patients at higher disability levels tend to deteriorate. Approximately 75% of MS patients are expected to live 25 years or more after diagnosis (as compared with 85% of persons at a similar age without MS).[15] Two thirds of all MS patients who survive 25 years or more after their initial attack remain active and functioning.

Diagnosis

Diagnosis of multiple sclerosis is difficult. There is great variability in location of lesions and time intervals between acute attacks. The clinical features of MS are rarely identical for any two patients. There is not a single reliable diagnostic procedure to prove the existence of the disease. MS is usually classified in one of three categories of confidence: clinically definite, probable, or possible MS:[42]

Clinically Definite Multiple Sclerosis
1. Relapsing and remitting course, with at least two bouts separated by no less than 1 month
2. Slow or step-wise progressive course over at least 6 months
3. Documented neurologic signs attributable to more than one site of predominantly white matter CNS pathology
4. Onset of symptoms between ages of 10 and 50
5. No better neurologic explanation

Probable Multiple Sclerosis
1. History of relapsing and remitting symptoms, but without documentation of signs and presenting with only one neurologic sign commonly associated with MS
2. A documented single bout of symptoms with signs of multifocal white matter disease with good recovery, followed by variable symptoms and signs
3. No better neurologic explanation

Possible Multiple Sclerosis
1. History of relapsing and remitting symptoms, without documentation of signs
2. Objective neurologic signs insufficient to establish more than one site of central nervous system white matter pathology
3. No better neurologic explanation

The diagnosis of MS is dependent upon clinical criteria aimed at documenting the presence of multiple lesions in the CNS, specific episodes of neurological disturbances, and exclusion of other possible causes for the patient's signs and symptoms. By far the most important tool in establishing a diagnosis of MS is a thorough history and physical examination. Vague, recurring symptoms such as lack of energy, fatigue, depression, anxiety, and vague sensory complaints may precede the development of more specific neurological symptoms.[47] Infections reportedly precede the initial attack or a relapse in 40% of cases.[48] An important clue to diagnosis is the fact that neurological symptoms may worsen with overheating from any cause. Therefore, physicians should question patients about symptoms such as abnormal sensations, bladder problems, visual disturbances, and performance losses as accompaniments to episodes of overheating.

Although any area of the CNS may be involved, the optic nerve and chiasm, brainstem (especially medial longitudinal fasciculus), cerebellar white matter, and spinal cord frequently are affected. Table 11-2 lists some of the common symptoms and signs of suspected multiple sclerosis. Other premonitory signs are incoordination, dysarthria, spasticity, ataxia, slurred speech, intention tremors, extreme weakness, foot dragging, or staggering gait.

The great variability in sites of CNS involvement and temporal sequence of symptoms and signs, coupled with inconclusive laboratory diagnostic procedures, necessitates an appropriate differential diagnosis of MS and the exclusion of other disease states. It is especially important to rule out other disorders which, unlike MS, may be amenable to pharmacologic or therapeutic cures. Table 11-3 lists some diseases which should be considered when developing a differential diagnosis of MS. Table 11-4 lists some additional pathological states to be considered in developing a differential diagnosis of the progressive spinal cord form of MS (seen especially in older patients), which often mimics other diseases.

Although no laboratory tests provide a conclusive diagnosis for MS, certain tests may strengthen the clinical diagnosis. Analysis of the cerebrospinal fluid (CSF) may be a valuable diagnostic procedure, although it is used less with the availability of CT scanning. Any elevation in CSF pressure warrants consideration of other diagnoses.[53] CSF tests of importance include an evaluation of the

TABLE 11-2   Common Symptoms and Signs of Suspected Multiple Sclerosis

Symptoms	Signs
Blurred vision (hours–days)	Impaired visual acuity
Diplopia	Nystagmus
Vertigo or "labyrinthitis"	Color desaturation
Bandlike paresthesia	Internuclear ophthalmoplegia
Urinary retention	Marcus Gunn pupillary abnormality
Urinary urgency or eneuresis	Asymmetric, brisk tendon reflexes
Fecal incontinence	Babinski's signs
Impotence	Absent abdominal reflexes

(Reprinted from Hart RG, Sherman DG: The diagnosis of multiple sclerosis. JAMA 247(4):501, 1982)

TABLE 11-3 Differential Diagnosis of MS

Major Causes of Disease	Specific Disease Considerations
Congenital malformations	Platybasia
	Syringomyelia
	Arnold–Chiari
	Vertebral malformation
	Brain stem angioma
Hereditary	Hereditary ataxias
	Adrenal leukodystrophy
Inborn errors of metabolism	Wilson's disease
Vascular	Thrombosis
	Embolic infarction
	Brain stem infarction
	Cerebral vascular insufficiency, especially carotid-basilar
	(Hutchinson–Yates syndrome)
Nutritional	Vitamin B12 deficiency (subacute combined degeneration)
Neoplastic disorders	Pontine glioma
	Acoustic neurinoma
	Spinal cord tumors, especially at foramen magnum
	Metastatic disease
Bony mechanical entrapment	Cervical spondylosis
	Radiculopathy
	Cord compression
	Arterial compression
Infection and inflammation	CNS syphilis
	Arachnoiditis
	Subacute sclerosing panencephalitis (SSPE)
	Progressive rubella panencephalitis
	Progressive multifocal leukoencephalopathy
Postvaccinal and postinfectious syndromes	Postinfectious encephalomyelitis
	Postvaccinal encephalomyelitis
	Guillain–Barré syndrome
	Acute transverse myelitis
Autoimmune diseases	Systemic lupus erythematosus (SLE)
	Polyarteritis nodosa
	Temporal arteritis
Intoxication	Triorthocresylphosphate
	Alcoholism
Unknown	Amyotrophic lateral sclerosis (ALS)
	Primary lateral sclerosis
	Leber's optic atrophy
	Sporadic Schilder's disease
	Subacute necrotizing myelitis
Functional syndromes	May be present to some degree in all patients; occasionally symptoms may be secondary to CNS dysfunction

(Veterans' Administration: Multiple Sclerosis: Guidelines for Diagnosis and Management, Pub. No. 1B 11-70. VA Neurology Service, Washington, Department of Medicine and Surgery, 1980)

TABLE 11-4 Differential Diagnosis of Spinal Cord MS

Related to bone and joint pathology
  Cervical spondylosis (root entrapment, cord compression, vertebrobasilar insufficiency)
  Median herniation of cervical disc
  Odontoid process abnormalities
  Basilar impression
  Arnold–Chiari malformation
  Vertebral malformations (spina bifida or Klippel–Feil) with associated cervical spinal cord
    abnormalities
Tumor
  Meningioma
  Neurofibroma (neurolemmoma)
  Glioma
  Granuloma
  Metastasis
  Congenital extradural cyst
  Chordoma
  Cholesteatoma
  Multiple myeloma
  Lymphoma
  Arteriovenous malformation
Metabolic or toxic
  Subacute combined degeneration (vitamin B12 deficiency)
  Toxic (anticholinesterases, *e.g.,* triorthocresylphosphate
  [TOCP]
  Diabetic myelopathy
Transverse myelitis
  Viral myelitis
  Syphilis (Erb's spastic paraparesis)
  Arachnoiditis
    Postinfectious
    Postirritant
  Remote effect of cancer
  Idiopathic
Collagen diseases
  Polyarteritis
  Lupus erythematosus
Motor neuron disease

(Veteran's Administration: Multiple Sclerosis: Guidelines for Diagnosis and Management, Pub. No. 1B 11–70. VA Neurology Service, Washington, Department of Medicine and Surgery, 1980)

protein content, the number and types of white blood cells and the amount of IgG. CSF total protein is usually normal or slightly elevated.

Fragments of myelin can be detected in approximately 70% to 90% of MS patients by electromicroscopy or immunological methods. The myelin basic protein (MBP) increases transiently after acute episodes but returns to normal levels in the majority of patients within 1 to 2 weeks. Elevated levels of this protein also have been found in patients with CNS lupus, central pontine myelinolysis, CNS infarct, encephalitis, leukodystrophies, metabolic encephalopathies, and other conditions reflecting tissue destruction and active demyelination.[19,32]

Immunological studies, including variations in T and B cell distribution, may also be helpful. For example, the number of T cells remains unchanged during the long-term course of MS, but a slight decrease in the total number of T cells has been reported during acute exacerbations. Other reported histological changes include a decreased production of interferon by lymphocytes in response to viruses and an increase in antibody-dependent cellular toxicity.[32]

In nearly three quarters of patients with definite MS, the gamma globulin fraction of total CSF protein level is elevated more than 12% without any corresponding increase in serum gamma globulin.[1,19,32] Increased gamma globulin fractions, however, are not specific for MS and can be found, for example, in patients with neurosyphillis, acute Guillain–Barré syndrome, and several other neurological diseases, infections, or connective tissue disorders.[19,40] There is about a 40% to 60% correlation between elevated IgG amounts and a diagnosis of definite MS. Occasionally IgM and IgA also may be elevated. Approximately 90% of MS patients have oligoclonal bands, which can be measured by agar-gel electrophoresis methods. These are not used commonly in diagnostic testing, but will correctly identify more than 90% of patients with MS; unfortunately, as many as 16% may prove to be false negatives with this technique.[40]

Computerized tomography (CT) may be useful in identifying lesions in the white matter, many of which may be multiple and clinically silent. Routine use of the CT scan is not encouraged, however, because the test is expensive and has limited usefulness. Although the CT scan can demonstrate lesions in periventricular and subcortical areas, it is unable to reveal lesions in the optic nerves, brain stem, or spinal cord unless they are extremely large.[40] Most abnormalities identified by CT scan are found in patients with definite MS and are less likely to be identified in patients with early, nondisabling MS.[19] Poser[40] suggests that the CT scan be reserved for cases in which a mass lesion is a serious consideration in the differential diagnosis. The newer method of magnetic resonance imaging (MRI) promises to reveal smaller and earlier lesions than the CT scan is able to reveal.

Evoked potentials, recordings of the brain's electrical responses to sensory stimuli, provide another means for establishing the existence of multiple CNS lesions. The evoked responses measure the integrity of myelinated axons. In demyelinating diseases, transmission is slowed and the waveforms are distorted. Three types of stimuli are used clinically. *Visually evoked responses* (VER) test the optic nerves, tracts, lateral geniculate bodies, and optic radiations. These are abnormal in 42% of MS patients without visual symptoms and in almost all patients with a history of visual symptoms.[26] *Brain stem auditory evoked responses* (BAER) test the integrity of the cochlear nuclei and auditory pathways in the brain stem. These results are abnormal in 37% of MS patients with symptoms or signs of brain lesions and 21% of MS patients without them.[26] Even minute MS plaques can cause a marked conduction abnormality. *Somatosensory evoked potentials* (SEP) evaluate the dorsal column pathway, thalamus, and corticosensory relay paths. They are abnormal in more than half of MS patients, including those having no clinical signs of sensory loss.[26]

Clinical procedures also can be used to support suspected diagnoses. Poser[40] describes two standard diagnostic procedures—the test for color blindness and the "hot bath" test. Special color blindness testing (*e.g.,* using pseudoisochromatic plates) may elucidate a subclinical optic neuropathy caused by a lesion of the optic nerve, even when visual acuity has not been affected.

Sometimes this test is useful in detecting a second site of lesions for confirmation of the MS diagnosis when clinically observable signs are absent. The hot bath test requires that the patient be in a bath at 40°C. Because MS symptoms often increase with heat, symptoms not previously present may appear, including visual impairment, weakness, paresthesia, reflex changes, and so on. The signs or symptoms quickly disappear as soon as the patient cools, so the test is reportedly harmless. This test does not assist the evaluator diagnostically. Rather it is useful only in demonstrating additional lesions. Increasing severity of already established symptoms may be experienced in neurological disorders other than MS.

Lhermitte's sign (also known as the "electric sign") is most commonly caused by MS, although it can occur in other conditions affecting the cervical cord such as cervical spondylosis, tumor, and trauma. This symptom, produced by active or passive flexion of the neck, is usually described by patients as an electric feeling, a "tingling" or a "vibration." The feeling is usually fleeting and does not occur upon repeated flexion of the neck. Frequently the abnormal sensation is referred down the back, and occasionally in the legs or front of the thighs; rarely, the patient feels it traveling from the trunk to the upper arms, or as an electric jolt from the toes to the head.[31] Lhermitte's sign possibly may be caused by a lesion of the cervical region of the cord causing segmental paresthesia when the neck is flexed[31] or increased mechanosensitivity of damaged axons.[54]

Sensory signs also may signal MS lesions. Earliest changes usually involve superficial sensation, but eventually two-point discrimination, vibration sensation, and postural sensation also may become impaired and spread over increasingly wider areas. These are examples of some of the clinical examinations that may be used to support a suspected diagnosis of multiple sclerosis. Continued observation and use of certain ancillary procedures may be necessary before a final diagnosis is established.

Mental Alterations

Mental alterations are known to occur, but the specific types of intellectual and cognitive deficits associated with MS vary from individual to individual, since the lesions are usually scattered and diffuse rather than discrete and focal as in stroke. Not all patients experience intellectual deterioration. Although there is not objective evidence to support such a conclusion, it is estimated that approximately 25% to 35% of people with MS experience some degree of cognitive deficit. Values as high as 75% have been reported.[23] Although cognitive deficit may progress (even when motor incapacities stabilize), only a small percentage of MS patients reach a stage of profound deterioration. In fact, the relatively low incidence, frequently late onset, and minimal severity may account for the finding that changes in the intellectual state are less critical than many other symptoms of MS.

Marsh[29] found that the severity of neuropsychological impairment is associated with duration but not with degree of physical disability, age of the patient, age of onset of symptoms, or verbal performance or full-scale IQ. Other authors concur that with increasing duration intellectual deterioration becomes more common and more severe. The most frequent intellectual impairment involves learning new information or new skills. Tasks with a motor component, especially those involving hand–eye coordination, frequently are affected. Short-term memory losses also are common. In some patients attention and concentration also may be impaired, but verbal concepts and numerical reasoning normally remain intact.

Because many lesions in the CNS may be of the silent type, and because cognitive impairment may not be obvious even to the patient, routine systematic evaluation of intellectual functioning may help detect early cognitive changes. Family members may report the patient's tendency to forget names, phone numbers, and everyday facts, alerting the physician to the need to evaluate mental status. Mental changes may help in the early identification of a "probable" or "definite" diagnosis of MS. Peyser and colleagues[39] suggest routine specialized psychological testing as part of the diagnostic evaluation of all patients suspected of having MS. The primary care physician routinely should perform at least a mental status examination by assessing memory, concentration, abstract reasoning, judgment, and orientation in all patients suspected or known to have MS. Anxiety and depression are common in patients with MS. The clinician therefore must be cautious about identifying changes of mental status as evidence of intellectual loss.

Psychosocial Implications of Multiple Sclerosis

Persons with MS are faced with a progressive course of deterioration of functional capacities. They must deal not only with physical changes, but also with alterations in social and psychological domains as well. Physicians' attitudes toward treatment have been shown to play a significant role in patients' acceptance of their illness and their interaction with others. MS strikes in the prime of life when a person has completed his education and has begun to assume responsibilities and to establish roles as spouse, parent, homemaker, breadwinner, and so on. By the time the MS symptoms occur, the patient is likely to have already established an identity as a "healthy, normal person." After the initial attack and before a final diagnosis is reached, many patients suffer from acute anxiety and psychological stress. Uncertainty about the disease and its course inhibits adjustment. Fear, resulting from not knowing what to expect next, may be so intense that some patients actually are relieved once the diagnosis is finally made. Afterwards, however, normally they have feelings of loss, confusion, depression, shock, and disbelief. Negative attitudes or preconceived notions about deformed or disabled individuals may already be engrained, adding to patients' difficulty in accepting the diagnosis.

Matson and Brooks[30] suggest that MS patients, as is true of patients with terminal illnesses, may experience a series of stages that include denial, resistance, affirmation, and integration, each of which will be described. Many patients in the *denial* phase avoid contact with other persons with MS or other disabilities, try to conceal their symptoms, and resist any change in normal activities. Patients become vulnerable and may go from physician to physician seeking a cure. Some amount of denial, however, may be helpful in preventing a patient from adopting an image of an invalid.

For many years hysteria was considered to be the emotional hallmark of individuals with MS, since lability may lead to poorly controlled outward expressions of emotion such as laughter. However, some early signs of MS (e.g., parasthesia, weakness, visual impairments) may be mistaken for symptoms of hysteria. Current literature suggests that, contrary to old beliefs, depression is far more common than hysteria. In a large number of cases, especially during the early stages of the disease, depressive states may predominate. In a study by Whitlock and Siskind,[56] MS patients were significantly more depressed than a group of control patients suffering from a variety of chronic neurologic syndromes matched for age, sex, and degree of disability. The depression is usually amenable to counseling efforts and group therapy. Physicians must be sensitive to the emotional significance of the illness.

The *resistance* stage is characterized by attempts to gain control over the disease. During this period, the patient seeks information about the disease and cures and even may be interested in contacting other people with MS to improve understanding of the disease and its progressive tendencies. It is very important that the physician tell patients of the diagnosis, when known, and teach them and their families as much as possible about the disease. Some physicians tend to be protective and to be unwilling to expose the patient to all that is known about a disease, which may prevent the patient from making a successful adjustment. Such an approach establishes a patient–physician relationship based on dependence, which may erode the patient's sense of self-control.

The alternative approach, which we recommend, requires that the physician promote a healthy optimism, stressing problems associated with MS that are preventable (e.g., overfatigue, overheating, and unresolved stress-provoking circumstances) or are treatable (e.g., bladder function and vocational disability). Since stress can accentuate the symptoms of MS, the diagnosis should be imparted with tact and sensitivity and without judgments as to the long-term course of the illness.

People who have MS must learn a lot about their symptoms. They must understand which ones are caused by demyelination and which may represent signs of other disorders. They must be able to differentiate side effects of drugs from symptoms of disease and know which side effects are expected as opposed to ones that require a change of drug or dosage. They must learn when they can manage their symptoms independently and when assistance from medical personnel is needed. They also need to know the pattern that their symptoms follow and whether new symptoms are appearing. Life styles may need redesigning in order to manage symptoms effectively.[9]

Affirmation involves confronting the fact that one has the illness and that changes will have to be made in previously established lifestyles. A patient may grieve for the former active and independent self during this stage but, eventually, integrates a new self-image as a person with MS. He may discuss more or less freely the disease with nonaffected persons. A number of factors may affect a patient's psychological and behavioral reactions to MS and therefore the ability to confront the illness. These factors include:[2]

- The nature and extent of dysfunction due to organic lesions in the CNS
- The severity of disability and its impact on life situations
- The patient's ability to adapt to his handicaps
- The premorbid personality

Miles[33] studied the psychosocial consequences for married couples when one of the partners has MS and examined the couple's mode of interaction with healthy people. According to Miles, persons with MS have two choices. If they choose *normalization,* they try to carry out their relationships with others based on pre-illness patterns and make no attempt to hide or disguise their symptoms, but determine instead to underemphasize them. If they choose *dissociation,* they turn away from former associates in an attempt to avoid the risk of being treated differently. Commonly both patient and spouse choose similar means of interaction. An interesting finding in this study was that nearly three fourths of those who chose the dissociation pattern claimed to receive no treatment for their MS or to have been told by their physicians that no therapeutic measures were possible. On the other hand, of those receiving physical therapy, occupational therapy, medication, testing, or diet regimens, two thirds chose normalization. These contrasting patterns of behavior suggest the *significant role physicians may play* in helping a patient assume a healthy outlook toward this disease.

Integration frequently takes a relatively long time to achieve, and it must be re-established after each exacerbation. The typical pattern of exacerbations and remissions, coupled with variable and unpredictable periods between attacks, requires the patient to adjust to the uncertainties of the disease and to cope with additional limitations as the disease progresses. During this stage the patient focuses less attention on the disease and more attention on matters other than illness and disability. Value systems may be reorganized as the patient acknowledges having MS. Some persons even may find an increased appreciation of life.

The physician can help the person make the transition from diagnosis to integration. Dependency and hostility are common. Some patients may use the diagnosis of MS as a means of perpetuating a sick role, even if symptoms do not warrant this attitude. Physicians should challenge patients with short-term tasks designed to keep them mobile as long as possible and that they can master. Relationships with people other than family should be encouraged. The patient should be made aware of community resources that offer support and practical aid. Referral to a local chapter of the National Multiple Sclerosis Society (205 E. 42nd Street, New York, NY 10017) can be invaluable. The Society publishes information for patients and their families and keeps them informed about new developments in research and treatment. It also provides numerous other services, including a course to teach friends and relatives to improve care at home, and equipment, supplies, and aids to perform daily living tasks. The MS Society also sponsors public education programs and offers social activities. The physician should encourage the patient to contact the Society and should inform the patient of any local chapters in the community. At all times physicians should assess the psychosocial state of the patient and should determine its role in promoting disability or interfering with the performance of daily activities.

Management of the Person With MS

The goals of a functionally oriented treatment program for MS should include the preservation of physical capacity, the prevention of complications, reduction in pain or discomfort, retention of optimal functional abilities (including utilization of body functions not yet affected, as well as compensation for deficits already present) and prevention of physiological and psychological deterioration. Functional capacities may be threatened by weakness, spasticity, incoordination, sensory deficits, and bowel and bladder disturbances. In addition to symptomatic treatment, supportive care plans should assure that the patient maintains good nutrition, gets adequate rest, and receives assistance with vocational and household management. Patients should be helped to establish a life pattern within the confines of their disability.

Granger found, in assessing 39 MS patients, that 41% had problems with self-care, 46% had problems with mobility, 55% had difficulty with control of bowel and bladder functions, 72% had limited use of transportation resources, 54% had reduced social activities, and more than 35% experienced depression or agitation.[17] Thus intervention planning for the MS patient must address not only medical issues but ones of transportation, recreation, social life, and vocation. A method of comprehensive assessment and an interdisciplinary approach to treatment are necessary to do so.

Graded assessments of functional abilities are helpful in pinpointing specific problems (thus assisting in a positive diagnosis of MS) and in designing treatment plans. According to Bauer,[2] an MS patient's ability to perform ADLs is most often limited by spastic paraparesis, followed by coordination disturbances, sphincter problems, cranial nerve impairments, sensation changes, and mental changes. Visual disturbances may also threaten performance. Rehabilitation measures should be based on the type of disease course and the current level of functioning. Patients with a benign course, for example, are likely to remain relatively stable and experience only minimal disability. Therefore they are good candidates for long-term training and vocational development programs. On the other hand, patients with a progressive form of MS would be better suited to a short-term training program that emphasizes adaptive devices, home services, and personal and financial counseling. In such cases the patient can be trained to be the homemaker, allowing the spouse to work. The majority of patients whose disease takes the exacerbation–remission course may find that with successive acute exacerbations previous levels of vocational skills are not retained. Therefore it may be important to establish vocational skill training that is adaptable to increasing disability. Patients should be given definite return visits for re-examination, education, counseling, detection of complications, and therapy. The use of the FASQ during visits should help clarify the current physical status of the patient and reveal the progressive state of the disease. It is important to keep in mind that MS patients are not immune to other diseases and that not all medical problems can be directly attributed to the MS illness. The mainstays of MS management include health maintenance, physical therapy, pharmacological intervention, and counseling.

Health Maintenance

Bedrest was the former prototypical treatment mode for acute exacerbations. Its efficacy has never been demonstrated, however, and it should be used only to avoid overfatigue. Often patients are admitted to an acute-care hospital for corticosteroid and adrenocorticotrophic hormone (ACTH) therapy, although hospitalization may not be required with less severe flareups. Graded activities should begin as soon as possible.

Onset or relapse of the disease is often due to one or more of the following:

- Increased body temperature (look for inapparent infection, *e.g.,* bladder)
- Emotional stress
- Overexertion or fatigue
- Trauma
- Immunization or surgical procedures

Physicians should discuss circumstances at work or home that might give rise to tension and suggest ways in which these can be lessened. When causes of anxiety are not clearcut, a psychologist or psychiatrist should be consulted. Poser[41] described a phenomenon of "psychologically-induced symptom recall," which may be responsible for the return of symptoms during emotional stress, physical trauma, pregnancy, intercurrent illness, or excessive fatigue.

Patients should be urged to pursue jobs that avoid or minimize the need for highly precise manual dexterity, physical exertion, tension, or demanding deadlines. Indoor jobs are preferable to outdoor ones in order to avoid temperature extremes. Short, multiple work periods are desirable; when this is not possible, the patient should take occasional short, scheduled rest periods. Patients should be cautioned against taking very hot showers or baths or swimming in heated swimming pools. Prolonged exposure to the sun also should be avoided and air conditioning should be used at home and in automobiles on hot days, whenever possible. Cool baths and jackets with pockets for carrying ice packs may decrease spasticity. Social activities that afford satisfaction and decrease anxiety levels should be encouraged.

Although reports conflict, pregnancy is not believed to affect adversely the course of MS. In some cases symptoms are accentuated during pregnancy or following birth, but it is not known whether this is due to the effect of pregnancy on the body, the emotional reaction of the patient to her pregnancy, or other factors. "Advice regarding the prevention or termination of pregnancy must be based solely on the patient's desire to have children and her ability to care for the newborn child."[41] Counseling regarding present and future aspects of parenting may be helpful in making a decision. Automatic sterilizations, as performed in past years, are unwarranted unless specifically desired by the patient.

Although no dietary management program is believed to affect the course of MS, diet programs may be of great assistance in preventing obesity, alleviating constipation, minimizing incontinence or nocturia, and controlling urinary tract infection. For example, constipation can be prevented through the ingestion of bran cereals, adequate water intake, and prune juice. Urinary tract infections can be minimized by maintaining an acid urine through consuming large amounts of cranberry juice, plums, prunes, and vitamin C; additionally decreased water intake at night may lessen nocturnal urges. A balanced diet should assist the patient in maintaining a sense of well-being.

Physical disabilities may prevent the patient from eating or drinking normally and may potentiate a nutritional or vitamin deficiency. A good daily multivitamin helps prevent complications due to vitamin deficiencies. Physicians should inquire routinely about an MS patient's dietary intake, especially as the disease progresses.

The MS Diet Book, by Roy Swank,[52] contains recipes, menus, and a diet based on limited fat intake. It is considered a healthy diet for MS patients, but its claims of preventing the negative course of the disease have not been proved.[49] The National MS Society distributes a booklet entitled *Nutrition and MS,* which is available upon request at no cost.

Sensory deficits may take the form of numbness, pain, paresthesia, or distortion of superficial sensations. Patients should be urged to take precautions to avoid injury, burns, or frostbite due to impaired sensations. Diminished sensory awareness, coupled with reduced mobility, potentiates dangerous skin breakdowns due to continuous pressure on the sacrum, buttocks, and heels in bedridden or wheelchair reliant individuals. Bed sores are a common cause of death in MS patients[31] and are therefore an important point of concern. (Tips for preventing decubitus ulcers are given in Chapter 9.) As a general rule, the longer the bedridden stage of the disease can be postponed, the less risk there will be of bed sores and urinary complications.

Physical Therapy

Physical therapy is an extremely important adjunct to case management of the MS patient. It should begin early in the disease when symptoms are minimal and be maintained continuously throughout the course of the disease, except during periods of acute exacerbations. Physical therapy is used in MS to increase muscle strength, improve coordination, improve and maintain motion of the joints, prevent contractures, assist in maximizing ambulation and transfer skills, and augment general health through a sense of physical and mental well-being. Exercise and other physical modalities will not return abilities lost because of pathological lesions but may help prevent weakness and contractures due to disuse accompanying motor loss. Physical therapy even has been said to delay the rate of deterioration, particularly in patients with the insidious progressive form of MS, although documentation is difficult.[8]

Spasticity, found in 90% to 95% of all patients during the course of the disease,[2,13] usually is severe in advanced stages. The spasticity is characterized by stiffness of extremities and hyperreflexia and may cause difficulties in walking or using the hands, even when normal muscle strength is present. Spasticity usually is combined with weakness of the antagonistic muscle group and progressive tightening of muscles and shortening of tendons, leading to decreased mobility and contractures. Spasticity often interferes with employment, sexual functioning, and hygiene. Sudden spontaneous contractures of the lower extremities are common during the night, disturbing sleep and increasing fatigue. Increased reflex spasms and increased muscle tone may present additional coordination problems.

Physical therapy maneuvers may significantly improve problems of spasticity. Daily passive stretching and active ROM help maintain strength and prevent loss of motion. Stretching exercises should be taught by an experienced therapist. Proper positioning in bed and relaxation exercises can also help. Ice packs are beneficial in reducing spasticity. In addition to physical therapy, antispasmodics such as baclofen are commonly used. Temporary relief may be available through nerve or motorpoint phenol injections. For severe spasticity that does not respond to medical treatment, surgical manipulations including the cutting of nerves (neurotomy) and the cutting of the spinal cord (myelotomy) may be considered. Brown and colleagues caution against such drastic procedures, however, unless the spasticity is extreme and has been present more than 2 years to be certain a remission will not occur.

Weakness, another bothersome symptom impairing motor function, may be present in varying degrees, from a feeling of "heaviness" to quadriplegia. Weakness also may be the result of fatigue or overuse of muscle relaxants, and it may vary from one muscle group to another and affect different muscle groups during different relapses and remissions. The imbalance between weak and strong muscles further limits mobility and contributes to a loss of joint motion and to deformity. Splints and orthotic devices may be prescribed to assist in activity or to prevent contractures. Physical therapy exercises and instruction can help to increase muscle power, to prevent further weakness because of disuse, and can help in technical training for use of mechanical aids and orthotics. Walking, swimming, and bicycling are excellent exercises for improving muscle weakness and cardiovascular capacities.

Ataxia, incoordination, and intention tremors occur not only in the extremities but also in the trunk. These symptoms are resistant to correction and are the most difficult to manage. Treatment, therefore, must focus on learning compensatory techniques. For example, weighted canes may help stabilize ataxic gaits. Weights can be placed on a variety of assistive devices or directly on extremities to decrease the velocity of the tremor and to increase stability. The use of weighted devices must be monitored, however; any increased fatigue is a signal to remove the weights.[35] Repetitive weight-bearing exercise may improve coordination in ataxic patients. According to Minkwitz,[35] techniques that facilitate contraction at proximal joints will improve stability during walking, transfer maneuvers, and neurodevelopmental sequencing.

A variety of physical activities serving different purposes are advocated for treating patients with MS, including active exercises for general conditioning, restorative exercises for specific deficits, and stretching exercises for relaxation and reduction of spasticity.[7] The most frequently suitable exercise for the patient with MS consists of an active muscle contraction that carries the affected joint through the full range of motion against low or moderate resistance. The movement should be repeated often enough to assure sustained endurance without causing overfatigue. For maximum benefit, the patient should expend active effort.

Health-care professionals have long been aware of the possible harmful effects of fatigue on the MS patient. Nonetheless, it may take considerable clinical judgment to decide whether fatigue is due more to physiological factors or to psychological ones. If the cause is largely psychological, more exercise is encouraged. If, on the other hand, the cause is primarily increased body temperature (*e.g.*, due to overexposure to the sun or use of heat in a physical therapy program), the patient may need to rest more frequently. Elevation of body temperature can produce a feeling of weakness or distress or a worsening of the patient's symptoms; it may even reveal subclinical deficits not previously apparent. Unduly subjecting the patient with MS to warm environments should be avoided.

Listed below are some points to remember when prescribing exercise. Patients should:

- Exercise in a relatively cool area
- Avoid fatigue by dividing the exercise period into several short daily sessions
- Make movements as smoothly and as completely through the range of motion as possible
- Avoid exercise that consistently causes pain or discomfort
- Stop if any unfavorable change occurs, such as progressive weakening or an acute exacerbation, and consult the physician

Pharmacologic Intervention

Although drug therapies may shorten the period of an acute exacerbation or decrease its severity, they have no proven effect on the long-term course of the illness. The two major types of drugs used in MS are ACTH and corticosteroids, both of which act as anti-inflammatory and immunosupressive agents. ACTH is believed to offer favorable results during exacerbations by decreasing the cellular response to antigen, offering anti-inflammatory and anti-edematous properties and stabilizing the basal membranes of blood vessels. Drug treatments usually are prescribed only on a short-term basis. Long-term drug courses have been reported, but there is not evidence to support claims of decreasing the frequency of relapses nor of slowing progression. Occasionally these drugs are alternated on a daily basis with synthetic adrenal glucocorticoids such as prednisone and prednisolone for severe cases in which a relapse occurs shortly after stopping short-term therapy. The synthetic adrenal glucocorticoids may decrease some of the undesirable effects of the ACTH or corticosteroids. This mode of therapy is still being investigated.

Some commonly used agents for symptomatic control include diazepam (Valium), which is believed to suppress brain and spinal cord multisynaptic reflexes and regulate muscle tension, baclofen (Lioresal), which has a similar effect at the spinal cord level, and dantrolene sodium, which affects calcium flux within the muscle cell and decreases the strength of the muscle contraction. Baclofen is widely used for decreasing spasticity. It significantly reduces painful spasms, uninhibited clonus, and severe adductor spasms that affect bowel and bladder care. It is effective and not very toxic in appropriate dosage strengths.[7]

Drug therapies must be regulated carefully, as complications include psychosis, infections, metabolic abnormalities, diabetes, "moon" face, exhaustion, negative disease course, increased weakness, and hypersensitive reactions, to name a few. Clinical evaluation of antispastic drugs is difficult because of the enormous range and variability in symptoms and signs of disease in different patients. Whenever feasible, patients should be urged to participate in determining adjustments in dosage levels of medication so that they feel in control and are more likely to comply, thus facilitating desired results.

Bladder

"More than 50% of MS patients will develop problems with bladder function during the first 5 to 10 years after diagnosis."[27] Also urinary bladder symptoms account for up to three fourths of morbidity in multiple sclerosis.[4] For many patients, this problem is the most disabling aspect of MS. Urinary frequency, urgency, and incontinence problems may result in loss of opportunities for work, recreation, and social life, and encourage the individual to become housebound. Bladder dysfunction in MS patients is normally due either to detrusor hyperreflexia (increased, inappropriate bladder muscle contraction) or resistance to outflow at the sphincter, with or without a flaccid bladder.

Early in the disease course most patients have detrusor hyperreflexia due to lesions high in the spinal cord. This condition is characterized by a sense of urgency, incontinence, or nocturia, with small amounts of accumulated urine eliminated. Since the patient is unable to coordinate contraction of the bladder, urine leakage can occur. Additionally, the bladder does not empty completely because of an inability to control the sphincter muscle. The retained urine is a medium for bacterial growth and recurrent urinary tract infections.

Treatment of spastic bladder may include anticholinergic medications, such as baclofen and Texas condoms for males. Indwelling catheters are used, if necessary, for females, but they perpetuate infections; therefore, intermittent catheterization is often the preferred mode. Self-catheterization is a technique generally taught to the patient provided there is adequate vision and manual dexterity. Urinary urgency and frequency often can be satisfactorily remedied with parasympatholytic drugs such as oxybutynin or propantheline, appropriately given when the patient wants to be independent (shopping, traveling, going to the movies, and so on).[41] Acidification of the urine by high intake of cranberry juice or high doses of ascorbic acid is relied on less than it used to be as a means of preventing urinary tract infections. A flaccid or hypotonic bladder may result from chronic overdistention of the bladder and should be avoided by appropriate early care of bladder emptying. Residual urine should be emptied by self-catherization rather than through the Credé maneuver or straining.

Bowel

Bowel dysfunction, secondary to spinal cord disease, may manifest with incontinence or constipation. Constipation, a major problem in over 50% of patients with MS,[38] is aggravated by medications that reduce bladder hypertonicity, but which also decrease bowel activity. Bowel disturbances are managed by encouraging adequate fluid intake, a dict rich in bran or other fibers, and use of stool softeners. Scheduled bowel training may be indicated.

Counseling

Counseling should focus on helping the patient to adapt to this unpredictable, progressive disease. The psychological impact, necessary vocational and home modifications, and changes in self-image and family roles must be subjects of counseling. MS is particularly stressful because patients face a prospect of progressive deterioration. It is no surprise that there is a high rate of divorce among patients with MS. Since emotional stress frequently aggravates the disease, counseling must be provided early to identify and overcome causes of stress.

Counselors, in conjunction with physical or occupational therapists, should help the patient accentuate abilities rather than disabilities. The patient can be helped to increase functional capacity. For example, a weighted cane or brace may help those with incoordination; weighted bracelets on the wrists may decrease incoordination in the upper extremities; weighted eating utensils may help in increasing independence in self-care. A ramp can be used instead of steps, and a stool can be placed in the shower (for those with intact balance and muscle strength). Buttons and hooks and eyes can be replaced by zipper fasteners on clothes, and furniture can be arranged to enable the patient to reach shelves or countertops. Widened doorways will provide greater wheelchair access. Many specially designed kitchen devices and aids for daily living are now available. Informing the patient of these simple environmental modifications may avert feelings of hopelessness or the perpetuation of the sick role.

Sexuality, a common problem of MS patients, usually is not discussed. In a 1976 survey of 306 MS patients, 91% of the men and 77% of the women reported a changed sexual life; nearly 50% reported unsatisfactory or discontinued sexual activity.[28] Many factors contribute to a less than satisfactory sexual life for the person with MS. Males may experience difficulty attaining an erection or ejaculating. Females often complain of decreased vaginal lubrication. Both sexes may suffer from decreased sensation and inability to achieve orgasm, resulting in diminished pleasure in lovemaking. A decreased libido coupled with easy fatigue may cause infrequent activity. Significant physical problems may further complicate sexual activity—weakness, contractions, and spasticity may limit positions or movements. Catheters, incontinence, frequent urinary tract infections, and decubiti may further inhibit sexual activity.

Psychosocial factors play an important part in a satisfactory sexual life. Decreased mobility, job loss, or self-consciousness may potentiate social isolation and limit the availability of sexual partners. Dependency and reversal of roles within a marriage may affect sexual relations, causing anxiety, insecurity about performance, and frustration. Feelings of guilt, anger, and depression can involve both social and physical relationships.

Management should be directed toward alleviation of as many physical problems as possible along with counseling to facilitate adjustment. Specific aids include penile prostheses, lubricating jellies, and antispasmodic drugs. Convenient and safe contraceptive methods should be prescribed. Insertion methods, such as a diaphragm, may be difficult for some MS patients to handle, and IUDs are contraindicated for women with impaired pelvic sensation. Other general management programs such as exercise, improved personal hygiene, care of pressure sores, and so on, can lessen some of the deterrents to satisfactory sexual activity. Counseling should deal with sexual options, improving communication between partners, and decreasing negative feelings. Since many MS patients may be reluctant to initiate the topic, physicians should question them about this special area. Open communication and a supportive demeanor by physicians and other health professionals will enable patients to discuss serious sexual problems as they arise. Family members must not be forgotten in counseling efforts.

> The person on whom the care of the patient mainly falls can be helped by being told that it is reasonable to want and to have a life of one's own without feeling guilty—that one does not have to sacrifice oneself, one's job, and self-fulfillment for the exclusive care of the patient. The physician should realize that not everybody is able or willing to accept the full-time care of a chronically ill patient. The physician should evaluate the personalities of the patient and of the responsible relative and their relationship to each other. The total home situation should be considered. In consultation with the family, the nurse, and the social worker, a decision should be made as to whether the patient can best be taken care of at home or whether he or she would be better cared for in an institution.[53]

A good review of the subject of therapy modes commonly used by MS patients can be found in the book *Therapeutic Claims in Multiple Sclerosis,*[7] published under the auspices of the International Federation of Multiple Sclerosis Societies.

> The single most important element in the long-term treatment of MS is the physician's attitude. Although it is important to involve physiotherapists, social workers, and other paramedical personnel in the treatment program, the patient must be able to retain close contact with the physician and should be assured of the continued support by and interest of the physician. Careful monitoring and immediate treatment of problems ranging from minor infections and water, electrolyte, and calcium metabolic alterations to decubiti and psychologic problems will lead to normalization of the patient's life and may actually retard the progression of the neurologic deficit.[41]

Summary

Multiple sclerosis is a chronic, disabling neurological disease, the cause and cure of which remain undiscovered. Clinical symptoms appear usually between the second and fourth decades of life, causing disturbances of motor, sensory, and excretory functions. MS, a demyelinating disorder that affects all parts of the central nervous system, is characterized by circumscribed areas of myelin loss, which are replaced by translucent plaques. The plaques harden forming sclerotic tissue that interferes with normal nerve conduction, distorting and blocking messages. Clinical symptoms vary from person to person depending on the size and location of demyelinated areas.

Although the clinical course varies, the four general patterns include: acute (rapid deterioration leading to death within months), benign (one or more mild bouts with relatively little resulting disability), progressive (continuous, gradual incapacitation) and exacerbation–remission (acute bouts followed by remission periods lasting 2 to 3 years resulting in variable disability). The latter course is the most common.

There is no single diagnostic test of multiple sclerosis. A definite diagnosis is dependent upon demonstrating multiple CNS lesions, separate episodes of neurological disturbances, and exclusion of other causes. Analysis of CSF for pressure, protein, and immunological factors can help support objective observations. Although the "hot bath" test is not recommended, other clinical techniques such as color blindness analysis and examination for Lhermitte's sign and sensory impairments are additional diagnostic aids, but none are exclusively typical of MS. A thorough history and physical examination are the major bases on which diagnosis depends.

Because of MS's variable and unpredictable course, coupled with the fact that it may take many years to establish a positive diagnosis, MS patients usually experience feelings of uncertainty, depression, and emotional distress. Aside from coping with the realization of eventual progressive deterioration of functional abilities, patients must deal with a series of acute phases and remissions, each of which adds to the sense of uncertainty and loss of control. Physicians who treat MS patients must pay attention not only to the physical changes but to the social and psychological accompaniments of the illness as well. Treatment must be aimed at preserving physical capacities and optimizing functional abilities, preventing physiological and psychological deterioration, and alleviating pain and discomfort. Mainstays of treatment include health maintenance, physical therapy, pharmacologic intervention, and counseling. Periodic functional assessments play an important role in keeping the physician informed as to the patient's changing abilities and disease course, and are required to assess treatment regimens.

References

1. Appel SH (ed): Multiple sclerosis. Neurol Clin 3(1):3, 1980
2. Bauer HJ: A Manual on Multiple Sclerosis, pp 4, 30. Vienna, Austria, International Federation of the Multiple Sclerosis Societies, 1977
3. Bender J: Exercise for multiple sclerosis. In Patajian JH (ed): Multiple Sclerosis Handbook p 49. Salt Lake City, Utah Chapter of the National Multiple Sclerosis Society, 1980
4. Blaivas JE: Management of bladder dysfunction in multiple sclerosis. Neurol 30(7PtII):12, 1980
5. Bordan RP: Sensory evoked potentials in multiple sclerosis. Neurol Clin 3(1):22, 1980

6. Brooks NA, Matson RR: Social and psychological adjustment to multiple sclerosis. Soc Sci Med 16:2129, 1982

7. Brown JR et al. Therapeutic Claims in MS. Vienna, Austria, International Federation of Multiple Sclerosis Societies, 1982

8. Cailliet R: Rehabilitation in multiple sclerosis. In Licht S (ed): Rehabilitation and Medicine. New Haven, Elizabeth Licht, 1968

9. Cantanzaro M: Nursing Care of the MS patient. Neurol 30(7ptII):44, 45, 1980

10. Caplan LR, Nadelson T: Multiple sclerosis and hysteria. JAMA 243(23):2418, 1980

11. Cook SD, Dowling PC: Multiple sclerosis and viruses: An overview. Neurol 30(7ptII):80, 1980

12. Cooper IS: Living With Chronic Neurologic Disease. New York, WW Norton & Co, 1976

13. Feld RG, Kelly–Hayes M, Fidler AT: Clinical Assessment of Disability of Patients with Multiple Sclerosis. In Multiple Sclerosis Update: Conference Proceedings from March 11, 1981. Boston University School of Medicine, MA 1981

14. Fischman HR: Multiple sclerosis: A two-stage process? Am J Epidemiol 114(2):244, 1981

15. Garibaldi R: Medical considerations in the management of multiple sclerosis patients with early disease. In Petajian JH (ed): Multiple Sclerosis Handbook. Salt Lake City, Utah Chapter of the National MS Society, 1980

16. Ghezzi A, Caputo D: Pregnancy: A Factor Influencing the Course of Multiple Sclerosis? Eur Neurol 20(2):115, 1981

17. Granger CV: Assessment of Functional Status: A Model of Multiple Sclerosis. Manuscript, 1980

18. Guerriero WG: Urologic management of patients with multiple sclerosis. In Appel SH (ed): Neurology Clinics 3(1):19, 1980

19. Hart RG, Sherman DG: The diagnosis of multiple sclerosis. JAMA 247(4):498, 1982

20. Illis LS, Sedgwick EM, Tallis, RC: Spinal cord stimulation in multiple sclerosis: Clinical results. J Neurol, Neurosurg Psychiatry 43:1, 1980

21. Jaffee C, Frankel D, LaRoche B, Dick P: Someone You Know Has Multiple Sclerosis. Waltham, MA, Massachusetts Chapter of the National MS Society, 1982

22. Kaplan S, LaRocca NG: Psychosexual aspects of multiple sclerosis. In MS Symposium, Vol. 5. Summit, NJ, Geigy CME Series, 1980

23. Kaplan S, LaRocca NG: Intellectual and emotional aspects of multiple sclerosis. In MS Symposium, Vol. 7. Summit, NJ, Geigy CME Series, 1981

24. Kraft GH: Multiple sclerosis. In Stolov WC, Clowers MR (eds): Handbook of Severe Disability. Washington, US Dept. of Education, Rehabilitation Services Administration, 1981

25. Kraft GH et al. Multiple sclerosis: Early prognostic guidelines. Arch Phys Med Rehabil 62(2):54, 1981

26. Lehrich JR: Diagnostic Criteria for Multiple Sclerosis. In Multiple Sclerosis Update: Conference Proceedings of March 11, 1981. Boston University Medical School, 1981

27. Lellidid N, Kwong P: Urinary tract problems in multiple sclerosis. In Petajian JH (ed): Multiple Sclerosis Handbook. Salt Lake City, Utah Chapter of the National MS Society, 1980

28. Lilius HG, Valtonen EJ, Wilkstrom J: Sexual problems in patients suffering from multiple sclerosis. J Chronic Dis 29:643, 1976

29. March GG: Disability and intellectual function in multiple sclerosis patients. J Nerv Ment Dis 168(12):758, 1980

30. Matson RR, Brooks NA: Adjusting to multiple sclerosis: An exploratory study. Soc Sci & Med 11(4):245, 1970

31. McAlpine D et al: Multiple Sclerosis: A Reappraisal. Baltimore, Williams & Wilkins, 1972

32. McFarlin DE, McFarland HF: Multiple Sclerosis. N Engl J Med 307(19):1183, 1982

33. Miles A: Some psycho-social consequences of multiple sclerosis: Problems of social interaction and group identity. Brit J Med Psychol 52:321, 1979

34. Millar JHD: Multiple Sclerosis: A Disease Acquired in Childhood. Springfield, IL, Charles C Thomas, 1971

35. Minkwitz J: Physical therapy. In Multiple Sclerosis Update, Conference Proceedings of March 11, 1981. Boston University Medical School, 1981

36. National Multiple Sclerosis Society: What Everyone Should Know About Multiple Sclerosis. South Deerfield, MA, Channing L. Bete, 1982

37. Ottenberg M: The Pursuit of Hope. New York, Rawson, Wade Publishers, 1978

38. Petajian JH: What Is Multiple Sclerosis? In Petajian JH (ed): Multiple Sclerosis Handbook. Utah Chapter of the National MS Society, 1980

39. Peyser JM et al: Cognitive functions in patients with multiple sclerosis. Arch Neurol 37(9):577, 1980

40. Poser CH: The Diagnosis of Multiple Sclerosis. In MS Symposium, Vol. 2. Summit, NJ, Geigy CME Series, 1980

41. Poser CM: Management of Multiple Sclerosis. Compr Therap 7(4):53, 59, 1981

42. Riley T: Overview of multiple sclerosis. In Multiple Sclerosis Update, Conference Proceedings of March 11, 1980, pp 2, 3. Boston University School of Medicine, 1981

43. Rose AS: Long-term care of patients with multiple sclerosis: A neurologist's perspective. Neurol 30(7ptII):59, 1980

44. Rose AS: MS: An overview. In Waxman SG, Ritchie JM (eds): Demyelinating Diseases: Basic and Clinical Electrophysiology. New York, Raven Press, 1981

45. Rusk HA: Rehabilitation Medicine, 4th ed. St Louis, CV Mosby, 1977

46. Schauf CL, Davis FA: Circulating toxic factors in multiple sclerosis. A perspective. Adv Neurol 31:267, 1981

47. Scheinberg L, Miller A: Clinical Problems of Multiple Sclerosis. In MS Symposium, Vol. 3. Summit, NJ, Geigy CME Series, 1980

48. Scheitzer L: Rehabilitation of patients with multiple sclerosis. Arch Phys Med Rehabil 59(9):430, 1978

49. Simmons JQ: Diet considerations in patients with multiple sclerosis. In MS Symposium, Vol. 9. Summit, NJ, Geigy CME Series, 1982

50. Slater RJ: Comprehensive long-term care of MS patients. Neurol 30(7ptII):37, 1980

51. Stockton V: Nursing and Multiple Sclerosis. In Appel, SH: Neurol Clin 3(1):22, 1980

52. Swank RL, Pullen MH: The Multiple Sclerosis Diet Book. Garden City, NY, Doubleday & Co, 1977

53. Veterans Administration: Multiple Sclerosis: Guidelines for Diagnosis and Management, p 9. Washington, VA Neurology Service, Dept. of Medicine and Surgery, 1980

54. Waxman SG: Clinicopathological correlations in MS and related diseases. Adv Neurol 31:169, 1981

55. Whitaker JN: Etiology and pathogenesis of multiple sclerosis. In MS Symposium, Vol. 1. Summit, NJ, Geigy CME Series, 1980

56. Whitlock FA, Siskind MM. Depression as a major symptom of multiple sclerosis. J Neurol Neurosurg & Psychiatry 43(10):861, 1980

CHAPTER 12

Back Pain

Ronald J. Kulich
Daniel W. Bienkowski

Low back pain remains one of the most commonly frustrating problems in primary care practice. In 1979 low back pain was reported to affect more than 15 million adults, and there is no indication that the problem is abating.[35] It has been estimated that 75% of adults will have at least one episode of low back pain by the time they reach their fifties.[21] Nagi and colleagues[26] also have noted that 44% of a stratified sample of 1135 community residents reported reduced job performance due to back pain within the past year, compared with 15% who reported reduced job performance without back pain. A national survey addressing office visit patterns reported that women 34 to 64 years of age, and men 25 to 64 years of age, list backache first as the reason for medical visits. This survey reported that 61% of patients with back complaints received treatment from a primary care physician.[10] The costs in terms of work loss, medical expenses, and human suffering are enormous.

When low back pain is acute, the primary care physician must rule out serious disease, reassure the patient, and provide suggestions for prevention of further injury. The exact cause of pain may not be readily determined, despite laboratory and radiographic studies. Fortunately, most acute episodes are disabling only briefly, and recovery can occur without active intervention.[25,28] Despite symptomatic treatment, a certain percentage of patients continue to experience subacute and chronic pain. In the presence of both acute and chronic back pain, the physician always must be alert to the possibility of another medical condition such as osteoporosis, visceral disease, blood dyscrasias, or metastatic disease. All of these must be diagnosed promptly. It is beyond the scope of this chapter to address these conditions further. Rather this chapter outlines a sequential treatment approach for patients with acute, subacute, and chronic low back pain of benign origin.

Causes of Benign Low Back Pain

Even now the causes for low back pain are not well understood. There is general agreement, however, on some antecedent factors. In young adults occasionally a congenital anomaly such as spondylolisthesis may give rise to pain. In adults of any age disc derangements can occur. The pain can be related to disc rupture or associated impairment of a nerve root. In the elderly patient arthritis of the facet joints of the spine may be added to the possibilities. In all age groups muscle spasm or ligament sprains can be a cause. Any of these patients can have continued symptoms and progress to experience subacute or chronic pain.

History and Physical Exam

As in any medical evaluation, a thorough history is important in low back pain. Often there is a clear history of trauma or overuse. Questioning the patient on postural effects on the back symptoms may help in making a specific diagnosis. The self-report instruments provided in this manual, by assisting the practitioner to assess functional activities, can help to clarify a diagnosis.

In prechronic or chronic back pain the history also should elicit the patient's activities at home and at work, as well as his understanding of and adherence to specific treatment recommendations. A review of the patient's functioning and lifestyle will help to give a picture of his activities and the likelihood of his complying with advice. An active person may have problems adhering to a regimen of extended bedrest with only bathroom privileges. Alternatively, a less motivated patient may abuse bedrest and avoid all activity.

A complete physical examination is necessary to assess the patient with acute low back pain, although the trunk and lower limbs are to be emphasized. The patient must be seen disrobed. It is better to avoid evoking pain in the beginning of the exam. Rather than testing straight leg raising and palpating sore areas, the patient's posture should be observed. Beginning with the standing position, the patient should be observed from the back and the side. Exaggerated lumbar lordosis or scoliosis should be noted. Either suggests structural or muscle origin. Again, palpation of sore points should be deferred until later in order to observe the patient's best level of function.

Next mobility of the lumbar spine is checked. Flexion and extension limitations should be noted. Although motion involves complex interaction at the discs and facet joints, some generalizations can be made: Flexion increases disc pressure.[25] A herniated disc will be associated with a loss of forward flexion of the spine. Extension loads the lamina and facet joints. Pain or limited motion may be found therefore in conditions such as spondylolisthesis or a facet syndrome. Disease of the facet joints may limit side bending and rotation, as well as extension. After posture and motion are checked, straight leg raising is recorded. It is positive only when it duplicates the patient's leg pain. Positive test results, as originally described by Lasegue, require that the pain be felt in the leg. Dorsiflexion of the foot[7] increases the stretch on the sciatic nerve and nerve roots as well and may help increase the validity of the results. Observations first noted on mobility may be helpful. Observations of patient discomfort while undergoing various examination maneuvers for specific functional limitations may help in directing an appropriate physical therapy program when treatment is planned.[27]

Kellgren[15] produced pain in the leg suggestive of sciatica by deep fascial and periosteal injections. Thus subjective complaints of radiating pain do not prove the patient has nerve root irritation caused by a herniated disc. It is also important to note that lumbar disc herniations above the level L4–5 are very rare.

Following the physical examination, specific diagnostic tests may be indicated.

Diagnostic Tests

Radiographs

Plain radiographs usually are not necessary in young patients with a reasonable cause for acute strain and no neurologic deficits. These patients should be followed with an expectation of a quick recovery.

For patients with subacute or chronic pain, or for patients with significant risk factors, plain radiographs, including anterior–posterior, lateral, and oblique views, may be advisable.

In considering diagnostic tests such as radiographs, abnormalities such as bone spur formation do occur in asymptomatic subjects. Other findings, such as degeneration of lumbar discs, are common in most older individuals. Torgerson and Dotter[32] compared radiographs of patients who had low back pain and patients who had radiographs to rule out urinary tract disease and found that spur formation was no greater in one group than in the other.

Laboratory Studies

Laboratory studies routinely done for back pain include a complete blood count (CBC), sed rate, and urinalysis. The sed rate may be elevated in organic illnesses. The CBC is used primarily to rule out other processes such as an acute abdomen. Even in certain infections of the spine, such as discitis, the CBC may not be elevated. Hematuria or pyuria may indicate an infection or a kidney stone. Occasionally specific studies such as the HLA-B27 may be helpful in identifying the patient with chronic low back pain who has ankylosing spondylitis.

Special Procedures

A *CT scan* is an adjunctive procedure to myelography for confirming the disc level causing symptoms in a patient with severe pain and radicular symptoms, as it is a noninvasive test with good specificity.

Myelography should be used only when surgical intervention is planned. Myelography should be done only in the face of a progressive motor deficit, bladder dysfunction, or intractable pain, since this invasive procedure can have significant complications. CT scans and myelograms should be interpreted in conjunction with clinical findings, since disc abnormalities are seen with both on occasion in patients without significant symptoms.

Technetium bone scans are helpful when a disc infection or bone tumor presents as acute pain. A scan can locate the problem before plain radiographs are positive. If a patient with spondylolisthesis has back or leg pain, a technetium scan may help to determine whether or not there is an acute process at the pars interarticularis. It is unlikely that a spondylolysis is the source of pain if the bone scan is negative. If that is the situation, other reasons for pain should be investigated.

Other Procedures

Electromyography (EMG) and *nerve conduction testing* are available to confirm or document radiculopathy. It is important that this testing be performed by a knowledgeable and skillful physician since this test requires interpretive skills.

Another diagnostic test that is being used to evaluate painful conditions is *infrared thermography*. According to Liao[19] and others, thermography offers a quantitative method for evaluating vascular flow changes. However, the predictive accuracy of thermography in clinical situations has not been clearly established.

Treatment

Frequently the patient with back pain is an enigma, since it may not be possible to pinpoint the exact cause of pain. This is illustrated by the many conflicting recommendations and treatment modalities suggested for low back pain. Most patients with acute low back pain will improve with time; thus, many diverse recommendations and treatments will offer "relief."[3] However, certain treatment recommendations are standard.

Time-Limited Bedrest

This is the mainstay of treatment for acute back pain. Biomechanically disc pressure is decreased by 30% to 40% in the supine position. Wiesel and colleagues[34] showed that bedrest will decrease the amount of time off from work by 50%. Limited standing may be permitted to allow the patient to attend to hygiene, but sitting should be avoided. Research has revealed that an unfortunate effect of bedrest is a 3% daily loss of muscle mass, and thus a time constraint on bedrest is important to consider.[4]

In general bedrest is not to exceed 1 to 2 weeks before beginning a physical therapy regimen. Physical therapy for a prescribed period of time is the most important source of rehabilitation as the acute back pain subsides. The physical therapist can be exceedingly helpful in performing a full evaluation of muscle strength and range of motion in the extremities and spine. The physical therapist also can help to supply the physician with some objective measures of gait, body mechanics, and posture, each of which should be addressed in an exercise and activity program with a goal of reducing pain and returning the patient to full functioning as soon as possible.

Medications

Medications can be used judiciously for the treatment of acute back pain. Aspirin, a satisfactory analgesic and anti-inflammatory agent, is very cost-effective for acute strains. Some patients are managed better with nonsteroidal anti-inflammatory medications than with aspirin. If the patient reports severe pain, narcotic medication may be used, but it should be tapered as soon as possible.

With time-limited use, management of medication for acute pain is not usually a problem. However, misuse and dependency often arise for patients at the subacute or chronic stages of their pain. A number of investigators and clinicians now recommend that we focus on the issue of management of pain medication when it is first used. It has been reported that physicians tend to *undermedicate* when a drug is used initially and *overmedicate* at the chronic stage.[23,24] At the acute stage dosage should be adjusted to provide adequate pain relief. There will be great variation among patients in the amount of medication required to relieve pain, and only the patient can judge his own level of pain. Medications should be prescribed contingent on time (non-p.r.n.) rather than pain. The patient will not then struggle with himself or the physician to tolerate the pain at the acute stage. If the patient does attempt to tolerate the pain at the acute stage, anxiety increases along with pain complaints, and the patient's self-report, as well as diagnostic issues, are impaired. In patients placed on a regular non-p.r.n. schedule medication dependency patterns are less likely to develop.

Physical Therapy

Physical therapy modalities have been reviewed in Chapter 5. Heat, ice massage, or ultrasound can be beneficial. These modalities decrease pain and muscle spasm so that mobilization can occur. In addition, the physical therapist is able to review body mechanics and precautions that the physician does not know well or cannot explain because of time constraints. Extensive instruction in appropriate body mechanics will minimize the chance of reinjury.

The physical therapy exercise regimen for the acute low back pain patient will emphasize flexion exercises to condition spinal and abdominal muscles. A written regimen with specific goals can offer optimal compliance. Prior to returning the patient to a work setting, the physical therapist also can add functional activity tasks to help the patient in bending, lifting, walking, and other activities the environment may require. Getting the patient to simulate the physical stresses of the work situation while still in a controlled environment can help him to develop confidence to return to work and other activities of daily living. A return to full activities or to a work setting before improving body mechanics, decreasing pain and spasm, and developing proper endurance and confidence can result in dismal failure for the patient and recurrence of injury. It is important, however, for a structured physical therapy program to include a termination date and provision for re-evaluation of the patient's level of pain and physical functioning. If few gains can be observed after 4 to 5 weeks of intensive therapy, the patient's status may be subacute or chronic. If that is the case, the alternative strategy may be management rather than active treatment.

"Back schools" represent a new and multifaceted treatment effort directed toward patients with acute back pain.[13] Goals of a back school typically include a prompt return to normal function and the cost-effective use of group training procedures. Many of the intervention strategies described in this chapter become part of the content, and patients undergo group instruction based on a protocol format. Content includes a review of anatomy and physiology, extensive instruction in proper body mechanics and posture, stress management and relaxation, appropriate exercise that can be integrated into the patient's lifestyle, and instruction on judicious, consumer-oriented use of the health-care system. Unfortunately, the physician must be aware that *no* extremely brief educational program can alter the ingrained lifestyle that leads to back problems. Every effort must be made to develop back education programs that promote both transfer of training to the patient's environment and practice of newly learned skills on a regular basis.

Conservative versus Surgical Treatment

Even acute patients with proven disc disease, with no progressive or serious neurological deficits, can be treated conservatively.[3] Because 80% of patients recover from an acute episode of back pain even if disc herniation is confirmed, conservative treatment is indicated in most cases. Long-term studies have shown that the results after 4 years, even for patients with recurrent symptoms, are approximately the same after conservative treatment as after surgical treatment.[11]

Surgical treatment is indicated in patients with a progressive neurological deficit, bladder dysfunction, or intractable pain. In patients with recurrent pain, surgery may also provide a quicker return to previous lifestyles. In patients with previous disc surgery, repeat procedures to excise the "recurrent" disc or to fuse an unstable area have less gratifying results. In most cases, the first surgical procedure should be considered the last. The patient considering disc surgery should appreciate that subsequent procedures offer a significantly decreased likelihood of success if initial surgical intervention does not provide pain relief.[20,29] Use of chemonucleolysis, which involves injecting chymopapain into the intervertebral disc, requires further experimental evaluation prior to widespread use.

It is important to rule out other acute processes when dealing with acute back pain. Fortunately the acute back pain from musculoskeletal disorders often resolves spontaneously, leaving the patient with no permanent disability. A reasonable, time-limited period of bedrest, followed by a structured physical therapy program, is often helpful in preventing the development of a subacute or chronic pain syndrome. Diagnosis remains the hallmark of the initial intervention, and a conservative approach must be coupled with educating the patient in appropriate self-care to avoid future injury.

The Subacute Pain Patient

If a patient has not displayed appreciable functional gains 5 weeks after the injury has been managed conservatively, potential chronicity should be considered. The physician should re-evaluate the patient, which he can do by reviewing a checklist such as the one presented below.

1. Does the patient have an underlying medical problem?
2. Does the patient require continued or increasing pain medication?
   - Recall that medication should be provided on a regular basis, and not as needed, from the earliest stage of treatment. The patient should be made aware that medication will be discontinued at a specific date. If pain persists and diagnostic tests are negative, consider a chronic pain management protocol (see following section). In the subacute stage, it is important to reassess other prescriptive needs (*e.g.,* medication for headaches, sleep difficulties, anxiety, dental problems, and so on).
3. Is the patient becoming dependent on regular contacts with the physical therapist for various pain relieving modalities?
   - As noted previously, physical therapy should be prescribed for a limited period of time. In particular, modalities such as ice, heat, transcutaneous stimulators, and massage should be applied on a time-contingent basis, as should prescriptions for medication. It is at this stage of treatment that the patient can become markedly disabled by chronic long-term dependence on strategies directed toward temporary relief.
4. Is the patient reluctant to return to work?
   - If so, additional assessment is needed to address concerns regarding return to the work setting. Secondary gain, social reinforcement, or issues of litigation also need to be addressed. Vocational counseling, work reassignment, or vocational retraining should be considered. If the disability is dealt with appropriately at the early stages, the patient is likely to be employable. When a lifestyle of disability becomes habitual, the likelihood of continuing vocational activity is reduced.
5. Have the recommendations for physical activity treatment been adequately integrated into the patient's home program?
   - Close cooperation with the physical or occupational therapist can assist patients to integrate activities into their daily lives or work settings. Often further assessment of the patient's lifestyle is needed. It is not uncommon for a physician who is unaware that a patient cannot swim, for example, to suggest returning to that activity.
6. Are the patients' self-reports of pain and disability corroborated by their levels of functioning?
   - Again, communication with the physical therapist, with the patient's spouse, and with personnel in the patient's work setting can provide insight into the patient's overall physical functioning. A valid assessment of the patient's functional activity as well as his level of functioning prior to injury and impairment is necessary.
7. Has adjunctive assessment with self-report instruments been considered?
   - In addition to the functional assessment questionnaire (FASQ) data, a number of other questionnaires have been developed to assist the physician in evaluating adjustment problems or mediating psychological issues. Presently the best short instrument available on a commercial basis is the Low Back Pain Classification Scale.[18] This computer-

scored questionnaire can provide the primary care physician with an assessment of psychological disturbance that can predict continued dysfunction. Research is being conducted on similar instruments that can be readily administered in the office and provide a basis for cost-effective screening.

8. Has the patient been given specific instruction about what he can and cannot do?
   - When multiple conservative interventions have been attempted and the patient's pain complaints persist, the physician may fall into the trap of continuing an ongoing search for new, potentially effective treatments to relieve pain. This process sends the patient mixed signals and fails to provide him with clear expectations about actual limitations or abilities. The patient may be unaware that he may lift 30 pounds, walk daily, or return to specific enjoyable activities. Fear of injury persists without a specified set of activity levels.
9. Has the patient obtained feedback from more than one physician, other health-care provider, or counselor since onset of injury?
   - Although the option of obtaining a second opinion should not be discouraged, patients should be discouraged from taking advice from multiple sources who may offer conflicting and therefore confusing recommendations. All treatment recommendations to the patient with acute or subacute back pain should be coordinated through one primary physician. Special consultants should supply the primary care provider with specific recommendations and information, rather than review detailed suggestions directly with the patient. Channeling all information through one primary care physician reduces confusion and anxiety, which may contribute to persistence of pain and disability.
10. If pain and disability continue, has the patient been referred for a comprehensive, multidisciplinary pain management program?
    - The ultimate criterion for such a referral rests on the patient's motivation to return to better functioning, often despite his continued level of pain.

The Chronic Low Back Pain Patient

Approximately 550 million work days are lost per year due to chronic pain; included in this number are 155 million days lost because of backaches, muscle pains, and joint pains.[31]

The typical patient has failed previously to respond to conservative treatment and more extensive interventions at the subacute stage. This patient might present himself to a physician complaining of constant and debilitating pain for 2 years after injury. He says that after multiple diagnostic and treatment attempts and two laminectomies he had limited gains from the second surgery and only several months of relief from his first surgery. A comprehensive interview will elicit from him that he has problems with walking, stairclimbing, and bending, and, not surprisingly, that he has severe restrictions in his lifestyle. He is scarcely able to tie his shoes, and his wife and two children now perform many of his activities of daily living. The physical exam may be unremarkable, and no apparent changes in reflexes are evident after reviewing the records from his three prior diagnostic evaluations. Results from a CT scan and myelogram conducted approximately 6 months ago suggest changes only secondary to prior surgical interventions and no new findings. The surgeon's report of a recent examination advises against further surgical intervention.

The patient's medical history includes an extensive list of treatments besides surgery, including three trials of physical therapy, 2 months each using William's flexion exercises, heat, ice, and various stretching exercises. The patient noted only temporary relief during these periods of treatment. Also, he may mention unsuccessful trials with a transcutaneous electrical nerve stimulation (TENS) unit, acupuncture, and visits to a chiropractor once a week, which "seemed to help a little." The patient now wears a back brace approximately 6 hours a day, uses a hydrocollator, and still sees his neurosurgeon on an intermittent basis for re-evaluations. Medication includes Valium 5 mg t.i.d., Percocet t.i.d., and (from his internist) amitriptyline (Elavil) 25 mg h.s.

The patient is resentful, markedly agitated, tearful, expresses helplessness and hopelessness, and is "looking for anything that might relieve the pain." He expresses marked anger at the medical profession because "everyone tells me different things . . . gives me drugs . . . and I'm not sure who to listen to." Over the last 2 years increased marital and family distress also has ensued, and the spouse now assumes most activities of daily living and has taken a fulltime work position to alleviate the financial pressures on the family. The patient also reports anxiety symptoms including occasional hyperventilation, shaking, and feelings of panic. He admits to feeling depressed because of his pain, but he is not suicidal. He has no significant personal or family psychiatric history; he is adamant that the pain is "not psychological," and he believes his life would improve measurably if "just something could be done about the pain." Sleep has become a significant problem, although Elavil has offered some assistance. The patient may self-medicate by taking approximately 10 aspirin per day and a small tumbler of wine "to help with sleep and relaxation."

The patient freely admits that his family situation has deteriorated to the point of multiple arguments. He uses medication on an as needed basis to reduce more intense pain; he spends approximately 5 hours per day lying on the couch, and he has adjusted his living situation by bringing a small bed downstairs to avoid painful stairclimbing. He perceives almost any activity as a possible precipitant of reinjury or exacerbation of pain. His wife and children assume that any increases in physical activity are potentially harmful, and they discourage the patient from attempting any activity. Communication between the patient and spouse center primarily on pain relief, and sexual or intimate activity has ceased, with the exception of daily back massages administered by the wife during the most acute periods of distress.

Financial pressures also complicate the picture, since he has been out of work for approximately 2 years and has had numerous difficulties with Workmen's Compensation regarding his disability status. An attorney is involved, but no settlement has been suggested since the patient is still looking for ultimate cures that may resolve the family's dilemma.

The many contacts with various treatment resources recommending conflicting forms of treatment have left the patient frustrated. Although bedrest and relaxation are strongly encouraged during severe episodes of pain, the patient also was told to exercise and swim and has received insufficient instruction about whether to undertake specific activities.

The patient admits to being extremely fearful of a significant reduction or elimination of medication.

Role of the Primary Care Physician

The role of the primary care physician in dealing with the situation just described is markedly different from his role during the acute phase of treatment. The physician must recognize that although many diagnostic procedures have been performed and many treatment modalities have been recommended, neither a specific cause nor any relief has been found for this patient with chronic, benign low back pain. Also, the physician must convince not only the patient but himself that continuing the attempt for a cure is not going to be effective. Instead the primary care physician with a rehabilitation perspective must view the patient as having a chronic condition requiring consistent and multifocused contacts on a long-term basis. The following is one approach to managing this problem patient.

1. If possible, all prior medical records should be acquired because the patient may forget to outline other significant chronic pain or disability episodes that predated the most recent, acute injury.
2. After a review of the medical history, examinations, and evaluation procedures, the patient is informed that all recommendations will be coordinated through the primary physician or another physician such as a physiatrist. An effort will be made to eliminate conflicting messages from various treatment sources.
3. The diagnostic interview for the chronic pain patient should include psychosocial and disability assessment.
4. The spouse or significant other who can make helpful contributions regarding the patient's physical and psychological functioning should participate in the diagnostic interview. The presence of the spouse also can provide insight into secondary gain or social reinforcement issues, as well as specific changes that have occurred in the patient's lifestyle since the onset of pain.
5. Prescription and nonprescription drugs must be evaluated. This includes all medications for *all* purposes, since it is not uncommon for patients to present with polypharmacy for multiple pain complaints. A typical example includes the chronic low back pain patient who may fail to mention the Fiorinal q.i.d. for chronic migraine headaches and the recently prescribed Percocet for dental difficulties.

Following the diagnostic interview, an outline of specific deficit areas as they relate to physical and psychosocial functioning can be developed. The physician should encourage the patient to be a collaborator in the development of a problem list, since the patient–physician interaction no longer involves dispensing a cure for a problem. The physical therapist can assist in providing further specification in functional areas, but specificity in describing problems and goals should be emphasized.

Management of the Chronic Low Back Pain Patient

Patients with chronic pain should be managed rather than treated aggressively. Consistency in care is important, and the physician must avoid aggressive pharmacologic or treatment interventions during periods of significant exacerbation of complaints. Following is a series of management suggestions:

1. The primary care physician should attempt to share the problem, as well as the proposed pain management plan, with the patient. Written instructions should be provided to enhance compliance with activities, exercises, and so on between visits. Visits to the primary care physician should not be scheduled on an as-needed basis. Otherwise the patient with chronic pain must have severe symptoms and complaints to receive feedback and suggestions from the physician. The noncrisis visit is especially therapeutic for the patient because it permits the physician to reinforce activities and coping strategies that the patient is doing right. Diagnostically the noncrisis visit is of particular value, since the physician can view the patient at a period of higher functioning, and the patient can view the physician as a supporter of well behavior rather than of pain behavior or crisis intervention. The physician should focus on what the patient is doing right during all visits, although no physical complaints can or should be summarily ignored.

2. Short-acting benzodiazapines and narcotic analgesics are contraindicated in virtually all cases of chronic benign pain. Nonsteroidal or anti-inflammatory agents should not be prescribed on an as-needed basis. Prescription of any drug on an as-needed basis markedly increases the likelihood of drug misuse and dependency. The first drug of choice often is a tricyclic antidepressant. A number of clinical reports suggest that tricyclic antidepressants can improve pain tolerance.[1] In the presence of significant affective symptoms secondary to pain complaints, a therapeutic dosage of these medications is necessary. Although many inpatient chronic pain management programs maintain the majority of patients on antidepressants, fewer than 20% of the patients at the Lahey Clinic Outpatient Pain-Management Program are on antidepressant medication. We recommend a conservative pharmacologic strategy, which includes resisting a patient's demands for medication.

   Detoxification is a major problem for patients using large amounts of opiates, sedatives, and antianxiety agents. Pain management programs are often best suited for detoxification in the presence of polypharmacy. Outpatients must be followed extremely closely and their physiological responses to a gradual reduction should be monitored on an ongoing basis. Effective management of medication should include alternative treatment modalities. For example, patients requiring medications for muscle spasms or sleep difficulties often may reduce medications successfully when offered alternative coping and relaxation skills.

3. From the initial stage of assessment and throughout management of chronic pain, significant others should be involved. The spouse who understands the approach to the management of the patient with pain can help to point out problems before a major crisis occurs.[2,5]

4. In contrast to the management of the patient with acute pain, the patient with chronic pain is often afraid of activity because of fear of re-injury. Physicians often recommend that the patient work to tolerance, that is, until it starts to hurt. Instead, an exercise regimen with a chronic pain patient should involve working to task. Small amounts of physical activity can be added to an activity and exercise regimen on a daily basis. The goal of an exercise prescription for the patient with pain is not complete reduction of pain. The patient is unlikely to be responsive to a program of management that offers the same unrealistic expectations he has had before. Instead, the exercise program should be presented to the patient as a way to improve flexibility and tolerance for increased enjoyable activities.

Exercises should be selected that are compatible with the patient's lifestyle and that he can do with a spouse or significant other. Such a program may be aerobic exercises such as walking, swimming, or stair-climbing. The physician and family members should encourage the patient, once he has integrated the exercise regimen into his lifestyle, to increase activities on a daily basis despite episodic periods of significant pain.

A physical therapist also can offer much assistance in the development of an endurance-building exercise regimen. However, the focus on building endurance is quite different from the focus on pain relief. The regimen for endurance should be geared toward increasing physical functioning on a gradual basis rather than toward offering strategies aimed at short-term relief such as whirlpool, braces, or simple flexion exercises, which merely perpetuate a lifestyle of disability and a counterproductive dependency on the health care system. A typical regimen for chronic low back pain emphasizes gradual increases in activity despite pain. Each exercise regimen should have as its goal the functional activity to which the patient would like to return.

If the patient has experienced physiotherapy for a limited period of time, the gains achieved from treatment may be maintained at a health club, YWCA/YMCA, or other facility. Simply referring the patient to such a resource, however, is not sufficient. The patient must experience the supervision and confidence-building phase of treatment.

5. Although considerable clinical evidence has suggested potential benefit from TENS, there are no controlled investigations to substantiate its value. Wolf and Rao[36] recommend that referral of the patient with chronic pain for TENS evaluation should be made in the context of a treatment package. They note that "TENS should not be provided as needed, but, like other aspects of a comprehensive pain management protocol, should be offered within the context of a 'contract' between patient and clinician wherein certain functional goals must be met. . . ." Examples include increased "up time," decreased analgesic intake, and an incrementally increased work routine. Other sources are available for discussion of electrode placement.[22] Contraindications for the TENS also should be considered by the physician, and these have been listed elsewhere.[36] The TENS unit is not a panacea and does not have a major impact on the multifaceted problems of the patient with chronic pain; however, it may

be helpful in some cases. The physical therapist who instructs the patient in the use of TENS must be experienced and able to strike a balance between any potential pain relief and reinforcing disability or illness behavior by long-term use of this pain-relieving device.

6. If the patient is to improve his lifestyle, he must be encouraged to return to vocational and avocational activities. The present bureaucratic compensation system often fails to reinforce a return to work or activity. However, a state vocational rehabilitation facility often can offer the patient viable alternatives to his former occupation. Insurance carriers also offer specialized work assessment and training programs that can be coordinated with the primary care physician's recommendations or the recommendations of a comprehensive pain-management program.[14]

7. Although not necessarily the final phase of pain management, many physicians may consider referral to a comprehensive outpatient or inpatient chronic pain-management program. Physicians are finding increasingly that their patients benefit from coordinated followup at a rehabilitation facility of this type even at the earliest phases of the patient's injury. In fact, it may be preferable for pain management programs to admit patients 6 months after an injury rather than 2 years afterwards. The chronicity and inappropriate behavior patterns have not yet become ingrained after 6 months, and patients have not as yet developed a level of comfort with a disability lifestyle. These comprehensive programs also may help to reduce the high costs of pain management.[30]

Pain-Management Program

The primary goal of the pain-management program is to provide clinical services that will improve the patient's physical, emotional, and social functioning. An estimated 300 pain control facilities in the United States provide a range of services.[8] The Commission on Accreditation of Rehabilitation Facilities has moved in the direction of certifying outpatient and inpatient centers.[9] A multimodal rehabilitation effort generally has been recommended. Although the goals of various pain programs vary, the following often are considered important:

- Increased physical endurance and functioning
- Improved pain tolerance and ability to cope with pain
- Decreased pain behavior
- Elimination of unnecessary medications
- Improved relaxation and stress-coping skills
- Improved family and marital communication
- Return to recreational and social activities
- Return to work or vocational retraining
- Decreased utilization of unnecessary health care

Although orientations vary, most programs that meet the criteria outlined by the American Pain Society focus on rehabilitation treatment and discourage single modality pain clinics that fail to address the multiple deficits of the patient with chronic pain. The typical patient with low back pain is unlikely to improve in all areas of lifestyle and functioning after being treated with a single modality such as biofeedback, epidural blocks, or a TENS unit. For a multifaceted problem such as chronic low back pain, a multifaceted treatment approach is recommended.

The costs of pain management programs have ranged from $6,000 to $22,000. Prices depend on whether the program is offered on an outpatient or an inpatient basis, as well as on the treatments offered. In general, a comprehensive pain-management program should include these components:

Treatment agreement—Many programs include a plan written by the patient, spouse, and treatment team, which outlines specific step-by-step treatment components and comprehensive treatment goals. Various patients' treatment goals may vary depending upon particular needs and medical status. Typical goals might be a return to gardening, bowling, lifting grocery bags, and work, or an opportunity to be retrained to perform selected tasks.

Physical therapy—After the physical therapist performs a comprehensive structural and functional evaluation, he often establishes a highly structured general conditioning program meant to increase the patient's overall strength, mobility, and endurance and designed to help the individual meet activity goals such as bending, sitting, lifting, and walking. As part of the treatment regimen, patients are encouraged to transfer these skills to their own environments and lifestyles and to practice the exercises and activities in the home setting.

Occupational therapy—Although all programs do not offer occupational therapy, patients can benefit from instruction in body mechanics, energy conservation, pacing, and work simplification. The occupational therapist helps the patient to improve functioning at work and in social settings and to decrease pain behaviors such as limping, grimacing, and complaining about pain.

Relaxation training and biofeedback—Relaxation training, often an integral part of the pain-management program, teaches skills to improve flexibility and sleep and to achieve activity goals. Biofeedback techniques, employed by a certified biofeedback therapist, are offered as an adjunct to improve relaxation skills, particularly for the patient undergoing detoxification.

Detoxification—Inpatient programs provide structured detoxification. Lectures and instructions are offered along with "pain cocktails" containing gradually reduced narcotics or other active ingredients. Narcotic antagonists also are introduced sometimes to help in reduction of medication.[12] Typically outpatients are given daily prescriptions with a gradually decreased narcotic content.

Clinical psychology—Throughout the assessment and treatment phases at the pain center, the clinical psychologist is likely to be involved in helping the patient address the many personal and family difficulties associated with the experience of chronic pain. Many patients are seen with their spouses or families on a regular basis to set goals and achieve a more satisfying lifestyle. Specialized group programs also may be offered to deal with stress management, assertivenes training, weight management, and social skills training. Generally, patients are viewed as having developed psychiatric symptoms secondary to their pain problem and as needing better than average skills to handle a lifestyle of chronic pain.

Vocational rehabilitation—Individual vocational counseling in coordination with state and private rehabilitation facilities helps the patient to return to a former work setting or to receive work retraining. This must be a part of any pain-management program, as it fosters a carryover of skills acquired within the pain unit.

Followup Training—An effective pain-management program includes active followup with the patient to maintain gains acquired in treatment. Although active treatment in any chronic pain-management program should be carried out for a limited period of time, followup programs are needed to provide a support and education setting for patients who need lifelong help with the management of their pain. The primary care physician remains an integral part of followup after a chronic pain-management program. It is easy for a patient to deteriorate upon re-entry into a multisource medical system. One primary care physician should act as the coordinator after discharge. Regularly scheduled rather than as-needed office visits and encouragement to improve physical functioning must continue even after completion of the pain-management program.

Research and Treatment Outcome Data

Results of evaluations of the long-term effects of chronic pain-management programs are inconclusive.[33] Pain-management programs have existed for close to 20 years, but adequate management of chronic low back pain is in its infancy. Physicians referring patients to chronic pain-management programs should make sure that the program emphasizes the rehabilitation criteria outlined by the American Pain Society and the Commission on Accreditation of Rehabilitation Facilities. Referrals should be made to a comprehensive multidisciplinary treatment program for the chronic pain patient. Programs that are involved actively in evaluation and research efforts are preferred. Single-faceted programs that offer only psychological or anesthesiological intervention without adequate coordination and rehabilitation focus will probably be significantly less beneficial. Patients with a benign pain problem particularly should avoid programs employing invasive strategies that may eventually do more harm than good.[6,16]

Summary

This chapter acquaints the primary care physician with critical management concepts with respect to acute and chronic back pain. In fact, many of the principles discussed are applicable to a wide range of pain-related disorders. Despite knowledge about the subject, training in the management of chronic pain is limited. Our health-care system may unintentionally promote increased disability and pain behaviors in the patients. Physicians with little to offer these patients at the chronic stage often dislike, mismanage, and avoid them. However, the primary care physician may be able to mitigate this confusing and stressful plight by helping these patients to enter into a coordinated treatment effort.

References

1. Adler RH: Psychotropic agents in the management of chronic pain. J Human Stress 6:13–17, 1978
2. Balis K, Kulich RJ, Peiser AH, Wright N: Family factors in the management of chronic pain. Paper presented at the American Psychological Association, Toronto, 1984
3. Bell GR, Rothman RH: The conservative treatment of sciatica. Spine 1:54–56, 1984
4. Bigos S: Chronic low back pain. Workshop presentation, #663, Internationl Association for the Study of Pain. Pain (Suppl 2), 1984
5. Block AR: An investigation of the response of the spouse to chronic pain behavior. Psychosom Med 43:415–422, 1982
6. Bonica J: Management of pain. Postgrad Med 53:56–57, 1973
7. Breig A, Troup JDG: Biomechanical considerations in straight leg raising test. Spine 4:242–250, 1979
8. Brena SF: Pain control facilities: Roots, organization, and function. In Brena SF, Chapman SL (eds) Management of Patients With Chronic Pain. New York, Spectrum, 1983
9. Commission on Accreditation of Rehabilitation Facilities: The Standards Manual for Facilities Serving People with Disabilities. 2500 North Pantano Road; Tucson, AZ 85715
10. Cypress BK: Characteristics of physician visits for back symptoms: A national perspective. Am J Public Health 73:4, 389–395, 1983
11. Fahrni, WH: Conservative treatment of lumbar disc degeneration: Our primary responsibility. Ortho Clin North Am 6:93–103, 1975
12. Greenstein R, Arndt IC, McLellan AT, O'Brien CP, Evans B: Naltrexone: A clinical perspective. J Clin Psychiatry 45:9, 25–28, 1984
13. Hall H: The Canadian back education units, Physiother 66:4, 115, 1980
14. Hammonds W, Brena SF: Pain classification and vocational evaluation in chronic pain states. In Melzack R (ed): Pain Measurement and Assessment. New York, Raven Press, 1983
15. Kellgren JH: Conditions of the back stimulating visceral disease. Proc Royal Soc Medicine 35:191, 1941–42
16. Keps ER, Duncalf D: Treatment of backache with spinal injection of local anaesthetics, spinal and systemic steroids: A review. Pain 22:33–47, 1985
17. King JS, Langger R: Sciatica viewed as a referred pain syndrome. Surg Neurol 5:46–50, 1979
18. Leavitt F: Comparison of three measures for detecting psychological disturbance in patients with low back pain. Pain 13:299–305, 1982
19. Liao JJ: Thermography for chronic pain. Presented at the Second Meeting of the American Pain Society, New York, September, 1980
20. Loeser JD: Low back pain. In Bonica JJ (ed): Pain. New York, Raven Press, 1980
21. Loeser J: Chronic low back pain. Workshop presentation #663, International Association for the Study of Pain. Pain (Suppl 2), 1984

22. Mannheimer JS: Electrode placement for transcutaneous electrical nerve stimulation. Phys Ther 58:1455–1462, 1978
23. Marks RM, Sachar EJ: Undertreatment of medical inpatients with narcotic analgesics. Ann Intern Med 78, 2:173–181, 1973
24. McCaffrey M, Hart LL: Undertreatment of acute pain with narcotics. Am J Nurs 76, 10:1586–1591, 1976
25. Nachemson AL: Disc pressure measurements. Spine 6:91–97, 1981
26. Nagi SZ, Riley LE, Newby LG: A social epidemiology of back pain in a general population. J Chronic Dis 26:769–779, 1973
27. Paris SV: Anatomy as related to function and pain. Ortho Clin North Am 14:475–489, 1984
28. Roland M, Morris R: A study of the natural history of low back pain, Part II. Development of guidelines of treatment in primary care. Spine 8:145–150, 1983
29. Rothman RH, Booth R: Failures of spinal fusion. Ortho Clin North Am 6:299–303, 1975
30. Sarkar S: Pain center: An alternative for management of chronic pain. Health Care Manage Rev 7:4, 77–84, Fall, 1982
31. Sternback RA: National Pain Survey, Lou Harris & Associates. Presentation at American Pain Society (unpublished), October, 1985, Dallas. Scripps Clinic & Research Foundation, La Jolla, CA 92037
32. Torgerson WR, Dotter WE: Comparative roentgenographic study of the asymptomatic and symptomatic lumbar spine. J Bone Joint Surg 58A:850–853, 1976
33. Turner JA, Chapman CR: Psychological interventions for chronic pain: A critical review. I, Relaxation training and biofeedback. Pain 12:1–21, 1982
34. Wiesel SW, Cuchler JM, Deluca F, Jonas F, Zeide MS, Rothman RH: Acute low back pain: An objective analysis of conservative therapy. Spine 5:324–330, 1980
35. U.S. Department of Health, Education and Welfare, Public Health Service, National Institutes of Health, National Institute of Neurological and Communicative Disorders and Stroke, 1979. HE.20.3517.N.39.3. National Research Strategy for Neurological and Communicative Disorders, pp 82–99, 1979
36. Wolf SL, Rao V: Transcutaneous electrical stimulation: Use and misuse. In Brena SF, Chapman SL (eds): Management of Patients with Chronic Pain, p 189. New York, Spectrum, 1983

CHAPTER 13

Visual Impairments

Man is highly dependent on his senses. Through his senses come the sensations which constitute his experience. Upon the information he receives from his senses he builds his world, his world of perception and conception: of memory, imagination, thought, and reason.[27]

Nearly half a million Americans are legally blind, and a much larger percentage have varying degrees of visual impairment. Unlike some neurological disorders, if diagnosed in time many visual impairments can be cured or at least corrected. Even if nothing can be done for the visual disorder itself, there are many low vision aids, rehabilitation programs, educational materials, and community services available about which a knowledgeable physician can inform the patient to enable a more productive and satisfying life.

Most physicians have limited contact with blind or deaf people in their ambulatory practices, however, almost every physician treats patients with some form of visual or auditory impairment. Unfortunately, many children are not diagnosed as having sensory disorders until they are identified by routine screening during school examinations. By then many of the detrimental effects have become irreversible. Many diseases, such as retinitis pigmentosa and Usher's syndrome, are congenital disorders that have progressive debilitating effects. Earlier intervention could better prepare these children for the future consequences of their disease.

Geriatric patients are at high risk both for hearing and visual impairments. Many elderly people, believing these disabling events are inevitable consequences of aging and "things they have to live with," do not seek medical attention until disabilities are fixed and even irreversible. Although the primary care physician may not be able to prevent the deterioration brought about by aging, he may help the patient with a sensory impairment find needed services and enjoy a more fulfilling life.

Definitions of Blindness and Visual Impairments

The visually impaired are a highly heterogeneous group whose one and perhaps only common characteristic is some degree of visual loss. Some are totally blind while others are able to distinguish between light and dark or even see a couple of feet away. Individuals with tunnel vision have good sight for distance but are handicapped by very narrow visual fields. Others have such a high degree of photophobia that, even with minor visual impairment, they are restricted in certain activities. These persons all function differently in their environment. It is not surprising, therefore, that it is hard to define who is not handicapped by visual impairment.[2]

Fuzzy vision, vision only out of the corner of the eye, vision that fluctuates with different lighting environments, as well as vision that is better some days than others, are characteristics of visual impairment or blindness. Because the characteristics are so varied it is difficult to define this group of sensory impairments.[13] In 1934 the Illinois Department of Public Welfare, wanting a standard upon which to determine eligibility for public assistance due to visual deficiencies, prevailed upon the American Medical Association (AMA) to define blindness in functional terms. The Ophthalmologic Division of the AMA provided the following definition, which remains to date one of the most widely used standards in industrialized countries for determining legal blindness:

Blindness is defined as visual acuity, in the better eye with correction, of not more than 20/200 or a defect in the visual field so that the widest diameter of vision subtends an angle no greater than 20 degrees.[18]

Most legally blind persons can see to some extent. Some can follow sidewalks as they walk, see a traffic light, or even read large print books if assisted by magnifying devices.[5] According to Ashcroft,[2] 75% of those who are legally blind have a visual acuity of approximately 20/200, 12% see only light and dark, and another 12% are totally blind—unable to see anything at all. At present, approximately 2 of every 1000 persons qualify as "legally blind." The designation as legally blind enables a person to be eligible for public assistance programs, tax exemptions, free educational materials, and many organizational services, but being labeled legally blind has drawbacks. One is the prevalent misconception among the general public that legal blindness is synonymous with total blindness. The term blindness may initiate an attitudinal bias in some sighted individuals. Phrases such as, "I could do it with my eyes closed," or "even a blind man could do it," conjure negative images of the blind person's abilities.

Equally important, the AMA's definition of legal blindness may have a twofold disadvantage for visually deficient individuals. First the definition is more applicable to adults than to children. Accurate diagnosis of distance visual acuity rarely can be estimated until the child is at least 3 years of age, and it may take even longer if possible at all, with a multihandicapped child.[18] The difficulty of making the diagnosis may deprive the child of services, corrective devices, or financial assistance in their early developmental years, when they are most needed. Second the present legal definition, although advantageous to those falling within its limits for special privileges and services, may prevent individuals who have different problems but are equally impaired from obtaining these services. Because of the negative aspects of legal blindness, there have been many attempts in recent years to define blindness in more functionally meaningful terms. The American Foundation for the Blind recommended the term "blindness" be reserved solely for those with complete loss of sight; all other degrees of visual loss should be referred to as "visual impairments."[5]

Types of Visual Impairment

Low Vision

The most common cause of impaired vision is a refractive error—the failure of light rays to focus with a clear image on the retina.[36] The resultant conditions include myopia (nearsightedness), hyperopia (farsightedness), and astigmatism. Most refractive errors can be compensated for with prescription glasses or contact lenses. There are, however, people with significant visual impairments due to pathology in the eye, in the visual pathways to the brain, or in the receptor areas of the occipital cortex. Impairments caused by these pathologies are not receptive to corrective refraction devices. People whose impairments are not amenable to corrective lenses are considered to have low vision (or equivalently, to be partially sighted). Their pathological processes may affect distance acuity, near acuity, or both. People with low-vision impairments may see blurred and distorted images, only parts of an object, or the object at only certain angles, or they may need to be extremely close to the object to recognize it.[34] People with low vision have a visual acuity between 20/70 and 20/200. Without special aids, the person with low vision is unable to perform visual tasks adequately.

People characterized as having low vision, like those who are blind, are a heterogeneous group. The prevalence of low vision is unknown, partly because there are no satisfactory guidelines for defining low vision disorders, and because many visual impairments short of blindness are never diagnosed. Children, encouraged to make the most of their remaining partial sight, can improve their visual efficiency,[3,18] thus complicating the definition of low vision by numerical measures alone.

Considerations of comprehensive care are often overlooked in treating the patient with low vision. Yet they can have problems uniquely related to their condition. Persons with low vision may have *more* difficulty in accepting their visual problems than totally blind persons. They are caught in an identity conflict—unable to consider themselves either totally blind or totally sighted. They frequently fear eventual total blindness while simultaneously hoping (sometimes unrealistically) for future improvement. Although low vision aids, courses of instruction, and counseling are available to individuals who might benefit from them, many are unaware of their existence. The primary care physician, in conjunction with the ophthalmologist or optometrist, should make sure that patients with low vision are informed of the many resources available to them, which will be discussed later in this chapter.

Residual Vision

Residual vision is any degree of vision that can be described clinically, although, like legal blindness, it cannot be described in numerical terms. A person with residual vision only cannot see any of the letters on a standard visual acuity test chart, even with correction, but does have minimal ability to perceive light and objects. A person with residual vision can discriminate or recognize certain objects within a limited visual range.

Remaining Vision

Remaining vision includes both residual vision and any near acuity vision. Low vision is sometimes described in terms of the amount of the remaining vision.

Etiology

Each year over 30,000 Americans lose their sight.[36] Physiological conditions (*e.g.*, insufficient blood supply to the brain), disease (*e.g.*, diabetes), and trauma to the eye contribute to loss of sight. Causes of blindness change over time. The incidence of glaucoma, for instance, has declined in recent years due to earlier detection, better medical procedures, and a more informed public. On the other hand, the increasing percentage of elderly people in our population has been associated with a concomitant rise in disorders that affect primarily older people. Descriptions of some of the more common causes of blindness follow.

Cataract, a progressive opacity of the normally clear lens of the eye, causes decreasing vision as opacity increases. Normally cataracts are not a problem in their early stages and may require only a prescription for glasses; however, if the opacity is permitted to progress untreated, blindness can result. The treatment for significant cataract disease is surgical removal of the defective lens with an option for replacement with an artificial one. The success rate for such a procedure is about 90% to 95%.[39] Unfortunately, many patients fear the operation so much that they continue to live with the disease. Preliminary research is currently being done to develop a filter which would enable the individual to see through the cataract tissue,[39] but such a device is not yet available.

Glaucoma is caused by an increase in intraocular pressure resulting from a greater amount of fluid entering or being formed in the eyeball than can escape through normal channels. As a consequence, the outer fibers of the optic nerve are unable to function, causing a loss in peripheral vision. If uncontrolled, tunnel vision may become so severe that only a tiny spot of central vision remains; eventually total blindness may result. Glaucoma is diagnosed by tonometry. At present, endstage glaucoma is the second leading cause of blindness in this country.[26] Although surgery is needed occasionally, glaucoma can be controlled usually with eyedrops.

Diabetic retinopathy is due to vascular changes that can cause hemorrhaging in the retina, which results in spots in the visual field. Frequently the blood reabsorbs and good vision can return; however, sudden permanent blindness due to retinal detachment is also a possibility. Diabetic retinopathy is a growing concern because of the increasing number of diabetics.[10] All patients with diabetes should have regular ophthalmological examinations to detect potential retinal changes and to allow time for early treatment. Since diabetes may start during pregnancy, all pregnant women should be watched for ocular changes.

Spots before the eyes may be due to several severe eye impairments, but *retinal detachment* is the most serious. Contracting fibrous tissue replacing blood clots in diabetes or other causes, such as trauma, may cause the retina to detach. The first sign of detachment is a flooding of "floaters," or spots in the eye. The next stage involves loss of a partial field of vision. In the final stage, the retina tears away and results in a loss of vision described by one author as "pulling a shade down over your eyes."[36] Immediate consultation and surgery are needed with the appearance of the earliest symptoms. Once total sight is lost, the prognosis is poor.

Optic nerve atrophy accounts for approximately 9% of blindness.[39] Although it has several causes, optic nerve atrophy is due primarily to interruption of blood supply to the brain, occlusion of the central retinal or ophthalmic artery, or inflammation of the ophthalmic artery.

Senile macular degeneration, a condition affecting many elderly persons, is of unknown etiology. The condition affects the central part of the retina where vision is clearest, and it is believed to involve vascular changes, perhaps arteriosclerosis. Senile macular degeneration usually begins as impaired reading ability, but it can progress to a marked visual loss with time. This disorder rarely causes total blindness; affected persons may not be able to read or drive a car, but they usually can get around satisfactorily. Completely painless and unrelated to other eye symptoms, this condition usually progresses in spite of treatment.

Presbyopia is a normal degenerative visual impairment in older people affecting adults between the ages of 45 and 50, sometimes as early as 40 years of age. It is due to relaxation of the ligaments of the lens, which prevents the lens from altering its shape in order to accommodate for near distance tasks. The resultant effect is a decline in near object visual acuity. Treatment usually involves a prescription for reading glasses.

Retinitis pigmentosa, an inherited, progressive condition, usually begins in childhood but often produces its most detrimental effects in the teenage and early adult years. Dystrophy of the rod-shaped cells in the retina causes this bilateral, peripheral field visual loss. Night blindness is one of the first symptoms, but as the disease progresses, tunnel vision results. By age 50 there is almost total bilateral loss of all useful peripheral fields.[26] Subcapsular cataracts may be present, which decrease or even eliminate the remaining useful vision. Although no cure is known, cataract surgery may lessen the loss of central vision. Because of the likelihood of visual loss in later life, patients with retinitis pigmentosa should be referred to organizations that serve the blind and handicapped to learn about rehabilitation that may be needed eventually and to obtain emotional support for the patient and family.

Screening Examinations

Early diagnosis of a visual disorder is often essential for the restoration and maintenance of sight.

Although definitive management of the problems often may require referral to an ophthalmologist, there is much to be gained by early detection. If early examination results in recognition of strabismus or discovery of congenital glaucoma, the gain may be conservation of sight. If it allows recognition of retinoblastoma, the result may be preservation of life.[30]

The family physician or pediatrician is in an ideal position to detect eye problems—especially in infants and children. Early diagnosis does not require the primary care physician to be an expert in the difficult technique of eye examination, but to be alert to the possibility that visual impairment exists. In order to be so alerted, a physician needs to have at least a cursory knowledge of the causes of blindness and visual impairment and a working familiarity with some basic techniques of eye examination.

Although total blindness should be easy to detect upon physical examination, some of the less obvious impairments may be more difficult. The FASQ may be an important instrument in detecting such losses. Review of activities that the patient has "a lot of difficulty" with or is "unable" to do should alert the physician to possible sensory impairment. Once visual impairment has been diagnosed, the physician can use the FASQ to determine functional areas with which the person is having the most difficulty and refer him for special assistance with these tasks.

An eye examination should begin with an evaluation of quantitative vision. Two tests that should be performed by primary care physicians are visual acuity testing (far and near) and peripheral field determination.

Testing Visual Acuity in Young Children

Accurate assessment of visual acuity usually cannot be performed on infants and very young children. Instead other eye functions, such as visual fixation and eye movement, can be evaluated.[36] By the time the infant is 2 months of age, he should be able to fixate and follow an object of visual interest. The physician can use a brightly colored toy or flashlight. Since acuity, *per se,* is not being tested, the size of the object and its distance from the child are unimportant. As the examiner moves the object back and forth in front of the child, he watches to see if the child's eyes turn toward it and follow its movement in the visual field. Eye movements should be smooth, free of nystagmus, and well aligned. The corneal eye reflex should be tested. If the child is not able to fixate by 4 months of age, or if any of the functions described are impaired, further evaluation should be done. Absence of pupillary reaction to light (sometimes difficult to detect in infants, since the pupil size is so small) usually implicates an abnormality of the retina or optic nerve.

Although preferential looking tests (used to determine an infant's preference for plain versus patterned stimuli), nystagmus tests, and cortical evoked potentials can be used to estimate an infant's visual acuity, they are not usually offered in the primary care practitioner's office. A 1-month-old infant has an estimated visual acuity of 20/300, and a 6-month-old infant has an estimated acuity of 20/100.[30]

Subjective testing of visual acuity is usually possible in a 2½- to 3-year-old child. Determination of acuity can help detect ocular disorders, neurological problems, and systemic diseases. Various methods have been developed to test young children, illiterate adults, and mentally retarded individuals.[8,18] For instance, picture cards can be presented to the child at increasing distances, testing each eye separately by use of eye patches; the distance in feet at which these cards can be identified is compared with the normal distance an adult needs to see them (20 feet). Another test used with younger children is the *STYCAR method*. The child is asked to match four letters, F, H, V, and O—on a distance chart with similar letters printed on flash cards in his hand. Still another method, and perhaps one of the simplest to use with children over 3 years old, is the *E test*. Capital Es in diminishing size are turned in various directions. The examiner asks the child to point in the direction of the "legs" of the Es. Using these methods it was found that 3-year-olds have a visual acuity of about 20/40, 4-year-olds have an acuity of 20/30, and 5- or 6-year-olds have an acuity of about 20/20, which is normal adult vision.[30]

Testing Visual Acuity in Older Children and Adults

The *Snellen chart* (Fig. 13-1), the most widely used test today for evaluation of visual acuity, can be used to test school age children and adults. This chart has a series of letters or numbers decreasing in size to be read at a set distance. Visual acuity is reported as a fraction: The numerator is the number of feet or meters the person being tested is from the chart; the denominator is the number of feet or meters from the chart a person with normal vision would need to be to read the same line. Table 13-1 indicates the corresponding English and metric equivalents.

A person who wears glasses should be tested both with and without the glasses. If he can read the 20/20 line, his vision is considered "normal." If a person cannot see the 20/20 line but can see the line above it, his vision is less than average; if he can read the line below the 20/20 set of letters, his vision is 20/15—better than average.

Patients who measure between 20/70 and 20/200 with the better eye with correction are termed "low vision," or "partially sighted." As previously mentioned, many services and aids are now available to help these patients make the most of their remaining sight. Patients who cannot see even the largest letter on the Snellen chart with corrective lenses are considered to be "legally blind." If this is the situation, gross additional testing should be performed to determine the extent, if any, of remaining vision. First the examiner should hold up two or three fingers from across the room and gradually move toward the patient until the patient motions that he is able to identify the number of fingers extended. The examiner should measure and record the distance he is from the patient. This is called "counts fingers" (CF). For example, acuity might be recorded as CF at 7 feet or CF at 10 inches, if vision is extremely impaired. If the patient's vision is so poor that he cannot discriminate any fingers, he is asked to observe the movement of the examiner's hand (hand movement—HM) or the movement of a large object (object movement—OM) as it is passed in front of him. If the patient cannot detect either of these, the examiner holds a flashlight above or below the patient's eye and asks him to identify the direction from which the

85 ₁

293 ₂

8754 ₃

63952 ₄

428356 ₅

3746285 ₆

7264793 **7**

3875264 **8**

693 7 4 2 5 **9**

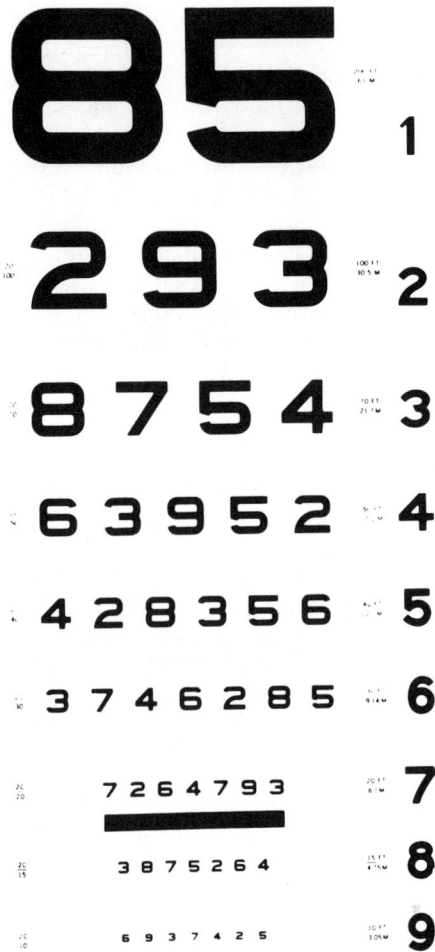

Figure 13-1. The Snellen chart. (Reprinted with permission from Miller D: Ophthalmology: The Essentials, p 33. Boston, Houghton Mifflin, 1979)

light is coming (light projection). Finally, if the patient cannot discern the direction of light but can recognize that a light is on, the degree of blindness is recorded as light perception (LP). This person would be almost totally blind. These legally blind individuals should be referred for further evaluation, as well as be informed of local organizations serving the blind and visually impaired. One point to keep in mind is that as children develop, maturation and an increase in intelligence enable them to use their remaining sight more efficiently; thus an infant diagnosed as having light perception only, may have more usable vision later on.

After measuring distance visual acuity, near visual acuity should be tested. Because near vision decreases with increasing age after the fourth decade of life, it is especially important to test for near acuity in older adults. Testing near acuity may also help the practitioner detect refractive errors due to hyperopia (farsightedness). Snellen and Jaeger are the two major testing systems used to assess near vision. Table 13-2 compares these methods. The Jaeger system,

TABLE 13-1 Snellen Conversion Table Used for Measuring Distance Visual Acuity

English (feet)	Metric (meters)
20/20	6/6
20/30	6/9
20/40	6/12
20/50	6/15
20/64	6/20
20/100	6/30
20/200	6/60

(Jan JE, Freeman RD, Scott EP: Visual Impairments In Children and Adolescents. New York, Grune & Stratton, 1977)

consisting of 20 different sizes of ordinary printing type in increasing gradations, is one of the most popular. The patient reads from a card held at a normal reading distance, and the smallest type that can be read is noted. Vision is normal (20/20) if the patient can read the smallest line of print on the card.

Several points should be kept in mind when testing for visual acuity:[22]

1. Psychological factors can influence the evaluation of visual acuity. Therefore, many patients can increase acuity with encouragement.
2. Increasing or decreasing illumination in the test room can substantially affect acuity scores; it is advisable to use different levels of illumination before arriving at a final numerical determination.
3. Examiner bias may skew some scores.
4. Misaligned, inadequate, or dirty spectacles can interfere with accurate results. Acuity sometimes can be improved just by cleaning the lenses.

TABLE 13-2 Jaeger Notations for Near Vision Testing, with Snellen Equivalents

Jaeger	20/20 System	Examples of Corresponding Printed Material
J1	20/20	
J3	20/30	Telephone directory
J5	20/40	
J6	20/50	Magazine text
J7	20/60	
J9	20/85	Typewriter type (pica)
J11	20/120	
J12	20/130	Large type children's books

(Adapted from Miller D: Ophthalmology: The Essentials. Boston, Houghton Mifflin, 1979)

If the patient requires glasses, has blurred vision, pain, or associated headaches, he may need to be referred to an ophthalmologist.

Testing Field of Vision

The second subjective visual test measures field of vision. Visual fields can (and should with low vision patients) be mapped. The amount of peripheral field loss, as well as its location, is important. For example, lesions involving the superior retina result in the patient's tripping and bumping into objects; loss of vision in the superior field, due to inferior retinal lesions, may result in the patient's incurring head injuries from hanging objects.[14] Once the type of field loss is determined, physicians should warn patients to take special care in preventing such problems. Also the pattern of field loss determines the effectiveness of magnification devices and may affect a person's ability to travel as well as education and job potential.[14]

Visual defects are often concomitant with old age or failing health, and long examinations may not be well tolerated. The usual method for visual field evaluation can be performed both quickly and effortlessly. The examiner positions himself directly in front of the patient and instructs the patient to maintain fixation on one of the examiner's eyes while the examiner's fingers, or some small object such as a pencil, is brought into view from the unseeing periphery. The patient is asked to let the examiner know as soon as the object is seen. This point is noted. Different meridians can be tested in a similar manner. To make the test more comprehensible for younger patients, a child can be asked to grab the wiggling finger or point to a particular toy as soon as it comes into sight. Normally each eye is tested separately with the other eye covered. If both the examiner and the patient have normal visual fields, the test object should be seen by each at about the same point. If any peripheral field deficits are suspected, referral to an ophthalmologist for more detailed testing is indicated.

When examining infants and young children, the primary care physician should keep in mind that the congenitally blind child's development may be retarded by a lack of maternal binding and normal child–parent interactions. The baby's inability to visualize and respond to human faces may result in a lack of appropriate expressions and body gestures. The blind child may smile less frequently than a sighted child and develop bizarre or awkward facial movements, known as "blind mannerisms," which can initiate ridicule in sighted children and can make adults feel uncomfortable. Children learn largely by imitation. If parents and others have not talked to a blind child, he may be markedly delayed in developing communication skills and socializing abilities. Development may lag in other areas as well. Curiosity, which triggers motor activity, is not as great for blind children as for sighted ones; as a result, severely visually impaired children tend to move less and be more passive. Hypotonia, resulting from physical inactivity, may also be present. If an infant is left on his back in the crib too long, trunk and head control may be delayed. Further, congenitally blind children have no visual memory and must depend totally on description by sighted persons for their perception of the world. It is very important for professionals to realize that, although mental retardation is much more prevalent in visually impaired children than in the general population, deprivation of stimulation and inadequate opportunities to learn certain skills may cause a blind child (especially a congenitally blind child) to appear to be retarded when he is not. Also EEGs of visually impaired children normally are different from those of sighted children and may result in a misdiagnosis of mental retardation.[18] Inaccurate diagnoses may cause anxiety, suffering, and irreparable damage; it is therefore extremely important for the physician to assess a child's mental status carefully before arriving at a final conclusion.

Management

Role of the Physician

Both ophthalmologists and primary care practitioners can play an extremely important role in the management of visually impaired patients. Knowledge of the implications, as well as the physical causes, of blindness and low vision is essential to the provision of comprehensive care.

Early diagnosis of visual impairments is vital in preventing further deterioration or in restoring sight. Often the parent is the first to suspect that something is wrong with the infant's vision. A suspicion is sufficient reason for performing a thorough eye examination. If the primary care physician is unsure of the pathological condition, he should make a referral to an ophthalmologist or low-vision clinic. Once the physician has made a diagnosis, both the diagnosis and its implications should be discussed with the family in clear terms.

A study questioning parents of visually impaired children about the helpfulness of their physicians during the initial diagnostic period revealed that nearly half of the parents said that the physician was *not* helpful in providing information about the cause of the impairment or in discussing possible hereditary factors involved. Sixty percent felt the physician was inadequate in giving the parents any idea of what to expect in the future, and many others felt there was little assistance in providing the family with outside sources of help.[18]

A diagnosis of irreversible blindness or severe visual impairment in their child can be shocking to parents. Therefore it is helpful if both parents can be present when the diagnosis is discussed. Also the child may have other handicapping conditions as well.

> Nearly three quarters of mentally retarded children have eye defects and over one half of patients with cerebral palsy show various types of ocular problems. Similarly, blind children commonly have neurological handicaps, such as cerebral palsy, mental retardation, seizures, hearing loss, hydrocephalus, and others.[18]

Realization of additional impairments may be even more traumatic to the parents, who may begin to perceive their infant as a bundle of imperfections and defects. Physicians should take great care in talking with parents about a multi-impaired child, balancing the negative aspects of the disorders with information about current services and aids available to help normalize the child's life. A sensitive attitude and positive interaction with the affected child can demonstrate to parents that it is possible to pick up, cuddle, and enjoy a child with many impairments.

Informing the patient and family of the facts about visual loss, especially blindness, can be very difficult for the physician. Doctors receive their training largely in acute care settings and have little exposure to handicapped children or chronic disorders such as blindness and deafness. The ophthalmologist, especially, may feel that he has failed the patient once treatment is no longer productive and may not report the case of blindness to state authorities. The ophthalmologist's contact with the patient may cease. Because primary care outpatient services generally are not structured to serve patients with many handicaps, these patients may receive fragmented evaluations from many specialists and may be delayed in referral to helping agencies. The primary care physician can alleviate the impact of some of these negative experiences by coordinating referrals, by remaining involved in the patient's progress through correspondence with the other physicians and therapists, and by continuing to see the patient in followup visits.

Infants and young children with subnormal vision are at risk for developing strabismus and amblyopia and therefore should be examined frequently. If needed, treatment should be devised to equalize their vision and increase binocularity. As the child gets older, the physician should continue to educate the youngster about his visual problem, its prognosis, and any hereditary implications. According to Marmon,[25] for example, between 60% and 90% of patients under the age of 20 with retinitis pigmentosa have visual acuity of 20/40 or better; by age 50 the percentage declines to 25%. Visual loss typically progresses from 20/40 to 20/200 within 6 years. Patients should be aware of the potential additional loss of vision. Simultaneously, however, the hopeful aspects of the prognosis should be explored; for example, 25% of patients with retinitis pigmentosa are able to retain good reading vision throughout their lives.

Occasionally, commonplace suggestions can help eliminate potential problems.

For example, children with albinism, congenital achromatopia, aniridia, congenital glaucoma, or corneal opacities are extremely light sensitive. Sunglasses are difficult and expensive to obtain for infants and toddlers. Many of them are helped by wearing a hat with a brim to protect their eyes from overhead and direct glare. For older children, a tennis visor, baseball hat or cap will be acceptable in addition to sunglasses or tinted lenses. When buying school supplies, parents of children with subnormal vision should look for bold-line paper, rulers with well-contrasted markings, large protractors, etc. As simple and obvious as these solutions may seem, many nonvisually oriented people never think of them.[38]

Even though many ocular conditions are not conducive either to cure or to correction, blind patients or those with visual impairments should continue to be seen at least once yearly. As Marmon states, "Medical management of the child with subnormal vision begins at the time of diagnosis and continues for the rest of his or her life."[25]

Primary care specialists also can make a significant difference by devoting their efforts not only to the rehabilitation of the visually impaired youngster, but also to the adverse effects the impairment has upon other family members. The ability of the family and school to cope with the impaired child's needs should be re-evaluated periodically. During the physical examination the physician should inquire about the siblings' adaptation to the impaired family member. The primary care physician should find out how many, if any, additional demands are being placed on the other children to care for the impaired brother or sister. When children are of school age, it is the physician's responsibility to inform the school or teachers of the child's problems. A letter should be written to the school indicating the nature of the visual impairment, specific requirements for its management, and helpful suggestions for more efficient learning experiences.

The primary care physician can be a vital and positive influence in helping the older patient accept a diagnosis of blindness or visual loss. When dealing with the adult patient, the physician's relationship with the patient, understanding of the patient's turmoil and grief, and informed knowledge about blindness can be a comfort to the patient. The physician also can offer valuable advice by negating false stereotypes about the blind, by alerting the individual to the many rehabilitation services available, and by helping to alleviate the patient's fears. The physician can help the patient gradually accept the diagnosis of blindness and can offer assistance in making realistic decisions about vocational training, educational experiences, and family responsibilities.

Physicians can tell their patients about many adaptive techniques developed by other patients. Many partially sighted people who have difficulty crossing streets, for example, due to their inability to perceive all but the yellow traffic lights, have found it useful to watch the light which is at a right angle to them. Its turning yellow indicates that it is almost time to cross. Door frames at home painted in bright colors can help to avoid accidents. Stimulation of the visual sense, through use of bright clothing and placement of attractive pictures at eye level in the home, is also helpful. When impairment is sufficient to limit functioning, patients should be encouraged to attend formal rehabilitation programs.

It might be helpful to consider some "tips" adapted from Gallagher's suggestions for establishing a harmonious doctor–patient relationship:[11]

1. Identify yourself whenever you meet a blind patient, especially if he is hospitalized.
2. When walking with a blind person, offer your elbow for guidance and walk a half step in front. This method can be used also on stairs, going through doors, and circumventing obstacles in hospital corridors.
3. Talk directly to the person, not to a third party. The blind person has a visual impairment, not a hearing disorder.
4. Always tell the person when you are leaving so he can avoid the embarrassment of continuing to talk as though the doctor were still present.
5. If not sure about the approach to make when offering assistance, ask the person himself.

Psychosocial Aspects of Blindness

A distinction helpful in assessing the psychosocial effects of a severe visual impairment is whether the condition is congenital or acquired.

> Whatever the handicap, the reactions of parents to all varieties of handicapped children have much that is similar. Reactions will be influenced by whether the handicap is evident at birth or becomes evident later, after the parents have "fallen in love" with the child. . . ."[18]

When a child is disabled at birth, many parents have universal reactions: shock, disbelief, depression, grief, and a sense of loss of the perfect child they had expected. Concomitantly, they may express anger toward the doctor, the hospital, and even toward friends who have healthy children. Many of these reactions are intensified if the impaired child is the first child or has multiple handicaps. Because many visually impaired children also have other medical problems, there may be a long period of separation before the newborn infant can go home from the hospital, further straining the development of a normal parent–child relationship.

After the initial reactions have subsided, new ones often emerge. A congenitally blind child faces many obstacles to normal bonding, most importantly the loss of eye contact between infant and mother. The mother may feel rejected if the child does not look at her or may feel reluctant to stimulate the baby because of fear or denial of the handicap. Parents may become frustrated and anxious about how they will raise a blind child. They often experience guilt, feeling that they failed the child or that the child's blindness is punishment for their sins. In addition, the infant's many demands may give them little time for normal grieving. As they become aware of the additional burden of care needed and the possibility of more years of dependency than they had anticipated, parents may become overwhelmed. Some may retreat from their responsibilities by sleeping excessively or by engaging in activities outside the home. On the other hand, continued overprotection as the child grows older will eventually contribute to the child's future sense of helplessness, self-devaluation, and dependency.

Most parents need some professional guidance in dealing with the visually impaired youngster. Cohen suggests four states parents pass through in the process of accepting their child's handicap:[37]

1. Experiencing a period of grief
2. Acknowledging and learing to handle their anger
3. Dealing with anxieties related to the child's handicap
4. Making adjustments for the sake of the whole family unit

Although almost any reaction can be considered normal if expressed for a short period of time, the physician should be alert to prolonged indications of abnormal reactions. Some of these include:[18]

1. Suicidal attempts
2. Inability to find anything nice to say about the child (when asked)
3. Difficulty controlling impulses to harm the child or set behavior standards
4. Unwillingness to take the child out in public
5. Impending marriage breakup, related to the child
6. Absence of reaction to the diagnosis lasting for a period of weeks

It is extremely important that the family physician be aware of the parents' feelings and reactions. Many authors concur that parental attitude is the most important aspect influencing adjustment of the child to a visual impairment.

Although those with acquired blindness far outnumber those who are congenitally blind, persons with acquired blindness are de-emphasized in rehabilitation and patient management. Acquired blindness may come suddenly or gradually. The way it is acquired will have an impact on the person's acceptance of it and motivation for rehabilitation. Age at onset is also an important factor. Children tend to adjust to disability more easily than adults. Their ability to comprehend what has happened to them is limited by their age, inexperience, and lack of preparation. To an adult, loss of sight is usually a bewildering and fearful experience: They may have great doubts about their futures; a previously stable personality may show signs of instability; newly blinded adults are likely to question their ability to function as an effective parent or spouse; sensory deprivation may cause aggression, hostility, withdrawal, or boredom.

Acquired blindness also affects a person's self-esteem. If the blinded person's self-concept was centered around something he can no longer do (*e.g.*, artistry, professional sports), blindness will be even harder to accept. A study of those with acquired blindness and those with congenital blindness showed that those who became blind after having had sight often had a greater sense of loss and found adjustment more difficult than did those who had never had vision.[6]

Rehabilitation of The Blind Patient

Carroll[6] has enumerated some of the losses associated with blindness. These include losses in the areas of psychological security, basic skills, communication appreciation, occupational and financial status, and losses to the whole personality. Many of these issues are addressed in the comprehensive training programs offered by state associations for the blind, which cover areas such as home management, personal care, use of medication, identification of money, orientation and mobility, sensory retraining, use of the telephone, tape recorder and typewriter, written communication, braille, low-vision aids, and counseling. A majority of the blind and severely visually impaired are elderly, and many live alone or are likely to live alone at some time. Several programs offer home training to maximize the transfer of learned skills to the home environment. Vocational training also is offered by most state agencies and requires sponsorship of the local Division of Vocation Rehabilitation. Although a referral from an ophthalmologist usually is required for acceptance into these programs, any physician can initiate the referral. Training courses to improve skills necessary for independent living are crucial to the rehabilitation process and should be encouraged in patients who are legally blind or who have a substantial degree of visual loss.

Visually impaired individuals perform no better than others on tactile and other sensory tasks, which suggests that development of the other senses does not occur naturally, but must be trained. Family members and other persons can provide sensory training outside the rehabilitation setting. Tactile and olfactory stimulation (i.e., holding a cookie in front of the child) can stimulate the visually impaired child and prevent some motor delays. Physicians should inform their patients of sensory exercises that can be used to obtain additional information from the environment and develop a heightened awareness of the information already being received through these channels.

Patients can be educated to increase acuity in the perception and interpretation of auditory information. The congenitally blind child needs to be taught to listen. Physicians should caution parents to restrain from deluging the blind child with loud sounds or constant auditory stimulation. Radios, televisions, and record players must be used for short periods of time, Too much background noise may irritate the infant, and he will tune out, cutting off his major source of contact with the outside world.[19] Older patients can improve their abilities to identify, localize, and discriminate sound through exercises that require them to identify and localize sounds or to pick out a sound from a noisy environment. A ticking clock in the home provides a stationary and constant source of sound which aids individuals with spatial orientation. Patients can be encouraged to exploit the binaural quality of the sound for localization, by turning their heads in the direction of a sound (or tilting the head so that one ear is above the other for the localization of sounds on a vertical plane). Reflected sounds or echoes provide an immense amount of information about the source of sound, the object or environment from which the sound is reflected. For example, a sound that echoes from a building provides information about the distance from and direction of the building. Echoes in a closed environment provide information about the size of the room and the number of people in it. Patients can be encouraged to wear metal heels or to snap their fingers to obtain this information. Alterations in sound quality also occur as sound reflects from an object without the time delay associated with echoes. For example, the sound quality of the voice changes as an individual approaches a wall, and the sound of footsteps as the blind person nears an object informs him of its presence and nature. 'Facial vision,' the perception of nearby obstacles, involves changes in background noise as it reflects from an obstacle. This sense can be heightened by presenting objects at varying distances to the body; a clothesline from which objects can be suspended and moved by a pulley is useful for training. All of these echo-detection techniques are useful for spatial orientation, mobility, and safety.

Training and practice in the home environment can heighten other senses. The awareness of pressure and pain, perceived through the tiny hairs on the skin, can be improved for safety purposes. Motor memory, on which the blind rely heavily, can be practiced to increase confidence and accuracy of movement.

Interpersonal communication is another part of rehabilitation programs. Physicians can help their blind patients improve communication skills. The blind person loses certain aspects of communication, which is frequently overlooked, due to his restricted mobility and to the altered experience of communication itself, such as facial expressions and gestures. Training and sensitization help the blind person develop the ability to interpret the rhythm and intonation of speech and infer, from pauses and voice quality, information concerning the speaker's age, personality, and feelings. Blind people cannot perceive that they are being addressed if other people are present. They cannot tell when a speaker has finished a sentence or ended a conversation. Training can improve interpretive powers. Family members can develop the habit of addressing the person by name when initiating a conversation, and they can provide auditory cues which indicate they are finished speaking. They also can use touch in their communication with the blind.

Rehabilitation of the Low-Vision Patient

The partially sighted frequently are neglected in rehabilitation efforts. Many low-vision people have the same problems of mobility, home and financial management, communication, and psychological insecurity as the legally blind.

Children with partial sight are often misdiagnosed, misunderstood, under-educated, and socially ostracised. They are neither blind nor sighted and frequently have difficulty fitting into society, which does not acknowledge their existence. It is next to impossible to overlook a child who has little or no useful vision, but it is very easy for a partially sighted person to be lost in the crowd. Because he sees some things, it is frequently assumed by parents, physicians and teachers that he sees everything and, therefore, the problems he may have are attributed to inattention, lack of ability, sheer perversity, or poor coordination.[18]

Because the partially sighted are likely to become legally blind, rehabilitation should take place at their present level of impairment. The type of visual loss and the amount of remaining vision are important in planning rehabilitation. A person who has central (macular), but no peripheral, vision sees quite differently than one who has only peripheral and no macular vision (Fig. 13-2). People with macular vision are able to perform near tasks; those who do not have macular vision will have difficulty with tasks dependent upon vision for detail, such as reading. People with good peripheral vision have the ability to maintain travel skills and orientation. Since mobility is important in maintaining personal independence, the person with central vision only may be severely limited. Physicians should encourage low-vision patients to use their remaining functional vision. They should make clear to the patient that eye strain does not damage eyes or add to deterioration of eyesight; on the contrary, continued use of remaining vision may increase optical circulation and even improve visual efficiency.[18]

Coping with visual loss requires more than visual aids and specialized training; emotional support is needed as well. Many organizations serve the needs of the visually handicapped by offering information regarding available resources

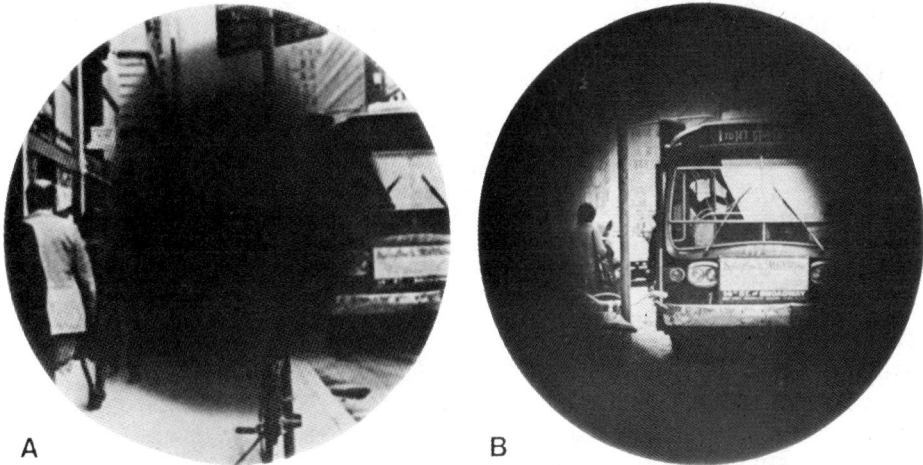

A   B

Figure 13-2. *A.* A central field defect interferes with reading ability and appreciation of fine detail, but not with ability to travel. *B.* A reduced peripheral vision defect interferes with a person's mobility and with his orientation to his surroundings.

and by providing opportunities for social interactions with other visually impaired persons. More specific information regarding these organizations can be obtained by writing to the American Council for the Blind, 501 North Douglas Avenue, Oklahoma City, OK 73106, or the National Association for Parents of the Visually Impaired, 2011 Hardy Circle, Austin, TX 78753.

Visual Aids

There are various aids which may help the blind or visually impaired individual: *nonoptical* aids, such as braille and large print books, recorded reading material, reading stands, and writing guides; *optical* aids, such as spectacles, contact lenses, telescopes, and handheld magnifiers; and *electronic* aids, such as closed circuit TVs and projection magnifiers. They vary in price; some are inexpensive, others can cost thousands of dollars.

The local or regional library can be one of the greatest resources for a blind or visually impaired individual. Talking Books lends recorded reading material and tape machines, at no cost, to eligible people as a service of the Library of Congress. Free bimonthly catalogs, which include braille and large print books and periodicals, are also available. Specialized musical scores and instructional cassettes for piano, guitar, and other instruments are available through the Library Service for the Blind and Handicapped. Eligibility criteria for these loan services are:[9] legal blindness (regardless of optical measurement); visual disability, which, with correction, prevents the person from reading standard printed material; or reading disability (inability to read or use standard printed material) as a result of physical limitations or severe organic dysfunctions. Eligibility must be certified by a competent authority such as a physician, optometrist, registered nurse, therapist, social worker, or welfare agency worker. If a person meets any of these requirements, all that needs to be done to obtain the free services is to get an application form from the local library and a letter of confirmation from the authority. If the referring agent is a physician, he should send a written statement on a letterhead or prescription form to the Library of Congress with a brief statement describing the reading disability. Even if the person with visual problems is unable to qualify for these services, a call to the library may inform him of other services available to everyone. One example would be the "Tips on Tape" program offered in some localities. An interested person can call a specified number to receive information on activities, services, and appliances for low-vision individuals.

Reading and educational materials can also be purchased from a number of private companies. The American Printing House for the Blind has educational materials, including a recorded adaptation of the World Book Encyclopedia; and Science for the Blind offers adapted technical equipment. The American Foundation for the Blind publishes the largest catalog listing these materials. A partial listing of the names and addresses of suppliers can be found in Appendix 13-1.

Besides printed materials, there are many other helpful nonoptical devices on the market. Reading stands (to hold books closer to eye level), wide-lined paper, felt-tipped markers, and braille typewriters are examples of visual aids which might be of assistance to low-vision students and careerpersons. Tape recorders can also be beneficial when rapid note-taking is needed. Braille dials, automatic needle threaders, and braille watches are examples of other nonoptical aids which make life easier for the individual with limited vision. Table 13-3 lists some of the nonoptical aids available.

Visual deficiencies should not prevent participation in healthful recreational activities. There are many physical education aids that can be suggested for use either in the local schools or private homes. For example, partner's belts, which connect a blind and sighted person, enable the blind person to pursue running activities: blind persons also can participate in long-distance track and field events by running their fingers gently along the ropes set up as a guide to track lanes. Training and tandem bicycles allow the individual with low vision to cycle on quiet streets. Special balls with bells attached and portable aluminum bowling guiderails are two more examples of the many recreational aids available today. More information on such aids can be obtained from the Playground Corporation of America in New York City or the American Foundation for the Blind.

Guide dogs may increase some legally blind individuals' mobility, but unlike the false popular notion about these animals, they are not trained to think for the sightless person, only to obey. Their usefulness is therefore proportional only to the competence of their master. Older persons often do not have the strength to keep the dogs in check or the ability to care for them. At present fewer than 2% of blind persons in the United States use guide dogs.[39]

TABLE 13-3   Low-vision Accessory Aids

Communication Aids	*Personal Care Aids*
Envelope guide	Sock clips
Signature guide	Dresser drawer dividers
Writing guide	
Check guide	*Leisure Aids*
Bold-line paper	Large-print cards and Bingo
Bold-line checks	Games adapted for visually impaired
Fiber-tip pens	Large-print magazines and books
Raised number and larger-number watches	Typoscope (reading slit)
	Book stands
Large-print standard and pushbutton telephone dials	Talking books or cassettes and machines
Wallets with dividers for coins and bills	*Homemaking Aids*
	Large-print or raised letter measuring cups, spoons, oven dials
Lighting Aids	Large print timers
Gooseneck or flexible arm lamps	Large-print cookbooks
Flashlights	
Health Aids	
Insulin devices	
Pillboxes	
Bathroom scales with large numbers	

(Hollander LL: Normal aging. In Logigian MK (ed): Adult Rehabilitation: A Team Approach for Therapists, p. 17. Boston, Little, Brown & Co, 1972)

Optical aids, which probably compensate most profoundly for visual impairments, come with a variety of filters and magnification. Although they do not restore normal vision, they allow visualization of many objects that could not otherwise be seen.

Many physicians don't see the importance of a particular optical aid. They realize that the magnification will not greatly improve the vision but don't always appreciate the fact that for this individual being able to do one task more easily is very important.[10]

The use of reading glasses, bifocals, or magnifiers can preclude the need for large-print books. Distance telescopes can be used to view bus numbers, street signs, aisle markers in the grocery store, blackboard assignments, and so on. Although they allow for distance vision, they also restrict the field of vision, limiting their use mainly to sighting. Some telescopic devices are too bulky for everyday use, but many smaller models that can be hung on a chain around the neck are now available.

Spectacles are portable, but have short focal distances. Teenagers and adults are often self-conscious about having to hold their reading materials at such close range. Instead they may use a small, less conspicuous handheld magnifier, although this is inconvenient to use if a large amount of material is to be read.

There are several general rules the physician should keep in mind when prescribing optical devices.

1. The least conspicuous device, which provides the most useful vision, will be most used.
2. If at all possible, devices should be prescribed before a child goes to school. Preschool children are less self-conscious and more willing to adapt than are teenagers or adults.
3. Except when glasses are prescribed for protection of remaining sight, children should not be forced to wear glasses all the time. Tongue[38] points out that extremely myopic children should be allowed, and even encouraged, to take off their glasses to do close work if it is easier. Infants, who tend to study objects at close range, also may find it easier without glasses.
4. Illumination can make a big difference in helping or hindering a vision disorder. Although bright illumination is usually beneficial, patients with retinal dysfunctions, albinism, and cataracts may prefer dimmer light. Generally, the person should be allowed to seek the type of lighting that is personally most comfortable.
5. It is important for the physician to try to find a low-vision aid that is acceptable to the patient. Once prescribed, there should be adequate followup.

Several electronic aids are now on the market, and there are hopes of more being developed soon. The Washington Ear provides radio receivers which are tuned to a station that reads newspapers twice each day. The Visualtek machine, which consists of a television camera, a monitor, and a zoom lens, magnifies written material and enables a person with a progressive impairment to read for a longer period of time than would otherwise be possible. Two new and more costly devices have been developed (the Visatoner and the Optacon), which read printed material aloud by converting visual images of letters into tonal or tactile forms, respectively. 'Talking' calculators offer the usual calculator functions but, in addition, convert input signals into audible responses. Electronic canes are being developed with laser beams or vibrating buttons to alert the owner to overhead obstructions and curbs.

Although some of the specific services and aids described may be quickly outmoded, the value of information about such resources will not be. National or state associations for the blind should be contacted for current information of this kind. The Directory of Agencies Serving the Visually Handicapped in the US, which is updated annually, contains the names, addresses, and low-vision services of most state, local, and federal agencies, schools, and organizations for the visually handicapped in the United States. It can be obtained for a fee by writing the American Foundation for the Blind, 15 W. 16th Street, New York, NY 10011.

Summary

Although most primary care practitioners have limited contact with totally blind patients, almost all will confront patients with varying degrees of visual impairment. In order to provide preventive, comprehensive care, the physician must be able to perform a visual screening exam, recognize common causes and symptoms of visual impairment, and provide appropriate referrals for low-vision aids, vocational and functional counseling, and training.

This chapter emphasizes the fact that, as of this date, there are no clearly established definitions of blindness or of other visual impairment levels. The American Medical Association's definition for legal blindness is used widely for determining legal compensation, social security benefits, and eligibility for training or educational purposes. However, the AMA's definition excludes many people who have substantial visual deficits. As a consequence, they are prevented from obtaining such benefits. Also, although categorizing a person as legally blind provides advantages for some, the label may hinder a person's acceptance and integration into a sighted society.

In addition to *legal blindness,* other terms such as *low vision* or *partial sightedness, residual vision,* and *remaining vision* are discussed. Some common causes of blindness are summarized. Basic examination techniques for testing infants, young children, and adults are described. The necessity for testing field of vision, in addition to visual acuity, also is addressed.

Some of the psychosocial aspects of blindness, including parental reactions to the diagnosis of blindness in a child, developmental barriers imposed by blindness, and the differing consequences of sight deprivation experienced by congenitally and adventitiously blinded persons, are explored. The primary care physician must be alert to methods of helping blind people improve developmental skills and interpersonal communication. To this end, some simple exercises for improving perception, identification, and localization of sound are presented, as well as some commonly useful suggestions for facilitation of communication.

Visual aids are described and references for further information about them are provided.

Finally, the role of the physician in case management of the visually impaired individual is reviewed. Physician responsibilities include: Early diagnosis of visual impairments with appropriate referral to eye specialists and periodic followup; provision of information to family members about possible hereditary or causative factors involved; a sensitivity to parental reactions, coupled with suggestions for adaptive techniques and assistive devices aimed at promoting acceptance of the handicap; and evaluation of the home environment and effect of the visual handicap on other family members.

References

1. Allen D: Orientation and mobility for persons with low vision. Visual Impairment & Blindness 71(1):13, 1977
2. Ashcroft SC: Social participation, citizenship and the visually handicapped. In Goldberg MH, Swinton JR: Blindness Research: The Expanding Frontiers, p 117. University Park, Penn State University Press, 1969
3. Barrago N: Increased Visual Behavior in Low Vision. New York, American Foundation for the Blind, 1964
4. Bauman MK: Dimensions of blindness. In Goldberg MH, Swinton JR (eds): Blindness Research: The Expanding Frontiers. University Park, Penn State University Press, 1969
5. Buell CE: Physical Education and Recreation for the Visually Handicapped. Washington, American Association for Health & Physical Education and Education Press, 1973
6. Carroll TJ: Blindness: What It Is, What It Does, and How to Live With It. Boston, Little, Brown & Co, 1961
7. Chapman EK: Visually Handicapped Children and Young People. London, Routledge & Kegan Paul, 1978
8. Davis CJ: Adjustment of the blind adolescent. In Goldberg MH, Swinton JR (eds): Blindness Research: The Expanding Frontiers. University Park, Penn State University Press, 1969
9. Department of State (Rhode Island) Library Services: Library Services to the Blind and Physically Handicapped, 95 Davis St., Providence, Rhode Island.
10. Dunham JR: Blindness and visual impairment. In Goldenson RM, Dunham JR, Dunham CS (eds): Disability and Rehabilitation Handbook, p 26. New York, McGraw-Hill, 1978
11. Gallagher WF: Rehabilitation of the visually impaired. In Licht, S: Rehabilitation and Medicine, p 73. New Haven, Elizabeth Licht, 1968
12. Geddes D: Physical Activity for Individuals With Handicapping Conditions. St Louis, CV Mosby, 1978
13. Goldberg MH, Swinton JR (eds): Blindness Research: The Expanding Frontiers. University Park, Penn State University Press, 1969
14. Goodlaw EI: Assessing Field Defects of the Low Vision Patient. J of Ophtham Physiol Optics 58(6):486, 1981

15. Hardy RE, Cully JG (eds): Social and Rehabilitation Services for the Blind. Springfield, IL, Charles C Thomas, 1972
16. Hoover RE, Blesdoe CW: Blindness and visual impairments. In Stolov WC, Clowers MR (eds): Handbook of Severe Disability: A Text for Rehabilitation Counselors and Other Vocational Practitioners and Allied Health Professionals. Washington, US Dept. of Education, Rehabilitation Services Administration, 1981
17. Hopkins HV: Principles and Methods of Physical Diagnosis. Philadelphia, WB Saunders, 1966
18. Jan JE, Freeman RD, Scott EP: Visual Impairments in Children and Adolescents, pp 18, 129, 161, 267. New York, Grune & Stratton, 1977
19. Kastein S, Spaulding I, Scharf B: Raising the Young Blind Child: A Guide for Parents and Educators. New York, Human Sciences Press, 1980
20. Keeney A, Keenery VT: A Guide to Examining the Aging Eye. Geriatrics 35(2):81, 1980
21. Kirtley DD: The Psychology of Blindness. Chicago, Nelson–Hall, 1975
22. Kleen SR, Levoy RJ: Low vision care: Correlation of patients' age, visual goals and aids prescribed. Am J Ophthamol Physiol 58(3):200, 1981
23. Leighton DA: Special senses: Aging of the eye. In Brocklehurst JC: Textbook of Geriatric Medicine and Gerontology. Edinburgh, Churchill Livingstone, 1978
24. Margo C, Brown B: Adjustment to visual loss. JAMA 248(10):1231, 1982
25. Marmon MF: Visual loss in retinitis pigmentosa. Am J Ophthamol 89:692, 1980
26. Miller D: Ophthamology: The Essentials. Boston, Houghton Mifflin 1979
27. Myklehurst HR: The Psychology of Deafness, p 1. New York, Grune & Stratton, 1960
28. Reinecke RD: Loss of vision: Eye pain. In Macbryde CM, Blacklow RS (eds): Signs and Symptoms: Applied Pathological and Clinical Interpretation. Philadelphia, JB Lippincott, 1970
29. Rhode Island Association for the Blind Literature, 1058 Broad St., Providence, Rhode Island.
30. Robb RM: Ophthamology for the Pediatric Practitioner, p 1. Boston, Little Brown & Co, 1981
31. Rosenfeld I: The Complete Medical Exam. New York, Simon & Shuster, 1978
32. Rusalem H: The role of motivation in the rehabilitation of the blind. In Goldberg MH, Swinton JR (eds): Blindness Research: The Expanding Frontiers. University Park, Penn State University Press, 1969
33. Schow RL, Christiensen JM, Hutchinson JM, Nerisonne MA: Chronic Disorders of the Aged. Baltimore, University Park Press, 1978
34. Stern EJ: Helping the person with low vision. Am J Nurs 80(10):1788, 1980
35. Sullivan MG: Understanding Children Who are Partially Seeing: A Classroom Teacher's Guide. Washington, Special Child Publications, 1974
36. Taylor RB: A Primer of Clinical Symptoms. New York, Harper & Row, 1973
37. Thompson RP: Parent and child relationships. In Goldberg MH, Swinton JR (eds): Blindness Research: The Expanding Frontiers, pp 37, 55. University Park, Penn State University Press, 1969
38. Tongue AC: Medical Management of the Child With Subnormal Vision. Pediatr Annals 9(11):428, 1980
39. Vaughn D, Ashbury T: General Ophthamology. Los Altos, CA, Lange Medical Publications, 1980

APPENDIX 13-1 Source Listing

Name of Supplier	Large-Print Books, Newspapers, Magazines	Talking Books, Cassettes, and Machines	Other Accessory Aids	Optical Aids	Absorptive Aids	Educational Materials
American Bible Society P.O. Box 5677 Grand Central Station New York, NY 10163	X					
American Foundation for the Blind 15 W. 16th St. New York, NY 10011			X	X		X
American Optical Corp., Inc. Optical Products Division Southbridge, MA 01550				X		
American Printing House for the Blind 1830–1839 Frankfort Ave. Louisville, KY 40206	X		X			
Apollo Lasers, Inc. 6357 Arizona Circle Los Angeles, CA 90045				CCTV*		
Bausch & Lomb, Inc. 635 St. Paul St. Rochester, NY 10146				X		
Designs for Vision, Inc. 120 E. 23rd St. New York, NY 10010				X		
G. K. Hall & Co. 70 Lincoln St. Boston, MA 02111	X Book club					

(continued)

Organization						
Howe Press, Perkins School for the Blind, 174 N. Beacon St., Watertown, MA 02172				X	X	X
Keeler Optical Products, Inc., 456 Parkway, Broomall, PA 19008			X			
Library of Congress, Division of the Blind and Physically Handicapped, 1291 Taylor St. NW, Washington, DC 20542			X		X	X
Lighthouse, N.Y. Assn. for the Blind, 111 E. 59th St., New York, NY 10022	X	X	X	X		
Luxo Lamp Corp., Monument Park, Port Chester, NY 10573				Lamps		
National Assn. for the Visually Handicapped, 305 E. 24th St., New York, NY 10010	X		X			X
National Soc. for the Prevention of Blindness, 16th E. 40th St., New York, NY 10016	X					
New York Lighthouse Aids Service, 32–02 Northern Bv., Long Island City, NY 11101			X		X	

APPENDIX 13-1 (Continued)

Name of Supplier	Large-Print Books, Newspapers, Magazines	Talking Books, Cassettes, and Machines	Other Accessory Aids	Optical Aids	Absorptive Aids	Educational Materials
New York Times 220 W. 43rd St. New York, NY 10036	X					
Pelco Sales 351 E. Alondra Blvd. Gardena, CA 90248				CCTV*		
Readers Digest Pleasantville, NY 10570	X					
Recreational Innovations, Inc. P.O. Box 203 Saline, MI 48176					X	
Selsi, Inc. 40 Veterans Blvd. Carlstadt, NJ 07072				X		
Visualtek 1610 26th St. Santa Monica, CA 90404				CCTV*		
Volunteer Services for the Blind 919 Walnut St. Philadelphia, PA 19107	X					

* CCTV = Closed circuit television
(Hollander LL: Normal Aging. In Logigian MK (ed): Adult Rehabilitation: A Team Approach for Therapists, pp 12–13. Boston, Little, Brown & Co, 1982)

CHAPTER 14
Hearing Impairments

Hearing disorders are among the most common chronic impairments in the United States. Total deafness, the inability to hear speech even with amplification, is rare. A wide range of difficulties, many of which can benefit from treatment, is common, however. Many people neglect telling their physicians of symptoms of hearing difficulties; consequently, their problems continue undiagnosed and untreated. The type and extent of hearing loss must be assessed so that appropriate comprehensive care can be offered the patient and his family.

> A person with mild or moderate hearing loss will differ greatly from someone with a more severe hearing loss—in terms of speech and language development, choice of communication systems, educational history and general life experiences.[28]

The primary care physician can play a crucial role in the early detection of hearing disorders, referral to appropriate specialists, education, alleviation of anxieties about hearing impairments, and provision of information about resources.

Definitions and Classifications of Hearing Impairments

Degree of Hearing Loss

The degree of hearing impairment is normally determined by an audiogram, which measures the amount of hearing loss over a range of frequencies. Hearing losses are measured in terms of loss of decibels (dB). The higher the decibel loss, the greater the degree of impairment.

Various terms are used to describe persons with hearing loss. Terms such as *deaf, hard-of-hearing,* or *hearing impaired* are all too often used incorrectly or interchangeably. Such inappropriate usage can lead to overgeneralizations about all hearing loss disorders and can impose unwarranted limitations or expectations on the affected individual. The following definitions have been adapted from lecture material provided by the Rhode Island Department of Social and Rehabilitation Services.[28]

Hearing Impaired. Covers a broad spectrum of hearing losses, ranging from moderate to profound. Although the term identifies a person as having some type of hearing loss, it neglects to discuss the limitations in terms of severity, type (conductive, sensorineural, or mixed), or configuration (frequencies at which hearing sensitivity is compromised) of the hearing loss.

Hard-of-Hearing. Pertains to individuals with mild to severe hearing loss, ranging from 25 dB to 85 dB, across frequencies important to speech reception. Most hearing impaired people fall into this category. Individuals who are hard-of-hearing usually have enough residual hearing to develop speech and language based on auditory reception, although there may be varying degrees of difficulty in achieving this. Although individuals who are hard-of-hearing often can function in a regular educational classroom, they may benefit from some form of amplification and special teaching techniques.

Deaf. Identifies individuals with a profound hearing loss of 85 dB or more in frequencies important to speech reception. People in this category have little or no residual hearing and may encounter problems in communication and employment. Educational programs for the deaf are usually specialized to meet their communication needs and provide the knowledge needed to function in a hearing world. It is likely that deaf persons will experience great difficulty in the development of speech and language through auditory means and may often seek a visual manual communication method. Many deaf and hard-of-hearing individuals choose not to use their voices, but few are unable to use it. For this reason, terms such as *deaf-mute* and *deaf and dumb* should be avoided.

Types of Hearing Loss

There are three major types of hearing loss: conductive, sensorineural, and mixed.

Conductive Loss

Conductive loss is a form of auditory impairment which involves a degree of difficulty or dysfunction in the conduction of sound to the inner ear by components of the outer or middle ear. Conductive loss involves defects in the external auditory meatus, tympanic membrane, eustachian tube, and auditory ossicles.

One of the most common of the many causes of conductive losses is excess accumulation of wax in the external auditory meatus. Foreign objects, such as pencil erasers or cotton wads, can also plug the auditory canal; careful removal of the obstruction will normally restore hearing. Congenital agenesis (absence or malformation) of the pinna or congenital atresia (occlusion) of the ear canal also contributes to substantial conductive hearing losses. Infection, a frequent cause of auditory problems initiated in the middle ear, is responsible for one tenth of the cases of severe deafness in adults.[9] *Otitis media,* the general term for inflammatory conditions located within the middle ear, may be due to infection of the upper respiratory tract, diseased tonsils, the common cold, other childhood illnesses, or allergic conditions. *Suppurative otitis media,* a specialized form, results from bacterial or viral infections in the nasopharynx escaping to the middle ear through the eustachian tube. Accumulation of pus, severe pain, elevated temperature, and a distended eardrum are all indications of suppurative disease. If not treated efficiently, this condition can become chronic and result in potential erosion of the middle ear structures, scar tissue formation, and substantial hearing loss. Additional causes of conductive loss include congenital malformations of the middle ear, as well as retraction, distention, or puncture of the eardrum.

Otosclerosis, a disease which turns normally spongy bone into hard bone, can cause malfunction of the stapes and mild to moderate conductive losses. A frequent site of otosclerosis is at or near the oval window. The incidence of conductive disorders can approach 25% in preschool and young elementary-school-aged children. Conductive disorders are less frequently a cause of hearing loss in adults.

A person with a conductive loss may present with the following symptoms[31]:

- A relatively soft speaking voice
- The ability to understand speech fairly well if spoken to loudly enough
- A tendency to have the same degree of hearing loss at all frequencies
- Tinnitus—a roaring, buzzing, or ringing sound in the ear

Treatment for conductive losses usually includes antibiotics, removal of obstructions or impactions, or surgery.

Sensorineural Loss

Sensorineural hearing impairments involve the inner ear, auditory nerve, brain stem or cerebral cortex. (Some authors include impairments occurring in the brain stem and auditory cortex in a separate category called central auditory disorders.) In the presence of sensorineural impairments, sound is conducted properly to the inner ear from the external and middle ears, but it cannot be perceived or analyzed properly. A sensorineural impairment, as with conduction losses, not only results in decreased auditory acuity, but also may cause difficulty with speech discrimination. Other disturbing conditions may accompany sensorineural impairment, including recruitment (the abnormal increase in the perception of loudness as the intensity of sound increases), hypersensitivity to intense noises, and a persistent, high-pitched tinnitus.

Sensorineural losses, similar to conduction losses, can have many etiologies. Some impairments are associated with congenital abnormalities resulting from genetic defects or damage to the embryo *in utero* by disease or drugs. Cytomegalovirus and some sexually transmitted diseases such as syphilis are known to cause neurologic and hearing loss damage *in utero.* One of the most feared occurrences, however, is the mother contracting rubella during her pregnancy. Approximately 12.5% of childhood deafness is due to rubella.[48] Nearly one half of rubella deafened children have at least one other serious physical, psychological, or neurological defect that increases their disability.[20,48] Nearly 5000 deaf–blind children are attributed to the 1963 to 1965 rubella epidemic alone. Sensorineural hearing loss also can be acquired after birth, from anoxia during the birthing process, head injuries, vascular disturbances, childhood illnesses, exposure to loud noises, toxic drug effects, aging, acoustic neuritis, otosclerosis, or Meniere's disease.

Patients with sensorineural impairments may present with the following symptoms[31]:

- Better hearing at low frequencies, and actual loss of hearing at high frequencies
- An awareness that someone is speaking, but no comprehension of what is being said
- A distortion of speech sounds
- A greater intolerance or discomfort for loud noises than the normally hearing person
- Tinnitus

With the exception of losses resulting from Meniere's disease, some vascular problems, and certain tumors or inner ear infections, which may be treatable, there is no known cure for sensorineural impairments. Proclaimed miracle cures such as fluoride treatments, vitamins, ear drops, ear massages, and acupuncture have no documented effect on hearing. Although neural implants may allow reception of some very gross sounds to the profoundly deaf, they have no value for the hard-of-hearing.

Mixed Hearing Impairments

Mixed hearing impairments involve both conductive and sensorineural lesions. The hearing loss may affect the external, middle, or internal ear and can result from one or any combination of causes previously discussed. Sometimes the conductive component can be treated by surgery or medication, but the resultant improvement, if any, will not exceed the amount of loss specifically attributable to the conducting defect.

Presbycusis *Presbycusis,* a normal deterioration in auditory functioning due to aging, may be the most common mixed hearing impairment. It has been reported that from the third decade of life on, the threshold for normal hearing adults begins to rise as a result of age.[12] Difficulties in hearing become 1½ to 4 times more frequent with each additional decade of life, compared with the preceding one. By age 65 nearly one in four adults reports hearing impairments;[5] of these, 10% are deaf and cannot use their hearing for communication.[37]

Earlier researchers described age-related impairments as solely sensorineural in nature. Now, however, aging is known to affect both sensorineural and conductive systems. A number of functional impairments are associated with age-related hearing loss. Impaired sensitivity is one. High-frequency hearing is affected first, and this loss results in difficulty in speech discrimination. Abnormal loudness perception due to recruitment and hypersensitivity is another functional limitation. Impaired sound localization causing increased difficulty hearing in noisy environments is a third. Tinnitus and occasionally, vertigo, are other age-related impairments. However, the diagnosis of presbycusis should be made only when no other specific cause of hearing loss in the older adult can be found. It is important to rule out systemic disorders, which can produce hearing loss so similar as to be mistaken for normal aging patterns of presbycusis. Once diagnosed, the physician should not shrug off age-induced hearing dysfunction as something the elderly individual has to expect and learn to live with. Presbycusis and its accompanying psychosocial effects, including potential social isolation and sensory deprivation, may present as a major medical management problem. A knowledgeable physician can offer the aging patient helpful advice on hearing assistive devices and assess the need for further intervention by other members of the interdisciplinary team.

Listed in Table 14-1 are some of the common causes and types of acquired hearing loss.

TABLE 14-1   Common Causes and Types of Acquired Hearing Loss

Causes	Type of Loss (Sensorineural, Conductive, or Mixed)
Brain Conditions	
Meningitis	Sensorineural
Encephalitis	Sensorineural
Tumors, vascular circulatory diseases	Sensorineural, including central
Concussion, central auditory area damage	Sensorineural, including central
Fracture of the temporal bone	Sensorineural or conductive
General Infectious Diseases	
Scarlet fever	Mixed
Measles	Sensorineural
Mumps	Sensorineural
Pertussis	Sensorineural
Varicella	Sensorineural
Influenza	Sensorineural
Pneumonia, viral and pneumococcic	Sensorineural
Typhoid fever	Sensorineural
Diphtheria	Sensorineural
Syphilis	Sensorineural
Common cold	Mixed
Any disease causing high fever	Sensorineural
Infections of the Ear	
External otitis	Conductive
Otitis media, acute and chronic	
Nonsuppurative	Mixed
Suppurative	Mixed

(continued)

TABLE 14-1   (*Continued*)

Causes	Type of Loss (Sensorineural, Conductive, or Mixed)
Serous	Conductive
Mastoiditis, acute and chronic	Conductive
Physical Agents	
Impacted cerumen	Conductive
Foreign-body impaction	Conductive
Trauma, accidental	Mixed
Noise exposure	Sensorineural
Barotrauma	Mixed
Excessive growth of lymphoid tissue in nasopharynx	Conductive
Surgical interference	Mixed
Toxic Agents	
Quinine	Sensorineural
Nicotine (tobacco)	Sensorineural
Aspirin (salicylates)	Sensorineural
Streptomycin	Sensorineural
Dihydrostreptomycin	Sensorineural
Hydroxystreptomycin	Sensorineural
Neomycin	Sensorineural
Miscellaneous	
Psychogenic	
Hysteria	
Malingering	
Advancing Age	
Presbycusis	Mixed, but mainly sensorineural

(Adapted from Glorig A: Rehabilitation in impaired hearing. In Licht S (ed): Rehabilitation and Medicine, p 714. Baltimore, Elizabeth Licht, 1968)

Screening Examinations

A hearing problem may be confirmed initially by the primary care physician from the patient's subjective complaint, through observation, medical history-taking, tuning fork or other hearing assessment, or from analysis of the patient's responses on the FASQ. A referral then is made to an otologist or audiologist for further evaluation of hearing loss.

The process of hearing involves *sensitivity* (the ability to detect a sound), *recognition of pitch* (the ability to hear a pure tone), *discrimination* (the ability to detect a difference in pitch or loudness and to differentiate speech from background noise), and *tolerance* (the point at which a sound becomes uncomfortably loud).[6]

Crude testing provides only a minimal amount of information about hearing loss. Examples are the watch tick and the coin click tests. The *watch tick* test is a comparison between how long a patient can continue to hear a ticking watch as it is moved away from the ear and the distance a person with normal hearing can just hear it. The *coin click* test employs the dropping of a large coin on a hard surface and determining whether the patient can hear a ring—indicating normal high-frequency acuity—or only a thud—presumable high-frequency loss. The *conversational voice test,* when employed skillfully, may be useful in detecting gross deviations from normal hearing.

In administering the conversational voice test, the patient is placed at the prescribed distance form the examiner so that first one ear and then the other is directed toward the examiner. The patient plugs the ear not under test with his index finger. He is instructed to repeat words he hears the examiner speaking. Then, in a "normal" level of voice, the examiner speaks some numbers, simple words, and simple phrases. If the patient is unable to repeat these, the examiner moves toward the patient until he is able to repeat what the examiner is saying. A score of 10/20 means that the examiner had to move to a distance of 10 feet from the patient before he was able to repeat what the "normal" ear is supposed to hear at 20 feet.[31]

The obvious flaw in the conversational test is that the normal conversational voice varies from examiner to examiner and so lacks uniformity in assessing results.

The two most common methods of testing hearing function are the tuning fork and audiometric evaluations. Both methods test differences between air and bone conduction hearing, but the audiometric exam provides a more definitive picture than the tuning fork of the pattern and degree of hearing loss. Usually audiograms are performed by audiologists and evaluated by an audiologist or otologist.

Tuning forks of various frequencies are used for administering the standard tests. Normally the octave frequencies used are 128, 256, and 512 cycles per second (cps); otologists may also test at 1024 and 2048 cps, since a large percentage of hearing loss involves frequencies greater than 512 cps. The normal speech range refers to the band of frequencies found in the spoken language. Generally, the speech range is said to extend from 250 to 4000 cycles; the low-frequency vowels are found near the 500 cycle band, and the high-frequency consonants are located near the 3000 cycle band. The majority of speech sounds occur between the frequencies of 500 and 2000.

Approximately 15% of the speech sounds fall between 250 and 500 cycles, 30% between 500 and 1000 cycles, 40% between 1000 and 2000 cycles, and 15% between 2000 and 4000 cycles.[29] The most common diagnostic tests carried out with tuning forks are the Rinne, the Weber, and Schwabach.

The *Rinne* test is used to differentiate between conductive and sensorineural hearing loss. To perform the test a tuning fork is set into vibration, and the handle of it is placed against the patient's mastoid bone. As soon as the patient reports that the sound produced by the tuning fork is no longer audible, the vibrating fork is held close to the patient's external ear, and the patient is asked if he can hear the fork again. It is normal to hear airborne vibration longer than vibrations conducted by bone. If the patient still can hear the vibrating fork, he is said to have a positive Rinne. If the patient can no longer hear the fork, he is said to have a negative Rinne. If the Rinne is negative, it is likely that normal pathways of conduction (air conduction) through the external and middle ear are blocked; vibrations initiated by holding the fork against the mastoid bone bypass the obstruction and stimulate the inner ear directly (bone conduction). A negative Rinne usually is indicative of a conductive hearing loss.

The *Weber* test compares hearing by bone conduction in the patient's two ears. The handle of a vibrating tuning fork is pressed against the midpoint of the patient's forehead, and he is asked where the tone is heard. If both ears are equally stimulated, the patient will not be able to differentiate which ear hears the sound; instead, sound will appear to be heard as if it were in the center of the head. If there is a conductive loss on one side, sound is lateralized to the impaired ear. The sound is heard better by the poor ear because it is not distracted by background noise and so can detect bone vibrations better than normal. If there is a sensorineural loss, the sound is heard better on the normal side. In the presence of hearing loss, the inner ear or nerve is less able to receive vibrations coming from any route, including bone conduction, and therefore sound is heard better in the normal ear.

The *Schwabach* test assesses bone conduction. The examiner sets a tuning fork vibrating and then holds the handle of it against the patient's mastoid bone, noting how long the patient continues to hear the fork sound. He then compares that time with the amount of time a normal ear (usually his own) hears the sound in the same environment. The Schwabach test is described in terms of Schwabach shortened or Schwabach prolonged. If the hearing time is shortened, it indicates the patient's bone conduction is less than average and may imply a sensorineural loss.

Each of the tuning fork tests is subject to error. For example, on administering the Rinne test, if the conductive loss is very mild it may not differ from the normal enough to be detected. Some patients given the Weber test, not realizing that they should hear better in the worse ear, may reply that sound is heard in the better ear, because that is how they think they should be hearing. The assumption of the Schwabach test is that the physician doing the testing has normal hearing, which may not be the case. Although tuning fork tests provide information about the patient's hearing abilities at discrete frequencies, they are not designed to yield quantitative results. The pure tone audiometer, an electronic sound-generating instrument which can produce tones as pure as those of the tuning fork, can provide both quantitative and qualitative information about hearing loss, including the shape and severity of loss over the important parts of the frequency range.

In addition to the frequency and intensity controls, an audiometer includes an interrupter switch, which enables the operator to turn the test tone on or off immediately and noiselessly; a masking circuit, so that the ear not under test can be prevented from participating; a voice circuit, which enables the operator to amplify his voice for the patient, making communication possible in cases of extreme loss, and also providing for the administration of certain speech audiometric tests; and a patient-signaling device, usually a cord and pushbutton connected with a small lamp on the face of the audiometer, so that the patient can indicate silently when he is hearing the test tone.[31]

Most audiometers only include frequencies between 125 and 8000 hertz (Hz) or, equivalently, cycles per second (cps); this range includes approximately one octave above and below the normal speech range (Fig. 14-1). The auditory stimuli produced by the audiometer can be directed to either ear through a set of earphones. This part of the exam is an air conduction pure tone test. Stimulation also can be sent from the audiometer by bone conduction vibrations placed on the mastoid process, in order to test bone conduction hearing capacity.

The audiologist presents specific test tones (*e.g.*, 500, 1000, 2000 . . . cps) for a second or two at various intensities of 0 to 110 dB. The pure-tone audiometer measures (in decibels) the deviation of a patient's threshold of hearing from an arbitrary normal standard. Zero dB, the standard reference, represents the lowest intensity at which the average normal ear can detect the presence of the test tone 50% of the time. The patient indicates when he hears the tone by signals, such as pressing a button or raising a hand. The tester normally starts at frequencies above threshold and gradually lowers the tone until a point is identified at which the patient responds correctly about half the time. The results are then graphed, with bone and air conduction test results usually marked on the same paper. If one ear was masked (a noise was introduced into it so it would not participate in the test), this also may be noted on the graph. On the audiogram conduction thresholds are graphed by frequency and hearing level. Air conduction thresholds are recorded as "O" for the right ear and "X" for the left ear. The right ear is always graphed in red, and the left ear in blue or black, for easy identification; when reproduced in black and white, the different symbols enable the reader to distinguish the ear being evaluated. *Bone conduction* thresholds are recorded either as arrow heads (<>) or brackets ([]), because audiologists and otologists do not agree on which of these symbols to use. The direction of the symbol corresponds to the ear being tested. Very few persons have audiograms that fall exactly on the zero line at all frequencies. Each person's audiograms have some minor deviations from the normal line, which appear quite constant from test to test. Figure 14-2 shows some examples of normal, conductive only, sensorineural only, and mixed hearing loss audiograms.

A hearing loss is expressed as the number of excess decibels that the tone intensity must be increased in order for the impaired ear just to detect its presence. Impairment levels are summarized in Table 14-2.

Recommendations to a specialist for further evaluation should be made for children with losses of 25 to 30 dB; adults who have losses of 40 dB or more will have difficulty in hearing conversation and should also be referred. An audiologist can evaluate a patient's need for a hearing aid; however, if a conductive loss is present, a referral should be made to an otologist for a surgical consultation. The physician also should supply patients with moderate to severe

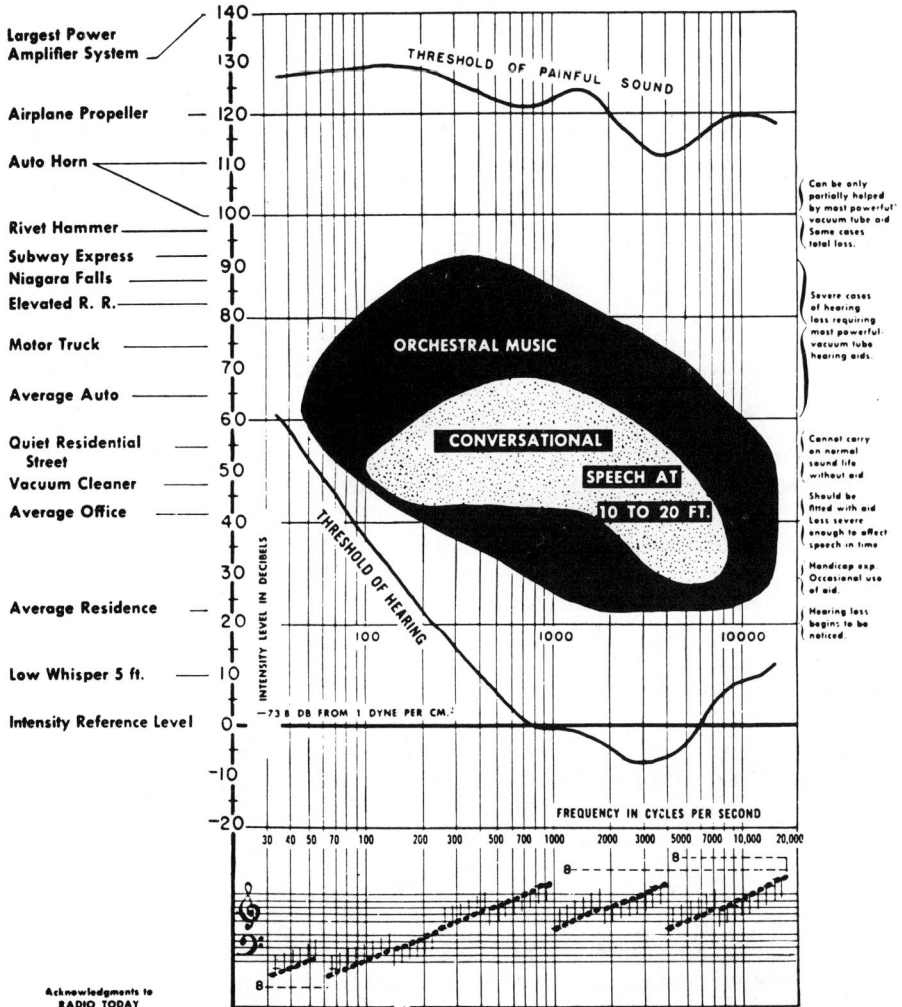

Figure 14-1. Human hearing, range in decibels and cycles. Schematic representation of intensity and frequency characteristics of the human ear and loudness of sounds. (Reproduced with permission from Watson LA and Tolan T: Hearing Tests and Hearing Instruments, p 8. Baltimore, Williams & Wilkins, 1949)

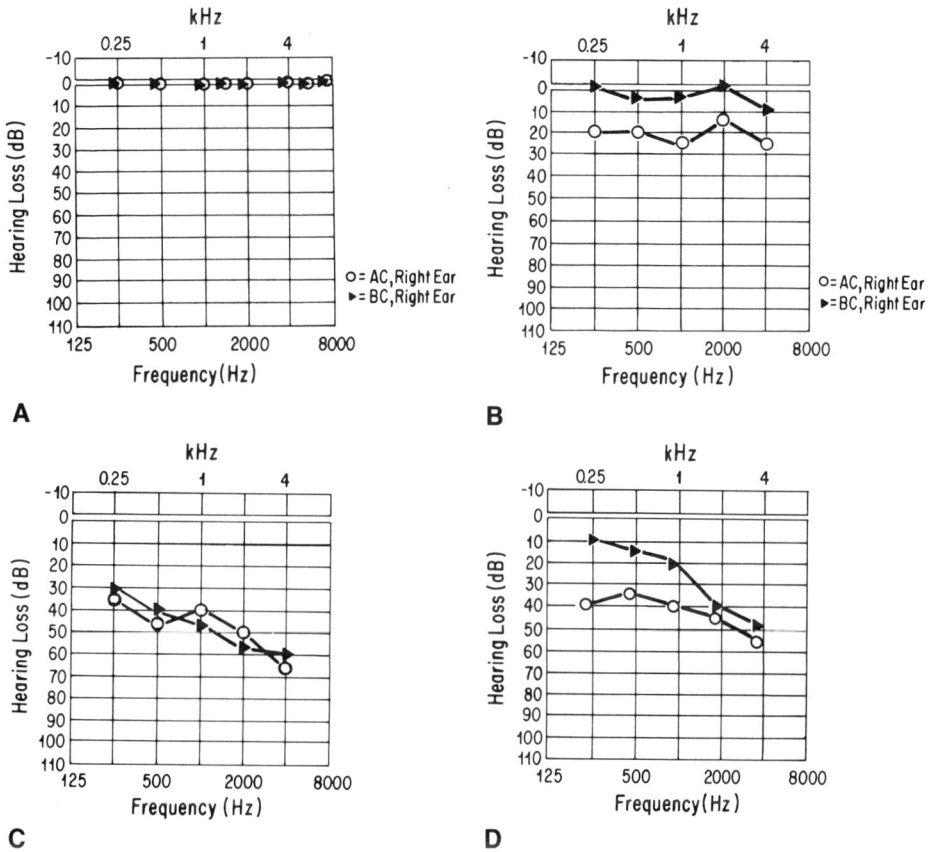

Figure 14-2. A. Normal hearing (air conduction, AC; bone conduction, BC). Straight line along 0 dB line; may deviate slightly from straight line. **B.** Conductive loss (BC, AC). Flat curve or curve with higher thresholds for lower frequencies, with progressively better hearing in higher frequencies (curve may drop off in high frequencies due to sensorineural involvement). BC results within normal or better than normal range, signifying intact inner ear function. **C.** Sensorineural loss. Greater loss at higher frequencies, with lower frequencies being at normal or slightly below normal threshold values. BC threshold pattern closely resembles AC threshold pattern, a diagnostic indicator of sensorineural loss. **D.** Mixed hearing loss. AC curves can exhibit a relatively flat hearing loss which drops off in high frequencies, or a slight loss in low frequencies, with a progressive drop over the entire range surveyed. BC may be better than AC for low frequencies and similar to AC at high frequencies. (Adapted from Heffernan HP, Simons MR, Goodhill V: Audiologic assessment, functional loss and objective audiometry. In Goodhill V [ed]: Ear: Disease, Deafness and Dizziness, pp 143–144. Hagerstown, Harper & Row, 1979; Wallensfels HG: Hearing Aids for Nerve Deafness, p 17. Springfield, IL, Charles C Thomas, 1971)

TABLE 14-2   Hearing Impairment Levels

Degree of Hearing Loss	Hearing Level (dB)
None	26 or less
Slight	27–40
Mild	41–55
Moderate	56–70
Severe	71–90
Profound	91 or more

impairments additional information about hearing devices and local organizations serving the hearing impaired.

The value of the pure-tone audiogram goes beyond determining the extent of loss; the shape of the conduction curve and type of impairment also are important. For example, Figure 14-3A represents a steeply sloping hearing curve, with normal hearing at low frequencies but severe impairment at higher frequencies.

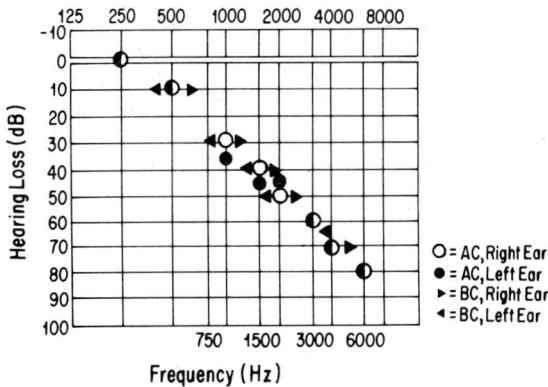

A

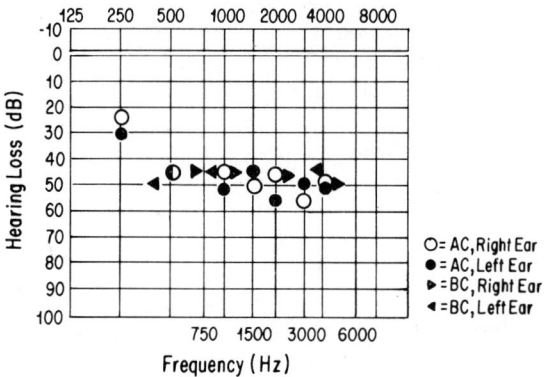

B

Figure 14-3. Shape of conduction curve (air conduction, AC; bone conduction, BC). **A.** "Ski slope" loss. **B.** "Flat curve" loss. (Adapted from Wallensfels HG: Hearing Aids for Nerve Deafness, pp 18–19. Springfield, IL, Charles C. Thomas, 1971)

The audiogram suggests that this patient can still hear many normal noises, such as doorknocks or traffic sounds (<700 cps); hearing, however, is impaired slightly for vowels (around 1000 cps) and is impaired seriously in the consonant range.

A common word like "cat" can easily be heard by this person but is not always understood correctly because there are many similar sounding words in our common everyday vocabularly, like "rat," "map," "sat" or "mat."[49]

Hearing aids may not provide much benefit to this patient since, with amplification, his response to different frequencies will not be equal. Figure 14-3B indicates a flatter curve. The patient who has this type of hearing loss can hear only when conversation is quite loud. The patient is likely to miss much spoken conversation, especially when listening to women with soft voices, and will have to pay careful attention in order to hear satisfactorily.

Although there is a strong correlation between sensitivity to pure tones and sensitivity to speech, pure-tone audiogram results do not provide perfect prediction of difficulties an individual will have hearing speech sounds, and tests measuring the response to words at above threshold frequencies are necessary to test speech sensitivity. A speech audiometer may be used to refine the evaluation of hearing loss further. Speech audiometry involves several different tests which are presented at controlled intensity levels. One such test is the *speech reception threshold* (SRT). To administer this test, two-syllable words are presented, and the patient is asked to repeat what he heard. The audiologist gradually decreases the intensity of the sounds until the point is reached at which the patient can repeat only 50% of the words. The results are then compared with those obtained through pure-tone audiometry. Another speech test evaluates *speech discrimination* abilities. A large number of single-syllable words are presented; the percentage of words correctly repeated by the listener from the original list of words is determined. For example, if a patient were able to repeat correctly 40 out of 50 words, the score would be 80%; 90% and above scores generally are found in the presence of normal or conductive hearing losses. Scores are usually lower in sensorineural loss. Tolerance for loud speech also can be measured with the speech audiometer. For medicolegal purposes, a percentage of impairment can be computed based on audiogram results. According to the American Academy of Ophthalmology and Otolaryngology's method,[31,47] hearing impairment is computed only on audiometric results within the speech frequency range, based on the principle that the handicap of a hearing loss is directly proportional to the effect the loss has on the patient's ability to communicate.

Although speech and hearing assessments are important elements of the otological exam, the primary care physician should be alert to other disabling conditions when examining a patient's ears. A patient should be asked about symptoms of dizziness, vertigo, and fainting. These usually are due to inner ear trouble, brain disease (*e.g.,* epilepsy), tumor, or arteriosclerosis. Sudden spells of dizziness, vertigo, tinnitus, and fluctuating hearing loss are characteristic of *Meniere's disease,* attacks of which occur in clusters. Between attacks, patients are symptom free. An anatomical finding associated with Meniere's disease is the distention of the membranous labyrinth. Although no definite cause has been established, one possibility is spasm or partial blockage of the circulation to the inner ear. Psychosomatic factors may also be involved. Meniere's disease usually involves a degree of permanent hearing loss.

Tinnitus may be caused by drugs (*e.g.,* quinidine, aspirin, streptomycin), high blood pressure, or Meniere's disease. It involves a rhythmic pounding, sometimes sounding synchronous with each heartbeat. No medicine is available to stop the noise and sometimes it is so severe that a psychiatric consultation is necessary. Hearing aids are said to offer relief to some by masking the noise. Tinnitus may clear suddenly; it may continue either intermittently or chronically. Since tinnitus is often a component of several ear diseases, it may be the first symptom to bring the patient to the doctor for diagnosis and treatment.

Otitis media is an inflammatory disease of the middle ear with subsequent accumulation of fluid. Twenty to thirty percent of cases occur in children between birth and 6 years of age,[46] making it the most common cause of acquired hearing loss in American children. For some children it is a chronic, recurring disease with serious consequences. Since the fluid in the middle ear may impede transmission of sound to the inner ear, otitis media often results in a conductive hearing loss. Children who acquire this condition during the critical stages of early development of speech, communication, and social relationships are at high risk for developmental problems. The child with recurrent otitis media may be mislabeled as inattentive or lazy, and delays in language acquisition will most likely result in poor academic performance. Social and emotional development may be delayed as well. Early diagnosis and frequent monitoring may prevent subsequent learning disorders from developing. An audiology consultation may be beneficial, as amplification aids may increase successful performance. Approximately one half of the patients have spontaneous resolution; the remainder need tube insertions to prevent adhesions and restore hearing.[4]

Usher's syndrome, which affects approximately 16,000 people in the United States, is a disease that begins with congenital deafness and then involves progressive visual problems. The initial symptom is the loss of some night vision around ages 6 to 12. Between the ages of 13 and 20, there is additional loss of night vision, and the beginning loss of some peripheral vision. The next stage of Usher's syndrome occurs during the early adult years and results in loss of most of the peripheral vision and some loss of central vision. By the middle adult years there is a continued loss of central vision. Approximately 1 out of every 25 congenitally deaf students has Usher's syndrome.[20] It is extremely important to identify these people before the disease progresses too far, in order to offer them psychological counseling, prevocational training, genetic counseling, information about potential disease symptoms, and preparation for progressive loss of sight. *Retinitis pigmentosa,* as discussed in Chapter 13, is a progressive, hereditary visual impairment disease; it may also be a significant cause of deaf–blindness, and children with deafness should be tested for it.

Ototoxicity

For many years it has been known that certain drugs and chemicals affect or damage the delicate structure and functioning of the auditory–vestibular system. With the proliferation of pharmacologic agents, there has been a concomitant increase in the number of potentially ototoxic medications. Today's physician must be aware of the potential dangers and take precautions to limit unnecessary hearing loss due to ototoxicity.

Table 14-3 presents a partial list of potentially otoxic substances.[30,42]

The risk of ototoxic damage is increased in patients with decreased renal function or pre-existing neurosensory hearing loss.[30] Very young and very old patients especially are at risk. Unfortunate experience has illustrated the detrimental effects that certain drugs can have when taken by pregnant women; the first trimester of pregnancy, especially the sixth or seventh week, seems to be the most vulnerable time for drugs to affect the developing fetus's ear.[42] In the elderly the frequency of ototoxicity is probably due to the large number of medications used by this age group and a possibly increased vulnerability to ototoxic agents. Prior exposure to ototoxic drugs may also increase sensitivity to further toxic drug effects. Even aspirin taken daily in high dosages (*e.g.*, to treat arthritis) has been incriminated as an ototoxic agent.

Symptoms of ototoxicity include tinnitus, neurosensory hearing loss, and vertigo, with or without nystagmus. "The otic changes may be unilateral or bilateral, permanent or transient, immediate or delayed, and dose related or idiosyncratic."[30] Patients should be carefully monitored when any potentially hazardous substance is prescribed, especially pregnant women, renal patients, and elderly people. A thorough medication history should be obtained to assess prior use of ototoxic drugs. Patients should be told to report any subjective

TABLE 14-3   Ototoxic Substances

Chemicals

Alcohol	Gold
Aniline dyes	Iodine
Arsenic	Lead
Benzene vapors	Mercury
Camphor	Nitrobenzol
Carbon disulfide	Tobacco
Carbon monoxide	

Diuretics

Furosemide
Ethacrynic acid

Antibiotics

Amikacin	Streptomycin
Chloramphenicol	Tobramycin
Gentamicin	Viomycin
Kanamycin	
Neomycin	

Miscellaneous Drugs

Antipyrine	Nitrogen mustard
Atropine	Novocain
Barbiturates	Quinine drugs
Caffeine	Salicylates (*e.g.*, aspirin)
Morphine	Strychnine

changes in hearing loss or increasing tinnitus. Frequent hearing evaluations should be performed to monitor any decrease in auditory ability. Drug dosages should be adjusted when decreased renal function is present, and drugs of lesser toxic potential should be used whenever possible. Once a therapeutic goal has been reached, any potentially ototoxic drugs should be promptly discontinued.

Noise-Induced Hearing Loss (NIHL)

Freedom from noise is growing harder to find. The reasons are many: growing urbanization; an enormous increase in transportation; new, larger, more powerful machines for work and recreation; and more people to use them. Americans may not notice the increase in noise around them—the total that acousticians call "community noise"—but it is there. Measurements of outdoor sound levels in areas whose residents might have considered them unchanged show an increase of 2 dB every 10 years. In neighborhoods that clearly have changed—rural to suburban, suburban to urban—the outdoor sound level may have increased as much as 10 dB or more.[23]

Hearing loss due to excessive noise exposure is of concern to all of us. Exposure to noise of a sufficient intensity and duration can injure the ear and produce a hearing loss. Developmental anomalies following exposure of gravid women to noise stress even have been reported.[16] Noise-induced hearing loss (NIHL) can be caused by acute trauma (*e.g.,* firecracker explosion) or chronic exposure to moderate sound levels. Hearing losses can be temporary, lasting minutes to days after termination of exposure, or permanent.

Acute acoustic trauma results from sudden overstimulation caused by a high-intensity, acute noise exposure such as an explosion or a gunshot. In such situations, either the tympanic membrane ruptures (acting as a safety valve) or the cochlea is damaged, resulting in moderate to total hearing losses. The patient with acute acoustic trauma presents to the physician with a history of a sudden onset of hearing loss and tinnitus related to a single incident or exposure to noise of short duration. Except in extremely intense sound exposures (greater than 160 dB sound pressure level), neither the outer or middle ear is likely to be involved in any permanent pathological changes; alternatively, the middle ear may protect the inner ear by the acoustic reflex, a delay between sound stimulation and muscle contraction that decreases hearing effectiveness, thereby lessening the damaging effects of intense noise. Although traumatic losses are more dramatic, the majority of persons experiencing permanent heavy losses are those impaired by repeated chronic exposure to hazardous noise.

Chronic noise-induced hearing impairment results from exposure over a period of time to less intense sound pressure levels (SPLs) than those causing acute acoustic trauma. According to Ward,[50] hearing losses among workers who spend 8 hours a day in a sound level no greater than 80 dB(A) (SPL measured with an "A" type sound level meter, which weights low and high frequencies less heavily than middle frequencies) are no greater than those found in non-noise-exposed persons: If the exposure is increased to 95 dB(A) for the same time periods, however, the incidence of noise-induced hearing loss becomes twice as great as it is in the general population. Duration of exposure is an important consideration, as damage occurs rapidly at first, then gradually slows down. Greater levels of intensity can be tolerated by the person, however, if exposure is intermittent or is interrupted by substantial recovery times. Rest periods away from a damaging noise may protect the ear from injury and hearing loss.[27]

Noise-induced hearing loss is hallmarked by several physical and physiological changes. Immediately after exposure, there is swelling and pyknosis of the outer hair cells, followed by deformation, swelling, and disintegration of the cell body. The basal cochlear turn is the most susceptible area and is normally involved in initial impairment. With progressive injury, there is additional involvement of the pillar cells, Deiters' cells and Heisens' cells, with internal hair cells affected and eventual cochlear neuron atrophy. In addition, histochemical and biochemical changes in the organ of Corti may occur, including a depletion of metabolites, which affect hair cell function. Vascular changes, including atrophy and spasm, result in anoxia. In acute acoustic trauma, rupture of the tympanic membrane and ossicular chain disruption may accompany or occur independently of hair cell loss.

Moderate changes may all be reversible, although acute acoustic trauma usually involves some permanent loss (permanent threshold shift). Temporary impairment (temporary threshold shift) tends to become permanent as time of exposure increases. According to Goin,[15] the degree of temporary or permanent threshold shift depends on:

Intensity of noise
Frequency composition of noise
Duration and frequency of exposure
Individual susceptibility
Pre-existing ear disease

Remarkably, noise-stimulation injuries characteristically involve a specific 8 to 10 mm region of the cochlea along the basilar membrane and result in hearing losses around 4000 Hz. An audiogram performed shortly after noise exposure shows a characteristic dip around the 4-kHz region, called a ''4-kHz notch.'' With progressive hearing loss, the notch spreads first into lower frequencies and then into higher frequencies, affecting the hearing capacity for ordinary speech (Fig. 14-4).

Noise-induced hearing loss can occur from traffic noise, construction work, firecrackers, firearms, airplane engines, and industrial machines, to name a few. Occupational noise exposure is the number one cause of hearing loss.[15] Infant incubators also have been implicated in hearing loss. The possibility that infants living in noisy environments may lose auditory nerve tracts or detectors either through lack of use (too noisy for verbal communication) or through overstimulation[27] is reason for concern. The effect of rock music on hearing loss is controversial. For example, one study of professional musicians failed to reveal any noise-induced hearing loss associated with exposure to rock music over a period of 5 to 10 years.[50] Other researchers apparently have found significant hearing losses in professional musicians playing loud music, utilizing powerful amplifiers, or sitting near brass and percussion instruments. In addition, loudspeakers

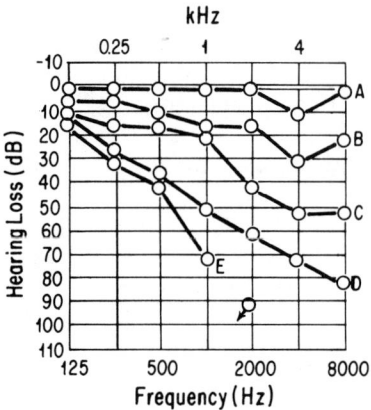

Figure 14-4. Five audiometric profiles in noise-induced hearing loss. **A.** Slight notch at 4-kHz. **B.** Widening and deepening of 4-kHz. **C.** Major hearing loss at 5 or 6 Hz. **D.** Deepening loss over period of years, with shift to left. **E.** Complete loss of high-frequency perception. (Adapted from Goodhill V [ed]: Ear: Disease, Deafness and Dizziness, p 521. Hagerstown, Harper & Row, 1979)

placed as close as one meter from the audience were found to result in a sound pressure level at the listeners' ears of 120 to 130 dB, far above the level known to cause damage.[16] Until further research is completed, children should be cautioned against continuous exposure to loud hard rock music without proper ear protection.

It is important to note that people are not affected uniformly by similar noise exposure. Studies have shown considerable variability of hearing loss among people working in similar noise environments.

. . . Even now, it is clear that structural details—the static and dynamic characteristics of the middle and inner ears—would indeed be expected to determine how much exposure to noise a given ear can tolerate before NIHL occurs. Such characteristics as the stiffness of the cochlear partition, thickness of the basilar and tectorial membrane, blood supply to the cochlea, rate of oxygen metabolism, density of afferent and efferent innervation must be important. . . .[50]

In addition to anatomical determinants, factors such as disease conditions or surgical procedures which lead to a loss of middle ear muscle reflex function cause a greater than normal threshold shift after noise exposure (especially in the low frequency ranges). Persons with hearing loss pre-existing to noise exposure, on the other hand, show less threshold shift, since the amount of sound reaching the sensory receptors in the cochlea is reduced (conductive loss) or damage already present accounts for a decreased differential in the amount of the shift (sensorineural loss). Certain drugs such as neomycin, kanamycin, salicylic acid, and certain mineral and vitamin deficiencies, may similarly reduce the ear's resistance to NIHL.

The diagnosis of noise induced hearing loss is based primarily upon a history of exposure to noise, coupled with a 4-kHz notch (and its variants) on the audiogram and no other significant otoscopic or x-ray findings. When assessing NIHL, differential diagnosis is important. Several other causes appearing separately or coexisting with NIHL can produce audiograms with comparable notches. These include head injuries, some genetic conditions, acquired cochlear lesions (*e.g.,* rubella, influenza, mumps), industrial chemicals, and ototoxic drugs. Thus a finding of NIHL does not eliminate the need for a complete otoaudiologic examination.

Initially the NIHL patient experiences only high-pitched tinnitus, perceived as more intense immediately after exposure to noise. Difficulty in hearing is not a usual complaint.[16] As additional frequencies are lost, however, communication becomes problematic, especially against background noise. Women's voices and other high-pitched sounds especially become hard to hear.

There is no medical treatment for noise-induced hearing loss, although temporary threshold shifts may occur that may be mistakenly attributed to coincidental treatments. Temporary threshold shifts are spontaneously reversible, whereas permanent threshold shifts are irreversible. There is no medication or vitamin supplement for curing either hearing loss or tinnitus; instead, management of the patient with NIHL must focus on prevention, reduction of further noise exposure, and auditory rehabilitation in severe cases.

Prevention may be aided through the employment of hearing protectors, such as earplugs or earmuffs; a combination of both afford the best protection. However, no device offers complete protection from the ubiquitous noises in our society. In addition, some people are unable to fit ear protectors properly (due to arthritis or other dexterity or anatomical problems), some people may not be instructed in the proper use of the devices, and some protectors in employment sites are poorly maintained (*e.g.,* seals are broken). Persons who have been diagnosed as having noise-induced hearing losses should limit their noise exposure by either changing jobs or wearing adequate ear protection devices. Patients also should be urged to avoid loud music, firearm use, loud engine repairs, and home workshop machinery.

Rehabilitative efforts should focus on improving communication. Once the source of damaging noise has been removed, there usually is no further deterioration. On the other hand, once hair cells have been destroyed there is little improvement expected, as hair cells do not regenerate. Ordinary hearing aids are of limited benefit, therefore, since they cannot restore perception to areas of receptor destruction; however, hearing aids may assist in masking the distressing ear ringing of tinnitus. Ward[50] discusses a new electronic instrument that drops all frequencies by a fixed amount (*e.g.,* a 4000 Hz tone becomes a 2000 Hz tone; a 3000 Hz tone becomes a 1500 Hz tone, and so on). Patients are retrained to hear only the shifted sounds with this device ; if feasible, this instrument may benefit persons with severe noise-induced high frequency losses. Lip reading should be advised automatically for any persons with far advanced hearing loss, and all patients should be cautioned about the possibility of further, permanent cochlear damage upon continued exposure to damaging noise levels.

Hearing Aids

Many types of conductive hearing loss, such as those arising from otitis media or otosclerosis, may be corrected through otological surgery. In other types of conductive hearing loss, and in almost all types of sensorineural loss, the impairment cannot be eradicated surgically and the major treatment is amplification of sound through hearing aids. Although hearing aids may not compensate entirely for a loss, especially one involving poor speech discrimination or hearing clarity, they do provide enormous help in making faint sounds louder and they can enable a person to make volume judgments and hear warning sounds in the environment.

Hearing aids primarily are useful in amplifying speech signals for people with intermediate hearing losses ranging from approximately 20 dB to 60dB.[41] Amplification with a hearing aid can establish speech at losses of up to 55 to 60 dB; even the smallest hearing aid can amplify sounds enough in conductive losses to increase conversational speech sounds by 25 to 30 dB.[40] If sufficiently motivated, a person with even minimal hearing impairment can benefit from its use; surprisingly, hearing aids provide many advantages to individuals with profound hearing losses as well.

Many children with profound early-life hearing impairments utilize acoustic cues from hearing aids to note presence or absence of a signal, to detect spectrum, timing and intensity cues regarding sentence type and emotional content, to monitor their own vocal level, and (within limits) to improve speech discrimination ability, particularly when combined with speech reading.[34]

The most important aim of amplification is to establish speech communication. For this reason, neither the degree of impairment nor the type of disorder should determine need and candidacy for a hearing aid. Rather, the decision should depend upon the amount of communicative difficulty the person experiences.[34] Once the need for a hearing aid has been indicated in a child, it is important that it be obtained as early as possible. Because most deaf neonates rarely receive amplification, the opportunity for sound awareness is denied for at least a couple of months. When the child is finally fitted, the infant must be taught sensory awareness.

There are many types of hearing aids, but they are all made up of the same three basic components: A *microphone* to pick up the sound signal and convert it to an electrical signal; an *amplifier* to magnify the signal; and a *receiver* to reconvert the electrical stimulus to a sound which is louder than the original (Fig. 14-5). Most hearing aids are equipped with a custom fitted ear mold which enables the sound to be transmitted into the ear canal. These molds are made by taking an impression of the concha and the ear canal, then sending this temporary mold to a laboratory, which makes a smooth, finished product. The purpose of this tight-fitting, individualized mold is to prevent sound from escaping the ear canal and re-entering the microphone, thus being further amplified. A whistling sound indicates that the ear mold is not fitting tightly enough, is not positioned correctly within the ear, or is damaged in some way.

Due to a larger microphone, amplifier, and power supply, the *body aid* is more powerful and provides better sound quality than the common ear level modes. It offers efficient amplification for the person possessing a severe hearing deficit. An additional advantage is that the controls are larger, enabling its use by people who are unable physically to manipulate the smaller controls on some of the ear types. Some of the body aids also provide their own recharging devices, which are helpful in eliminating the expense of replacement batteries. The main drawback to the body aid is that, due to its size, it is cosmetically unappealing.

Also available are hearing aids that attach to the frames of a pair of eyeglasses. This aid offers good fidelity for persons with mild to moderate hearing impairments. The spectacle-attached hearing aids are good especially for binaural amplification, since an aid can be placed on each temple of the eyeglasses. The eyeglass hearing aid should only be prescribed for people needing constant hearing aid amplification who also wear eyeglasses all the time.

By far the most popular hearing aid types are the ear models. Over 50% of all hearing aids sold are of the behind-the-ear type, which resembles a shrimp

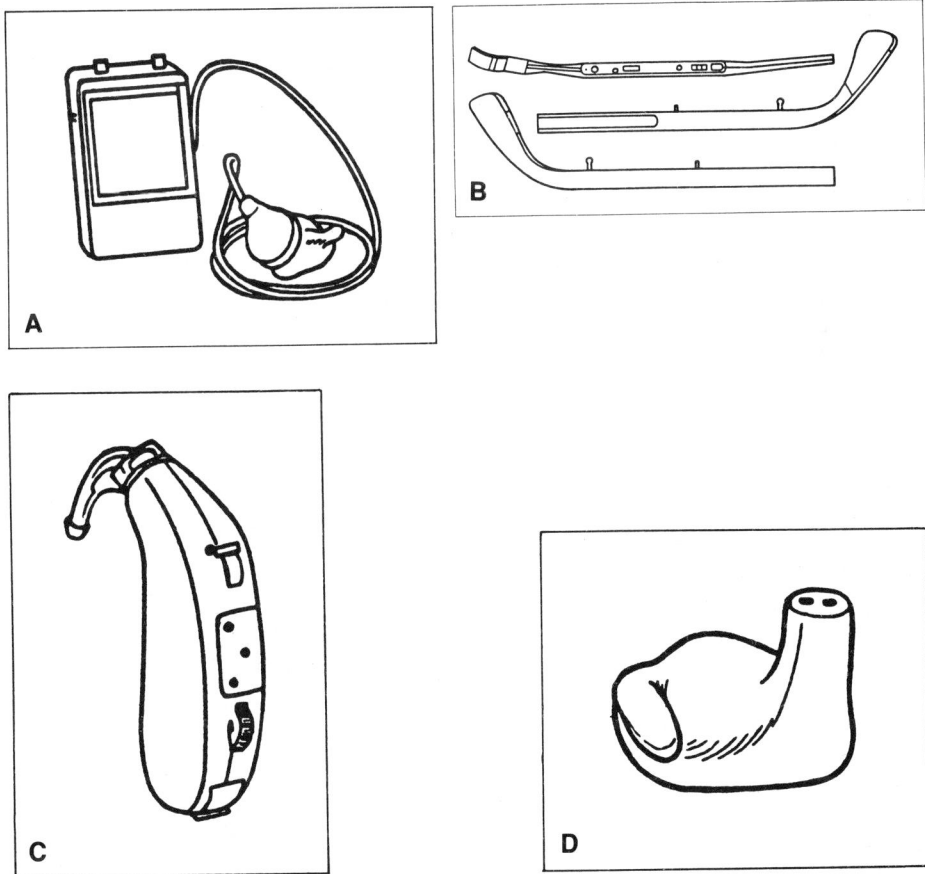

Figure 14-5. Types of hearing aids. **A.** Body aid, pocket version. **B.** Eyeglass aid. **C.** Behind-the-ear aid. **D.** All-in-the-ear aid. (From Elpern BS: Hearing aids. In Goodhill V [ed]: Ear: Disease, Deafness and Dizziness, pp 747–748. Hagerstown, Harper & Row, 1979)

and fits snugly around and behind the ear. Its small size makes it relatively inconspicuous and a good choice for the active person. This unit is also able to provide good amplification and fidelity for the moderately impaired. Some recent developments have made it possible even for some severely impaired individuals to wear this aid. A major consideration when prescribing the behind-the-ear aid is the person's ability to manipulate the small controls.

The *all-in-the-ear* aid is the smallest and least conspicuous of all the aids. It fits directly into the ear, is lightweight and has no external parts and, not surprisingly, is enjoying increasing popularity. Although its miniature size is cosmetically appealing, however, it is less efficient than the bigger models. Since some of the components of the larger size aids have been left out, the all-in-the-ear type may not possess the fidelity of other wearable types. Many models tend to whistle past 25 dB of amplification, making them impractical for anyone needing greater amplification. Their basic utility is for persons with mild to moderate losses. Another drawback of these aids is the miniature controls, which are extremely difficult for the elderly, arthritic, or physically impaired person to operate.

For those who work in one place for most of the day, desk amplifiers also are available. These are much larger than the portable aids, but provide a better sound quality. They draw their power from a wall socket. Many have multiple outlets and with modification can be used with televisions, radios, and recorded music.[12]

In addition to the style of a hearing aid, the need for a monaural (single hearing aid) or binaural (hearing aid in each ear) must be considered. Whenever possible, an attempt should be made to provide binaural hearing, which may provide many benefits, including:[49]

1. Additional loudness sensation of between five and eight dB
2. Improved speech discrimination
3. Increased speed of speech comprehension
4. Increased ability to understand speech in a noisy environment
5. Better localization of sound
6. More natural tones due to both ears being in balance

Binaural amplification should only be used, however, when the hearing function of the two ears is reasonably similar.[34] Major differences in threshold, tolerance, or speech discrimination prohibit binaural candidacy. The added expense of a second hearing aid and replacement batteries may cause some people to reject binaural amplification for financial reasons.

When a person has two equally aidable ears but rejects a binaural system, Peck[34] suggests it might be advantageous to alternate the single hearing aid between the two ears. He feels that it is important for each ear (especially in moderate or severe hearing losses) to become accustomed to amplification for several reasons: First, the usually aided ear could for some reason lose a great deal of hearing; second, a medical condition could develop, contraindicating continued use of the hearing aid in that ear; third, eventually the person may wish to try binaural amplification and, by using alternating ears occasionally, each ear would be accustomed to an aid. Peck observed that one-ear users tended to have markedly better speech discrimination on the aided side. If two aids were used, speech discrimination could be improved even more.

A Y cord arrangement splits signals entering from one microphone and delivers them to both ears. Although this arrangement provides two-ear stimulation, it does not provide true binaural amplification, since there is only one source of pickup and amplification.

The Contralateral Routing of Signal (CROS) hearing aid is a compromise between monaural and binaural. This device is designed for people who hear better in one ear than in the other. In the CROS model, a microphone and amplifier are placed in the "bad" ear, and a receiver is placed in the "good" ear. Sounds are picked up by the microphone near the bad side and then transmitted to the better ear. The CROS system's unique feature is that the receiver in the good ear is an open ear mold. This has several advantages over the normally closed ear mold:[34]

1. It allows people to use their natural hearing in regions in which they have good hearing (for example, in presbycusis, which involves the loss of high frequencies, a person can continue to hear the low sounds normally through the good ear, but use the hearing aid for high pitched sounds).
2. It minimizes the feeling of pressure from the hearing aid.
3. It offers a more comfortable fitting.
4. It can be used on persons with chronic otitis media or other conditions involving drainage from the ear.

There are several variations of the CROS system, including an ICROS (entire unit on one side, but ear mold on the other side), BICROS (separate microphones for each ear, but only one amplifier and receiver), and a MULTICROS (allows the individual to activate microphones in each ear separately).

Most hearing aids are of the air conduction type. There are bone conduction receivers, however, which transmit sound through the mastoid bone. These operate by sounding vibrations directly into the inner ear. The clarity of sound reproduced this way is poor; use of this type of aid is limited to persons with problems, such as infections or ear drainage, which prohibit a closed ear mold. Approximately 5% to 10% of people using hearing aids get better performance from a bone conduction aid than an air conduction aid.[42]

When buying a hearing aid, several performance features should be tested:[41]

1. Tolerability
2. Intelligibility of ordinary speech, faint speech, and difficult words
3. Freedom from internal noise
4. Aesthetic quality
5. Intelligibility under difficult (noisy) conditions

Regulations established by the Food and Drug Administration in 1977 require that a person have a hearing examination by a physician before buying a hearing aid.[11] The physician must state in writing that the patient's hearing has been evaluated within the past 6 months and that his medical condition will benefit from a hearing aid. If the person seeking the aid is over 18 years of age, a waiver may be signed to circumvent the exam. If the patient is under 18 years, the exam is mandatory. Hearing aid dispensers should give the patient written instructions for using the selected hearing aid. In many states the buyer has 30 days to test the hearing aid before the sale becomes final. Although hearing aids can be purchased by mail, it is suggested that the person with a hearing impairment have personal contact with the hearing aid dispenser and try different applicable models.

It is reported that one half of the hearing aids purchased end by not being worn.[40] There are many reasons for this. One is that expectations for the aid are unrealistic and therefore end in frustration and anger. "Hearing aids are never replacements for normal ears."[34] Individuals with moderate hearing loss can expect considerable improvements in their understanding of speech. Individuals with severe loss realistically might expect only to be alerted to sounds or to be aided in lip reading. Whether or not an aid will be worn depends on motivation. Hearing impaired persons often are pressured into buying an aid by family members who are tired of repeating themselves or speaking loudly. The person buying the aid must be willing to use it for his own sake, and not just to appease friends and relatives, for the aid to be effective. To some people, wearing an aid may seem a sign of aging or physical defect. They are embarrassed to acknowledge their need for an aid, fear ridicule or degradation, and choose to continue to have trouble understanding speech and hearing music rather than wear a prosthetic device. The physician or hearing aid counselor can play an important role in helping the hearing impaired individual accept the disability.

A hearing aid will never prevent the additional loss of hearing.[34] The aid will neither injure nor cure the abnormal ear, but rather will enable its user to make better use of the remaining hearing ability. More detailed information about hearing aids can be found in a booklet entitled *Facts About Hearing and Hearing Aids,* a joint publication of the National Bureau of Standards and the Food and Drug Administration (FDA). Free copies are available by writing to FDA/Hearing Aids, 8758 Georgia Avenue, Silver Spring, MD 20910. Another helpful source of information on this topic is the booklet, *Facts About Hearing Aids* (publication no. 03-250-73), published by the Council of Better Business Bureaus, Inc., 1150 17th Street, NW, Washington, DC 20036.

Hearing Impairments in Children

It is extremely important that physicians be aware of the potential threat of hearing impairment in infants and young children. An infant may appear completely normal—gurgling, crying, and babbling like any other child until the lack of auditory stimulation causes the infant to stop. Parents may begin to notice their child is different from other babies of the same age, or they may instinctively sense something is amiss even during the baby's first few weeks home from the hospital. Any suggestion or concern on the parent's part about possible deafness in the child should be thoroughly investigated. An intact auditory feedback system is important for learning speech and language. Children who hear muffled conversations or do not hear conversations at all are deprived of the optimal time for learning (age 3 or even younger). They will experience an irrevocable loss in the development of learning patterns.[28] Unfortunately, many hearing impaired children are not diagnosed until they are far beyond this stage, sometimes not until a routine school testing program recognizes a problem.

While developing speech and language, a child must hear the sounds he produces, as well as those produced by others, in order for speech to become a deliberate, planned, and self-controlled activity.[28]

The effect of hearing on this auditory feedback system is determined by a number of factors including time of onset (cogenital, prelingual, or adventitious), the degree of impairment (mild to profound), and the pattern of loss (including hearing sensitivity at a number of frequencies). A child's capacity to learn language has been suggested as the major criterion of his success or failure in general learning and development. Vocabulary development, auditory discrimination, and cognitive abilities of hearing impaired children all may be significantly retarded in comparison to hearing children. The congenital and prelingual hearing impaired child is at the greatest disadvantage. Prelingual hearing-impaired children have severe distortions in the production of their speech and intonation patterns and a great deal of difficulty in discriminating between speech sounds. Profoundly prelingually hearing-impaired children may not be able to learn speech and language skills through an auditory system and may depend completely upon visual and manual communication systems.

As just described, degree of hearing loss is one of the major factors affecting a hearing-impaired person's ability to develop language and communicate successfully. Age of onset is another important determinant in this development. Myklehurst has summarized the effects of age at onset of deafness on language and socialization skills:[29]

I. *Prenatal or before 2 years*—Loss of hearing in this age group has the greatest effect on ability to communicate, as well as implications on personality and emotional adjustment. Basic psychological processes, such as identification, are disturbed. When the deafness is profound, isolation is more apparent in these children than in any other group. Reliance on vision and taction may be marked. Specialized educational training is necessary.

II. *From 2 to 6 years*—There is evidence that if a child hears normally for the first 2 years of his life, he not only benefits verbally, but the psychological effects of his hearing loss may be lessened, particularly if onset occurs before 5 to 6 years of age. After 5 years there is a noticeable benefit verbally and a concomitant advantage to personality development and structure. When onset occurs after 5 years of age the classification of deafness is most useful, but this implies a profound degree of hearing loss.

III. *School years*—Language function is well retained for inner purposes and in other ways. The greatest effect is on personal and school adjustment; often special education is necessary. Friendships and identification with the majority group are difficult to maintain, but ego development and general emotional growth are less affected in this age group than in groups I and II. Children in this group who sustain profound deafness often become leaders in the deaf community.

IV. *Early adulthood*—The age range for this group is from 18 to approximately 30 years. Except for those deafened by disease such as meningitis, the degree of deafness often is moderate. Otosclerosis is a common etiology. Basic personality patterns are not altered, although undesirable traits may be accentuated. Disturbances of social relationships, including marital plans, educational programs, and vocational choices are often severe. Attitudes and patterns of behavior may be characteristic of other deaf persons. Choice of friends and social contacts may shift to others whose hearing is also impaired.

Almost all children attempt to test out different behaviors and personalities in the course of developing a satisfactory self-concept. Reactions from parents, teachers, friends, relatives, and others help them sort out which behaviors are socially acceptable, appropriate, and pleasing, and should therefore be maintained, and which bring disapproval and should be discontinued. Deafness may inhibit such feedback to a child, potentiating inappropriate behaviors and attitudes and possibly retarding social development. In addition, initial negative reactions to the deaf child, if unresolved, may hamper the child's social growth and adaption. Overprotectiveness may limit the development of independence and foster helplessness, further handicapping the child socially. The child's social, educational, emotional, and motor delays are compounded by parents' confusion about what sort of school they should send their child (*e.g.*, deaf students only or public school) and what mode of communication (*e.g.*, oral, manual, or sign) they should teach him.

Greenberg[17] identifies three family variables of importance to a deaf child's mental health: (1) degree of parental overprotectiveness, (2) development of unrealistic expectations, and (3) effectiveness of parent–child communication. Deaf children of deaf parents are better adapted than deaf children of hearing parents. They show fewer behavioral problems, more complex interactions, and better school achievement. Deaf parents, however, may find it difficult to fulfill the expected "good parent" role, since trying to call the doctor, to talk with teachers at school, or to communicate with other children's parents may be too difficult and frustrating. Hearing parents also have problems, but different ones. They are unable to relate to the experiences and difficulties of their hearing-impaired child and therefore are more likely to become apprehensive about their parenting roles.

All of these psychosocial factors are important for the primary care physician to keep in mind. Parents of deaf children should be offered emotional support and should be referred for appropriate counseling. Referrals to agencies serving the hearing impaired may provide additional support and ideas to help parents and patients cope with deafness. The International Association of Parents of the Deaf, 814 Thayer Avenue, Silver Spring, MD 20910, may offer some beneficial information and needed support services. Physicians should encourage deaf patients to exercise their independence and to compensate for their impairment by making full use of their other senses. Knowing the devastating effects on learning and language development that a hearing impairment brings, physicians should be alert to hearing impairments, especially in infants, and begin aural rehabilitative efforts as soon as possible, preferably before the baby has reached 6 months of age.

Mixed Sensory Impairments

"Of the 27 million persons in the United States who have impaired hearing and/ or vision, approximately 10% have both."[10] Most of these individuals are neither totally deaf nor totally blind but have varying combinations of hearing and visual impairments, ranging from slight to severe. It is estimated that there are close to 6000 deaf–blind children under the age of 21 in the United States and nearly the same number of deaf–blind adults.[20] These individuals will face many, if not all, of the problems mentioned in earlier parts of this chapter and Chapter 13, and additional problems as well. When occurring in combination, the disabling consequences of these two sensory impairments have more than an additive effect.

Since perhaps as much as 99% of acquired information and knowledge are learned through sight and hearing, being dually handicapped leads to severe educational and communication problems. The deaf child learns mainly by imitation and is heavily dependent on his vision; the blind child learns by verbal communication and is primarily dependent on auditory cues. The deaf–blind child is deprived of all these means of learning.

> The deaf blind child lives in a world of vibrations, air currents, temperature, changes, smells and a great many tactile sensations and sensations from within the digestive system, muscles, joints, etc.[8]

The degree of loss and age of onset are important determinants of future abilities in people with several impairments, as well as in those with single impairments. The person who is born blind and becomes deaf will have different problems than the person who was born deaf and becomes blind. Even different problems besiege the person who acquired both or who was born with both. In a study of probable causes of hearing loss in students who are both visually and hearing impaired,[20] maternal rubella was found to be the leading prebirth cause, followed by prematurity, hereditary factors, and pregnancy and birth complications. Meningitis was the most frequent single factor associated with hearing loss after birth. Other factors are high fever, otitis media, and childhood diseases.

Characteristics of the Multisensory Deprived (MSD) Child

> Parents of the multi-sensory deprived child are faced with a possibly mislabeled child who may evidence unusual sleep patterns; feeding, chewing and swallowing difficulties; adverse reactions to clothing . . . ; irregularity and

delay in toilet training; lack of ability to communicate leading to frustration and resulting in discipline problems; as well as lags in social, emotional and cognitive development. A low-functioning MSD child might be prone to head banging and other forms of self-stimulation, such as poking the eyes, waving the fingers before the eyes, rocking, or staring at lights.[25]

Because of a multitude of handicaps (physical, social, and developmental), the congenitally deaf–blind child often becomes an introverted, egocentric human being with little or no meaningful contact with the environment. The parent may feel the infant is nonsatisfying. This may be reinforced if the infant has a "tactile defensive mechanism reaction"—arching the back and screaming with the slightest touch. This reaction further interferes with attempts by the parents to handle and enjoy the baby and requires counseling efforts to teach parents ways to overcome it. The inability of the infant to perceive visual or auditory cues prevents him from anticipating changes. The youngster may be startled easily or frightened when any new change occurs. The lack of perception of his environment, as well as a lack of motivation and curiosity, can lead to developmental delays. Perhaps the most important deprivation of the multisensory handicapped child is a lack of love and affection. Often it is difficult for the child to develop an emotional bond with the parents, in part due to parental tensions and in part due to the absence of a return of emotional investment from the child.

Interventions

A thorough medical examination should be performed on any sensory-impaired child. Frequently, once a child has been identified initially as being blind, deaf, or retarded, little further evaluation takes place. Sometimes it takes years before additional handicaps are identified. If the physician suspects any possibility of multihandicaps, the child should be referred to a facility that can perform complete diagnostic examinations. If the mother was known to have rubella during her pregnancy the child should be referred automatically for evaluation. It is important to understand that some testing will be difficult because of the inability of the child to respond in understandable terms.

Once a visual–hearing impairment is identified, an attempt should be made to help the child use any existing residual vision and hearing. Parents should be encouraged to talk to the child when handling him and to stimulate the child with repetitive games and gustatory and tactile stimulation. Rehabilitation will follow many of the same courses of action as for the singly sensory-handicapped child (*e.g.*, mobility training and proficiency in self-care). To be an emotionally satisfied, social human being, the child will have to learn to communicate with the outside world. Parents should establish a communication cue with the child, such as a pat on the arm before beginning a certain activity. This cue should be used each time that activity, such as diapering, is to begin in order to enable the child to anticipate the action and be less fearful. At the end of an activity another type of cue should be given to indicate the activity is finished. At all times the baby should be encouraged to respond. Programming assistance for the multisensory-deprived child can be obtained from several sources.[25] The John Tracy Clinic in Los Angeles publishes a parental guide for young deaf–blind children.

The Perkins School for the Blind in Watertown, Massachusetts, has programs for the deaf–blind and will willingly share their knowledge and expertise. The Helen Keller National Center for Deaf–Blind Youths and Adults in Sands Point, New York, established in 1973, publishes a journal entitled *The Center News* for those working in the field of deaf–blindness.

The Role of the Physician

Specialities have evolved within the health care system to identify and diagnose deafness, offer therapy for remedial conditions of the ear, conduct hearing aid evaluations, develop and implement programs for the prevention of hearing impaired people. Such specialities deal principally with only one component of the health care delivery to the deaf patient—the ear and its dysfunction. However, the health care system is most frequently called upon to provide care for the deaf patient when the patient's complaint is unrelated to deafness. It is here that the system has the most difficulty adapting.[7]

Communicating With the Deaf Patient

Working with a deaf patient may be one of the physician's most difficult and challenging experiences. Deafness can interfere with the doctor–patient relationship, an important limitation on quality medical care. A knowledgeable and sympathetic physician must understand and overcome the many barriers, such as communication and education, to providing health care for the deaf.

Many deaf persons do not know their own medical histories.

The scenario is simple: All the information interchange when the deaf child is ill occurs between the parent and the physician. Later, no one takes the time to explain to the child what the illness was. It is not unusual for a hearing adult to know the medical history of his/her deaf sibling better than does that sibling.[7]

Even if the deaf patient knows his medical history, it may be difficult for the health-care provider to obtain accurate answers to routine examination questions, since many deaf individuals are ignorant of medical terminology or common health disorders. Some do not have good comprehension of the names of the different parts of their bodies or cannot understand what the doctor is trying to ask them. They may also refrain from asking questions and, if they do ask, may be unable to hear the responses.

Most physicians use regular speech, assuming their deaf or hearing-impaired patients have a functional lip reading ability. Speech reading is a very difficult skill, however, especially for the prelingually deaf, and not every hard-of-hearing person is capable of this mode of listening. Nearly 70% of English sounds are homophenous—either invisible or identical in appearance to other sounds on the lip—and a majority of English word sounds are produced from the back of the mouth and cannot be lip read. Poor lighting, anxiety, or the physician's mustache or beard may also increase the difficulty of speech reading.

Writing, an obvious alternative to speech, also has limitations. First, it is a slow process; the busy practitioner may not have the time to sit and write notes. Second, it is a tiring process; both the physician and the patient may tire and lose interest in the process of inquiry. Abbreviation or deletions in the explanation may result, increasing the deaf person's ignorance about his own health. Third, a large percentage of the deaf are educationally limited (some may not have more than a fourth grade education), complicating the physician's efforts to explain technical aspects of the disease.

Physicians can do several things to circumvent these problems. The most important step is to ascertain the best mode of communication for the patient. If the patient prefers speech reading, the physician should try to talk at a slightly slower rate; slowing speech too much or over-enunciating can distort speech. The physician also should supplement the talk with diagrams and models. If writing is the selected mode, some of the more detailed and lengthy explanations can be pretyped and given to the patient to take home. At all times, writing tools should be accessible. If the deaf person prefers to use sign language, an interpreter should be obtained. Physicians are cautioned against using family members in this role, as confidentiality may be compromised and emotional problems and subjective interpretations may lead to faulty information. Local chapters of the Registry of Interpreters for the Deaf can help. No matter which type of communication is chosen, the practitioner occasionally should ask the patient questions to verify comprehension. Many deaf persons characteristically nod their heads in agreement, even when they do not understand what is said.

As part of a survey aphasic patients were questioned about their feelings with respect to communication with health professionals during the course of their illness.[39] Many of their responses are applicable to the feelings experienced by deaf and hearing-impaired individuals as well. The aphasic patients:

1. Felt fear and anger would have been lessened if they had received reassurances and explanations of what had happened to them
2. Were insulted that professionals treated them as if they were not there or as if they were children
3. Were given few explanations because it was assumed they could not understand much
4. Were aware of nonverbal cues given by hospital workers indicating annoyance and impatience
5. Felt too many questions were asked, questions were repeated too rapidly, or they were not given sufficient time to respond

Responsibilities of the Primary Care Physician

The primary care physician plays an important role in the provision of good health care to hearing-impaired individuals. Early identification of hearing problems is a major responsibility of the pediatrician or family care practitioner. Attentiveness to parents' observations concerning the impairments of their children is crucial, as parents are most often the first to discover the hearing loss. This has been discussed in detail in Chapter 7. High-risk populations should be routinely screened; elderly patients should be checked annually, especially those in long-term care institutions where the incidence of hearing loss is higher than normal. Continued contact with the otologist or audiologist after initial referral is necessary for coordinated care of patients of all ages. Physicians have a responsibility to be aware of community agencies serving the deaf and deaf–blind and to make appropriate referrals if indicated. Since vision is the key remaining sense in deaf and severely hard-of-hearing individuals, it must be thoroughly assessed periodically. The physician should be alert to early signs of Usher's syndrome or retinitis pigmentosa, as discussed earlier in this chapter. All deaf children should be taught the fundamentals of good eye care to safeguard against abuse of this remaining sensory mechanism.

In order to deal effectively with the deaf or hearing-impaired individual, the physician should be sensitive to the psychosocial repercussions of hearing loss. Deafness is not an isolated phenomenon. It affects a person's development, mental state, and family and interpersonal relations. Depression, frequently noted in the adult following hearing loss, suspicions about people talking behind their back, and paranoid tendencies (sometimes to an intolerable degree) are commonplace. Many of these problems are due to society's handicapping attitudes toward the deaf. As Milroy describes,[28] deafness is low in the hierarchy of disabilities. Deaf persons suffer discrimination and disadvantages, as do other minority groups, but unlike the others they have no sense of "roots." It is unlikely that they have a sibling, parent, or friend with the same hearing problem. Deafness is also an invisible handicap; some of the courtesies or assistance extended to other minority groups are withheld from the deaf. Whereas some handicapped groups, such as the blind, receive accolades for extraordinary use of their remaining senses, characteristics such as slowness or dumbness are attributed to the deaf. As a consequence, the deaf person may be unhappy; he may have a sense of shame and a low self-concept and may deny the impairment.

Loss of the ability to communicate causes social isolation and withdrawal. The loss of warning signals in the environment and the deprivation of background noise causes uneasiness and discomfort and can contribute to paranoia. Friendships tend to decrease. Even when the deaf person does participate in social gatherings, the difficulty of hearing in group conversations, especially for the elderly hard-of-hearing person, limits the fulfillment derived from this sort of social interaction.

Primary care practitioners also should play a major role in preventing deafness:[7]

. . . by promoting vaccination against rubella, by promoting good maternal and neonatal health care, by cautioning patients about exposure to industrial noise, and other potentially damaging noise levels, and by supporting routine screening among preschool, school age and elderly populations.

Equally important is the physician's role in helping the patient accept a hearing loss and encouraging him to seek appropriate help. Physicians can be helpful in offering family members training in techniques that ease communication with the hearing-impaired individual. For example, the use of low tones in speech can alleviate some of the difficulty associated with high-frequency loss, and written communication should be encouraged. Musical games and exercises, such as tapping water glasses which are filled to various levels, can help with the identification of pitch and help stimulate the patient's auditory sense. Since much presbycusis involves difficulty in discriminating between figure and ground, the elimination of background noise is helpful, especially for those with hearing aids. Family members also should be made aware of the fact that the hard-of-hearing person may hear some sounds (*e.g.,* low-frequency voices) and not others (high-frequency loss with presbycusis); this may cause the family to charge the elderly or hearing-impaired persons with hearing only what they want to hear. Face-to-face communication should be encouraged, and speech should be less rapid than usual. Ample time should be allowed for the individual to respond. Family members also should be told to place the hearing-impaired person where he can easily read lips (well-illuminated, full view of the face), with the better ear turned towards the speaker. When a child has a hearing problem, getting down to the child's level when speaking (not just bending over) may help the child with listening and speech reading. Parents should be alert to the fact that the child is constantly straining to hear what is being said; they should be aware that the hard-of-hearing child may fatigue more easily some days than others; therefore, parents should encourage rest periods or shortened homework sessions.

The following list adapted from Schow and colleagues,[39] provides some helpful communication tips for talking with the hard of hearing:

1. Communicate with the hearing-impaired person in a quiet environment free from radio, TV, and other background noises. Visual distractions should also be reduced.
2. Since considerable information is available by watching the lips, facial expressions, and gestures, the faces of those speaking to the hearing-impaired person should be well lighted. Avoid gum chewing, eating, or covering the mouth while speaking.
3. Get the attention of the hard-of-hearing person before speaking, for example, by touching the shoulder.
4. Speak distinctly, somewhat more slowly than usual.
5. Give the person a clue as to the topic of conversation. Avoid sudden shifts in the topic and emphasize when changes are made.
6. Avoid long, involved sentences. Use appropriate gestures. When necessary to repeat, rephrase the sentence making it shorter or simpler, if possible.
7. When telling a long story or giving important instructions, wait to make sure the person understands before going on, and
8. Encourage the hearing aid user to wear the aid when you talk. Be knowledgeable about hearing aid function so that you can help if it is not working or if the user is having trouble with amplification. Do not talk too loudly or shout.

Services and Aids Available to the Hearing Impaired

Isolation, one of the most devastating results of deafness, is intensified by an inability to use a telephone, even for medical emergencies. Telephone companies now offer several adaptive devices to aid the hard-of-hearing in telephone communication. Phones are available that ring loudly and provide amplification through the receiver, although many hearing aid users are able to use a telephone satisfactorily by just holding the receiver very close to the hearing aid. Telephones that ring in a special frequency range, audible by most people with hearing problems, are also available. Another specialized type of phone, designed for deaf or severely hearing-impaired people, causes a light to flash each time the phone rings. Hearing-impaired people are encouraged to contact the local phone company to determine other special services offered.

Other adaptive devices for the hearing impaired include alarm clocks that light up or vibrate when the alarm goes off, a door bell rings, or a baby cries, and loud buzzers to replace normal doorbells. Headphones are available with built in volume controls for listening to television, radio, or phonograph; often these provide better results than hearing aids. Inductors are inexpensive devices for use with a hearing aid that substantially improve the clarity of television and recorded programs. Intercom systems, especially helpful with small children, can pick up the sounds in one room and deliver them amplified to another room, such as the bedroom, kitchen, or family room. For recreational enjoyment, full-length, Hollywood captioned films are now available, as well as special adaptors to receive captioned interpretations on television. For these and many other assistive aids that are available, the National Association of the Deaf, 814 Thayer Ave., Silver Spring, MD, or any local organization serving hearing-impaired individuals, should be contacted.

Aside from adaptive devices, many other services are available to persons with hearing problems. Individuals whose hearing cannot be corrected may benefit from a referral to a hearing aid dealer. The National Association of Hearing and Speech Agencies, also at 814 Thayer Ave., Silver Spring, MD, can provide a list of the hearing and speech centers in your area. The Registry of Interpreters for the Deaf, at the same address, can provide information on the art of interpreting and can refer the reader to local chapters for help in locating interpreters. Local or state health departments can provide additional information about nearby services for the hearing impaired. Many clinics offer intensive auditory training, hearing aid counseling, and specialized training in lip reading. The physician is urged to locate these services in the community and refer patients to them. Physicians, as well as patients, who have questions about hereditary hearing impairments are referred to the National Genetics Foundation, 250 W. 57th St., New York, NY.

Physicians may also be interested in reading *American Annals of the Deaf,* a periodical available at many libraries, which discusses education, rehabilitation, and other relevant problems, services, and new research developments in the field of deafness. The Alexander Graham Bell Association for the Deaf, with headquarters in 1537 S St., NW, Washington DC, offers free lists of pamphlets and books on speech reading, speech and auditory training, and information about education for the deaf. *Hotline,* which can be obtained by writing to Twin Vision, 18440 Topham St., Tarzana, CA 9135, is a magazine designed exclusively to keep the deaf–blind up-to-date with new events. Gallaudet College, Florida Ave. and 7th St., NE, Washington, DC, remains the only postsecondary institution catering entirely to the needs of deaf persons. The college also publishes a quarterly, *Gallaudet Today,* which includes articles about deafness and programs on higher education for the deaf. Complimentary copies are available upon request. The bookstore at Gallaudet contains nearly 200 publications related to problems concerning hearing loss, deafness, and hearing-handicapped children.

Summary

To provide comprehensive care to the hearing-impaired person, knowledge of definitions, causative factors, proper techniques of the medical examination, and aural rehabilitative measures is important. Fundamental information about audiogram interpretation and hearing aid selection is helpful as well. All of these are addressed in this chapter.

Age of onset, type of disability, and degree of disability are three main factors determining the effect of hearing loss on the individual. An especially important effect of hearing loss is lack of language development in the young child and adolescent. Intervention during the prelingual phase of development of the hearing-impaired child may prove critical to the establishment of normal communication. Early diagnosis is therefore emphasized as being critical, not only for the possible curtailment of progressive disease, but also for providing early intervention in rehabilitation services. In addition, physicians need a broad-based knowledge of aids, services provided locally and nationally, and publications related to sensory-impaired individuals.

Deafness as an invisible handicap presents many problems to the hearing-impaired person; a mixed sensory impairment provides additive complications. This chapter discusses some of the psychosocial issues with which primary care physicians should concern themselves when working with deaf and hearing-impaired individuals and their families. Since many medical conditions, such as Usher's syndrome and retinitis pigmentosa, are both mixed sensory impairments and progressive diseases, physicians are cautioned to be alert to visual as well as hearing deficits. Equally important, health-care providers must urge children and adults with hearing deficits to protect their remaining senses by proper eye care and using precautions to protect against damaging noise pollution. For this reason, a discussion about noise-induced hearing loss has been included. Finally, since substantial hearing deficits may cause difficulty in the execution or interpretation of a medical examination, some helpful hints for physicians are provided to aid in examining persons with hearing impairments.

References

1. Alberti PW, Abel SM, Riko K: Practical aspects of hearing protector use. In Hamenik RP, Henderson D, Salvi R (eds): New Perspectives on Noise-Induced Hearing Loss. New York, Raven Press, 1982

2. Bates B: A Guide to Physical Examination, 2nd ed. Philadelphia, JB Lippincott, 1979

3. Bradford LJ, Hardy WG (eds): Hearing and Hearing Impairment. New York, Grune & Stratton, 1979

4. Chui R: Otitis media. In Crumley RL (ed): Primary Care Clinics in Office Practice: Communication Problems of Ears, Nose and Throat. Philadelphia, WB Saunders, 1982

5. Hearing Aids. Consumers' Research Magazine 16(3), Sept 1979

6. Davis H: Audiometry: Pure tone and simple speech tests. In Davis H, Silverman SK (eds): Hearing and Deafness. New York, Holt, Rinehart & Winston, 1961

7. DiPetro LJ, Knight CH, Sans JS: Health care delivery for deaf persons: The provider's role. Health Care Deliv 4:106–107, 1981

8. Dunham JR: The Deaf–blind child. In Goldenson RM, Dunham JR, Dunham CS (eds): Disability and Rehabilitation Handbook, p 34. New York, McGraw-Hill, 1978

9. Dunham JR, Dunham CS: Hearing disorders. In Goldenson RM, Dunham JR, Dunham CS (eds): Disability and Rehabilitation Handbook. New York, McGraw-Hill, 1978

10. Durrant JD: Anatomic and physiologic correlates of the effects of noise and hearing. In Lipscomb DM (ed): Noise and Audiology. Baltimore, University Park Press, 1978

11. Hearing Aids. FDA Consumer Magazine 10(4), May 1980

12. Fisch L: Special senses: The aging auditory system. In Brocklehurst JC: Textbook of Geriatric Medicine and Gerontology. Edinburgh, Churchill Livingstone, 1978

13. Gerstman HL: Evaluation and management in auditory disorders. In Krusen FH, Kottke FJ, Ellwood PM: Handbook of Physical Medicine and Rehabilitation (eds). Philadelphia, WB Saunders, 1971

14. Glorig A: Rehabilitation in impaired hearing. In Licht S (ed): Rehabilitation and Medicine. Baltimore, Elizabeth Licht, 1968

15. Goin DW: Trauma of the middle and inner ear. In English GM: Otolaryngology. Hagerstown, Harper & Row, 1976

16. Goodhill V (ed): Ear: Disease, Deafness and Dizziness. Hagerstown, Harper & Row, 1979

17. Greenberg MT: Hearing families with deaf children: Stress and functioning as related to communication methods. Am Ann Deaf 125(9):1063, 1980

18. Harrison R: Current Concepts in the Management of Hearing Loss. Am Fam Physician, 19(1):138, 1979

19. Heffernan HP, Simons MR, Goodhill V: Audiologic assessment, functional loss and objective audiometry. In Goodhill V (ed): Ear: Disease, Deafness and Dizziness. Hagerstown, Harper & Row, 1979

20. Hicks WM, Pfau GS: Deaf–visually impaired persons: Incidence and service, Am Ann Deaf 124(2):76, 1979

21. Hopkins HV: Principles and Methods of Physical Diagnosis. Philadelphia, WB Saunders, 1966

22. Hull RH: Hearing Impairment Among Aging Persons. Cliff Notes, Lincoln, NE, 1977

23. Jensen P: Community noise. In Lipscomb DM (ed): Noise and Audiology, p 245. Baltimore, University Park Press, 1978

24. Lewis RG: The Deaf Child. In Goodhill V: Ear: Disease, Deafness and Dizziness. Hagerstown, Harper & Row, 1979

25. McInnes JM, Treffry JA: The deaf–blind child. In Jan JE, Freeman RD, Scott EP: Visual Impairments in Children and Adolescents, p 337. New York, Grune & Stratton, 1977

26. Melnick: Temporary and permanent threshold shift. In Lipscomb DM (ed): Noise and Audiology. Baltimore, University Park Press, 1978

27. Mills JH: Effects of noise on young and old people. In Lipscomb DM: Noise and Audiology. Baltimore, University Park Press, 1978

28. Milroy V: Personal lecture notes. Dept. of Social and Rehabilitation Services, Vocational Rehabilitation Services, Providence, RI

29. Myklehurst HR: The Psychology of Deafness, pp 25, 120. New York, Grune & Stratton, 1960

30. Nathan MD: Protecting the Elderly Against Drug-Induced Hearing Loss. Geriatrics 36(6):95, 1981

31. Newby H: Audiology, pp 60, 110. New York, Appleton-Century-Crofts, 1964

32. Noble WG: Assessment of Impaired Hearing. New York, Academic Press, 1978

33. O'Neill JJ, Oyer HJ: Applied Audiometry. New York, Dodd, Mead & Co., 1966

34. Peck JE: Uses and abuses of hearing aids. Ann Otol Rhinol Laryngol 89(5)pt 2 (suppl) 74:70, 1980

35. Rose DE: Audiologic Assessment. Englewood Cliffs, NJ, Prentice-Hall, 1971

36. Rosenfeld I: The Complete Medical Exam. New York, Simon & Shuster, 1978

37. Schein JD: Hearing impairments and deafness. In Stolov WC, Clowers MR (eds): Handbook of Severe Disability. US Dept of Education, Rehabilitation Services Administration, 1981

38. Schein JD: Childhood hearing loss: Epidemiology and implications. In Levin LS, Knight CH (eds): Genetic and Environmental Hearing Loss: Syndromic and Non-Syndromic. New York, Alan R Liss, 1980

39. Schow RL, Christiensen JM, Hutchinson JM, Nerbonne MA: Chronic Disorders of the Aged, p 39. Baltimore, University Park Press, 1978

40. Schubert EP: Hearing: Its function and dysfunction. In Arnold GE, Winckel F, Wyke BD (eds): Disorders of Human Communication. Heidelberg, Springer-Verlag, 1980

41. Schuknecht HF: Pathology of the Ear, p 327. Cambridge, MA, Harvard University Press, 1974

42. Schulman JB: Ototoxicity. In Goodhill V (ed): Ear: Disease, Deafness and Dizziness. Harper & Row, Hagerstown, 1979

43. Silverman SR, Taylor SG: Counseling about hearing aids. In Davis H, Silverman SR (eds): Hearing and Deafness. New York, Holt, Rinehart & Winston, 1960

44. Silverman SR, Taylor SG, Davis H: Hearing aids. In Davis H, Silverman SR (eds): Hearing and Deafness. New York, Holt, Rinehart & Winston, 1960

45. Smoorenburg GF: Damage risk criteria for impulse noise. In Hamernik RP, Henderson D, Salvi R (eds): New Perspectives on Noise-Induced Hearing Loss. New York, Raven Press, 1982

46. Stein DM: The hard of hearing child. In Goodhill V (ed): Ear: Disease, Deafness and Dizziness. Hagerstown, Harper & Row, 1978

47. Travis LE: Handbook of Speech Pathology and Audiology. New York, Appleton-Century-Crofts, 1971

48. Vernon M, Hicks D: Relationship of rubella, herpes simplex, cytomegalovirus and certain other viral diseases. Am Ann Deaf 125(5): 529, 1980

49. Wallensfels HG: Hearing Aids for Nerve Deafness, pp 18, 94. Springfield, IL, Charles C Thomas, 1971
50. Ward WD: Noise-Induced Hearing Damage. In Paparella MM, Shumrich DA (eds): Otolaryngology, Vol 2: Ear p 386. Philadelphia, WB Saunders, 1973
51. Watson LA, Tolan T: Hearing Tests and Hearing Instruments. Williams & Wilkins, Baltimore, 1949

CHAPTER 15

Organic Mental Disorders: Dementia

Organic mental disorders is the most recent nosological phrase used to describe disorders that are "psychological or behavioral abnormalities associated with transient or permanent dysfunction of the brain."[1] In the *Diagnostic and Statistical Manual of Mental Disorders (DSM-III)*, a distinction is made between organic brain syndrome and organic mental disorders. The latter category describes a problem with a known or presumed known etiology, whereas the former refers to signs and symptoms without reference to etiology.

As a rule, it is difficult to diagnose organic brain syndrome clearly and to identify the etiology of many of the cognitive impairments included under the rubric of organic mental disorder. In fact, one of the goals of this chapter is to explore the puzzling differential diagnostic and treatment issues within this classification category. In so doing, some of the reasons for the classification uncertainty will emerge.

An estimated 10% of persons over the age of 65 years, and 20% of those over age 80 have clinically important intellectual impairment.[24,38] In addition, more than half of the 1 million American nursing home residents are afflicted by chronic brain syndromes.[13,34] This is significant for the medical practitioner because of the increasing percentage of the United States population over age 65 who are at increased risk for senile dementia and other disorders involving a diminished mental status. Patients with dementia have a reportedly marked decrease in life expectancy. Depending on the age at the onset of symptoms, the number of years of survival is decreased 50% to 75% percent as compared with normal age-matched people.[23,34] Although senile dementia is rarely recorded as the primary cause of death, realistically it is believed to be the fourth leading cause of fatality in the United States.[13,34] One family in three will see one parent succumb to it.[13] Indeed, it has been stated that organic brain syndromes are among the most frequently encountered and undertreated psychological disorders in the contemporary teaching hospital.[37]

Historically chronic organic brain syndromes (OBS) were believed to be an exaggerated form of normal aging. Current literature suggests that cognitive dysfunction is not an inevitable concomitant of old age, however, since many elderly people do not experience significant memory impairment. Also, there is pathological evidence suggesting differences between the diffuse brain damage in dementia and the slowly progressive impairment that frequently occurs in normal aging.

Cognitive impairments may result from a number of organic origins. Contributing factors include:[19] (1) traumatic lesions to the skull and brain, (2) inflammation of the brain and its coverings, (3) benign and malignant neoplasms of the meninges and parenchyma, (4) vascular lesions, (5) toxic and chemical influences, and (6) degenerative processes. Approximately 29% of organic brain syndromes are reversible, or partially reversible, if recognized and appropriately treated;[36,38] the remainder produce chronic, irreversible dementia.

Dementia

As adapted from the diagnostic criteria established by the American Psychiatric Association, dementia refers to a mental state involving:[1]

1. A loss of intellectual abilities of sufficient severity to interfere with social or occupational functioning
2. Memory impairment
3. At least one of the following:
   - Impairment of abstract thinking, as manifested by concrete interpretations of proverbs, inability to find similarities and differences between related words, difficulty in defining words and concepts, and other similar tasks
   - Impaired judgment
   - Other disturbances of higher cortical function such as aphasia (disorders of language due to brain dysfunction), apraxia (inability to carry out motor activities despite intact comprehension and motor function), agnosia (failure to recognize or identify objects despite intact sensory function), "constructional difficulty" (*e.g.,* inability to copy three-dimensional figures, assemble blocks, or arrange slides in specific designs)
   - Personality changes, such as alterations in or accentuation of premorbid traits
4. State of unclouded consciousness, and
5. Either
   - Evidence from the history, physical examination, or laboratory tests of a specific organic factor judged to be "etiologically related" to the disturbance, or
   - In the absence of such evidence, an organic factor necessary for the development of the syndrome can be presumed if conditions other than organic mental disorders reasonably have been excluded, and if the behavior changes represent cognitive impairment in a variety of areas

According to the *Diagnostic and Statistical Manual* of *Mental Disorders (DSM-III)*,[1] dementia may refer to a progressive (Alzheimer's disease), static (anoxia), or remitting disease course (corrected metabolic disorder), so long as the symptoms listed above are present. In earlier editions of the DSM-III, however, and in much of the current literature, the term dementia is reserved for chronic, progressive disorders. In this chapter dementia refers to the chronic, irreversible form of cognitive impairments; reversible disorders involving global intellectual impairments will be referred to as "pseudodementia."

Etiology

There are relatively few disorders that cause irreversible dementia. Two of them account for 80% of dementias in the elderly: Alzheimer's-type and multi-infarct dementia.[2,38] Alzheimer's disease is often referred to as "presenile" dementia, since it affects individuals in the 40- to 60-year age bracket. It is characterized by a relentless, progressive dementia resulting in death within 5 to 10 years. Pathologically, the hallmark of Alzheimer's disease is a combination of neurofibrillary tangles, senile plaques, and granulovascular changes in the cells of the brain.

The *neurofibrillary tangles* are normally present mainly in the hippocampus and amygdaloid nucleus. These double helixed structures are found within brain neurons and partially displace normal cell structures in the cytoplasm, possibly interfering with cell metabolism and axonal transfer. *Senile plaques* are degenerated cell structures located at synapses between cells that may affect the conduction of nerve impulses across cells. A number of studies have demonstrated a correlation between the degree of intellectual deficit in Alzheimer's and an increasing number of senile plaques.[13,34] In addition, biochemical researchers have shown a strong association between loss of choline acetyltransferase activity and both senile plaque formation and mental test score deficits.[34] *Granulovascular bodies* are found in large amounts in the hippocampus of Alzheimer's patients. Although these bodies are also formed in normal elderly individuals, there is a 2 to 100 times greater incidence in persons affected by Alzheimer's disease.[34] Alzheimer's disease is also characterized by diffuse brain atrophy (especially in parietal, frontal, and temporal lobes), ventricular dilatation, and decreased cerebral blood flow, most likely due to reduced metabolic needs secondary to a decrease in cortical tissue.

Studies of Alzheimer's patients (under 60 years of age) and senile dementia patients (over 60 years of age) have shown that it is nearly impossible to distinguish histologically between the two disorders. One of the only significant distinguishing factors has been suggested by Larson,[23] who finds a familial trend in senile dementia patients suggestive of an autosomal dominant gene with age-related penetrance, which is apparently absent in Alzheimer's families. Current thinking suggests that senile dementia cases are, therefore, frequently referred to as "Alzheimer's-type" senile dementias.

The reasons for the development of the pathological changes in Alzheimer's-type dementia are unknown. Possible causes have included a genetic disorder, a slow-acting virus, metabolic dysfunction, or metallic (*e.g.*, aluminum, lead) poisoning.[34,41] As of this writing, Alzheimer's disease and Alzheimer's-type senile dementia can neither be cured nor reversed through medical means.

Multi-infarct dementia is a less common form of organic brain syndrome. Vascular disease accounts for between 10% and 20% of dementia cases and is more common in men. Hypertension or diabetes often are concomitants of the arteriosclerotic form of dementia. Mental impairment is most likely to appear if there are large areas of infarction in addition to the multiple small lesions. Major lesions may be caused by narrowing of the carotid, anterior, or middle cerebral arteries. Deficits occur in areas of sensory, language, and motor functions, and may be focal or diffuse. Recurrent cerebral infarction may result in cerebral "softening" leading to cognitive impairments in a progressive, stepwise course (in contrast to the gradual deterioration in Alzheimer's-type disease). When multiple infarctions occur in the basal ganglia, internal capsule, or pons, a lacunar state develops which may have clinical manifestations of rigidity, pseudobulbar palsy and hyperreflexia. Focal neurological abnormalities, dysarthria, and abnormal gait patterns (*e.g.,* short steps) often are present in the multi-infarct form of dementia. When the frontal lobe is involved, loss of spontaneity, social inhibition, and apathy may be present as well.

Other *degenerative neurological disorders* precipitating dementia include Pick's disease, Huntington's ataxia, and diffuse cerebral sclerosis. In addition, chronic alcoholism, normal pressure hydrocephalus, untreated hypothyroidism, and anoxia can cause varying degrees of irreversible dementia.

Disease Course

Stoudemire and Thompson[36] divide the course of clinical dementia into three progressive stages—*early* (characterized by subtle impairments in judgment, orientation, intellect, affect, and memory), *middle,* and *late* (characterized by drastic changes in the patient's personality, neurological changes, and progressive loss of consciousness leading eventually to death).

Early signs of dementia frequently are first noted by relatives, friends, or employers. Forgetfulness is a common finding. Patients may report difficulty in remembering names, appointments, phone numbers, or the placement of items. Frequently during the early stages, patients are able to deny or conceal their cognitive deficits successfully from physicians and family members. Behavioral or personality changes such as anger, restlessness, irritability, diminished drive, withdrawal, apathy, anorexia, mood swings, or depression may dominate during this period. Friends may say that the patient "is not acting like himself." Frontal lobe involvement may result in inappropriate jocularity or crying and laughing in rapid succession.

During the middle phase, other global intellectual deficits become more prominent. In addition to recent memory loss, judgment may become impaired. Patients may lose their appreciation of the social consequences of their actions and express sexual or other impulsive fantasies or paranoid behaviors. Pervasive intellectual impairments may interfere with the patient's ability to comprehend and integrate new information. Concretization of thought is a frequent finding, and patients may confabulate to compensate for memory losses. Patients also begin to lose their abilities for mathematical computation and other activities requiring attention. As the disease progresses, they may be unable to shop and carry out even simple tasks at home or in their place of employment, or they may be found stopping halfway through a task—not remembering what it was they set out to do (cognitive ambulia). Attention to dress and personal cleanliness may be lacking. Patients may become labile in mood. As the severity increases, patients may become disoriented to time, place, and person; they may fail to recognize immediate family members and may even forget their own birth date or name.

The late phase of dementia is characterized by marked changes in the patient's personality. Also, neurological signs such as gross defects in motor functioning, abnormal reflexes, ataxia, agraphia, and anomia, may occur. Patients also may develop urinary and fecal incontinence. Eventually the patient's level of consciousness may lead to obtundation, coma and, eventually, death.

Depression Versus Dementia

The differential diagnosis of depression is difficult. Depression can mimic dementia; in addition, depressive illness and dementia coexist. Twenty-five percent of patients with dementia may be concurrently depressed.[23] Not infrequently physicians mistakenly diagnose depressive disorders as irreversible dementia, thus denying the patient access to appropriate treatment. According to one study,[35] 15% of those referred for treatment of dementia are misdiagnosed and actually have depressive pseudodementia. On the other hand, Williamson reports that the general practitioners of 71% of depressed patients do not know that their patients are depressed.[21] It is extremely important for the physician to differentiate between these two disorders. Many elderly patients with depressive illness present with typical signs of a mild organic mental syndrome, characterized typically by defects in memory, abstraction, and calculating abilities. After recovery from the depression, however, the apparent organic symptoms may improve markedly or may clear completely.

In most cases, a differential diagnosis between depression and organic brain syndrome depends on the history. Both demented and depressed patients may present with memory loss, disorientation, paranoia, and behavioral changes. However, dementia usually has an insidious and relentless course, whereas depression normally has a more cyclic course, often with an abrupt onset (frequently associated with a particular stressful event, such as the death of a loved one), and may remit spontaneously after several months. The physician, however, should use caution in differentiating between the two disorders solely on this basis. Dementia may go unrecognized until a precipitating event brings it to the attention of the patient's family. For example, a family might report that the patient was fine until the death of his spouse, when suddenly he became forgetful; in reality the patient's spouse may have been compensating for the patient's progressive losses, which only become apparent after the spouse's death. Emotional lability and neglect of personal care also are common both to dementia and depression. Demented patients, however, may tend to wander, confabulate, and exhibit severe disorientation—symptoms not usually present in depressive illness.

Depressed patients, on the other hand, show vegetative signs normally absent in demented patients. These include loss of appetite, often accompanied by a substantial weight loss over several week's duration, disturbances of sleep, particularly during the middle and end of the night, diurnal variation with symptoms worsening in the morning, pronounced agitation, psychomotor retardation, consistent anhedonia (inability to experience anything pleasurable), complaints about petty issues, fatigue, decreased libido or aggressive drives, somatic symptoms such as headaches, and feelings of guilt, reduced self-esteem, and helplessness. Table 15-1 highlights some of the common clinical findings in depressive illness. Table 15-2 reviews some of the common features differentiating depression from dementia.

Depressed patients frequently have a history of depressive episodes and a possible family history of affective disorders. These two pieces of information are invaluable in developing a differential diagnosis. Fifteen to twenty percent of first-degree relatives of patients with recurrent unipolar and bipolar depressive disorders have a history of depressive illness; this represents a tenfold increase in incidence, as compared with the incidence of these disorders in the normal population.[33] A history of mood swings or previous depression may also aid in establishing the presence of an affective rather than an organic disorder. Depressive illness is marked by feelings of worthlessness, suicidal ideation (with intent), and reactions out of proportion to the realistic underlying problems. In addition, depressed patients with cognitive impairments usually exhibit mild

TABLE 15-1   Differentiation of Dementia from Depressive Pseudodementia

	Dementia	Pseudodementia
Onset	Intellectual deficits antedate depression	Depressive symptoms antedate cognitive deficits
Presentation of symptoms	Patient minimizes or denies cognitive deficits, tries to conceal them by circumstantiality, perseveration, changing topic of conversation	Patient complains vocally of memory impairment and poor intellectual performance, exaggerates and dwells on these deficits
Appearance and behavior	Often neglected, sloppy; manner facetious or apathetic and indifferent; catastrophic reaction may be evoked; emotional expression often labile and superficial	Facial expression sad, worried; manner retarded or agitated, never facetious or euphoric; bemoans or ridicules own impaired performance but no true catastrophic reaction
Response to questions	Often evasive, angry, or sarcastic when pressed for answers, or tries hard to answer correctly but just misses	Often slow, "I don't know" type of answer
Intellectual performance	Usually globally impaired and consistently poor	Often confined to memory impairment; inconsistent; if globally impaired, it is so because patient refuses to make effort
Sodium amobarbital interview	All cognitive deficits accentuated	Performance improved

(Kaplan HI, Sadlock BJ: Study Guide and Self-Examination Review for Modern Synopsis of Comprehensive Textbook of Psychiatry IV, 2nd ed. Baltimore, Williams & Wilkins, 1985)

TABLE 15-2   Differentiating Dementia from Depression*

Dementia	Depression
Patient attempts to hide cognitive losses, is apathetic or unaware	Patient complains of memory loss and other cognitive losses and is distressed
Symptoms progress slowly and insidiously; difficult to pinpoint onset	Symptoms are of relatively rapid onset
Approximate or "near-miss" answers are typical	"Don't know" answers are common
Patient struggles to perform well and is frustrated	Little effort to perform, apathetic
Affect is shallow or labile	Depressive mood is pervasive
Attention and concentration may be impaired	Attention and concentration are usually intact

* Adapted from Wells
(Reproduced from Stoudemire A, Thompson TL: Recognizing and treating dementia. Geriatrics 36(10):114, 1981)

memory disturbances and severe depression; the reverse is common in demented patients.

Depression is characteristically treatable, even in the presence of organic brain syndrome, and treating it successfully usually improves function even in demented patients. However, patients incorrectly diagnosed as depressed may receive medication (*e.g.*, tricyclic antidepressants) that can produce serious side-effects, such as orthostatic hypotension, cardiac arrhythmias, constipation, confusion, or interference with other medications. Patients incorrectly labeled as depressed also may become resentful of their physicians for erroneously accusing them of having "mental problems," when they are trying to cope well with the emotional strains of their physical disease.[9]

On the other hand, health-care providers must refrain from attributing all depressive tendencies to purely affective disorders. Certain medical conditions, such as hyperparathyroidism, Cushing's syndrome, and hypothyroidism produce mental changes which may include fatigue, reduced motivation, poor self-esteem, or significant depression. A lack of ambition or reduced participation in social activities, symptoms common to a depressive state, may be secondary to energy depletion resulting from medical or surgical procedures. Weight loss, similarly, may reflect swallowing problems resulting from postcerebral artery strokes or pseudobulbar palsy. Spasticity, ataxia, urinary and fecal incontinence, paralysis, and so on, make even the daily performance of simple activities a chore and frequently result in feelings of loss, frustration, and hopelessness. Rehabilitation patients may express suicidal ideation such as, "I wish I were dead," usually, however, *without* intent.[9] These feelings may fluctuate, depending on the patient's medical state, and they represent normal grief and reactional emotional displays as a consequence of changed physical status. Physicians must try to sort out normal, appropriate feelings of depression from depressive illness, medically induced mental disturbances, or symptoms of organic brain disease.

One approach to solving this diagnostic dilemma is to treat all dementia patients with antidepressants. As noted, however, there is some risk of complications with false positives. A more suitable approach is to repeat psychological evaluations in possibly demented patients within a 3-month interval. Demented patients invariably show some regression in psychological functioning during this period, whereas depressed patients are likely to improve or stabilize functionally.[23]

Often it is helpful in establishing a diagnosis for patients to undergo a battery of neuropsychological tests. Even patients who are severely depressed and display significant disorders in short-term retention and learning usually retain their perceptual–cognitive skills such as visual spatial discrimination, auditory receptive processes, fine and gross motor coordination, and somatosensory functions. In contrast, persons with organic brain syndrome (OBS) exhibit perceptual–cognitive difficulties. Neuropsychological testing provides data about perceptual–cognitive processes which permits the differentiation between organic brain syndrome and depression.

Delirium Versus Dementia

Delirium normally results from acute organic brain syndromes caused, for example, by high fevers, head injuries, seizures, anesthetics, systematic infections, hepatic or renal failure, metabolic or ionic disturbances, or drug or alcohol intoxications. Although delirium may present in any age group, it is more likely to occur in young children and adults over 60 years of age. Engle suggests that 10% to 15% of all patients hospitalized for acute medical or surgical services manifest an acute brain syndrome (delirium) of varying severity.[37]

As with patients with dementia, delirium patients have trouble sustaining attention and also may have memory impairments and disorientation. Behavioral changes such as anxiety, irritability, and depression may occur in both types of organic brain syndromes. However, delirium usually is typified by an abrupt onset, a short duration, and by fluctuating states of consciousness, in contrast to dementia, which is typified by an insidious onset and a stable and progressive course. A delirious state may last as long as a week, but rarely exceeds 1 month. However, delirium caused by reversible conditions such as pernicious anemia, myxedema, or cerebral insufficiency may develop more gradually and mimic dementia.

In addition to attention deficits and cognitive impairments, the hallmark of delirium is a disturbance of sleep–wakefulness. Delirious patients have decreased awareness of the environment–a "clouded consciousness," in contrast to the unclouded consciousness present in dementia patients.[1] Patients in a delirious state frequently experience misperceptions, illusions, or hallucinations. Symptoms seem to worsen during sleepless nights or in darkened areas. On the other hand, lucidity appears to improve in the morning. Disturbances of psychomotor activities are also involved in the delirium state; for example, patients may appear agitated (restless, hyperactive) or quiet (sluggish, catatonic). Delirium also may involve the accentuation of various underlying personality disorders or psychotic or neurotic reactions.[23] In severe cases, delirium may progress to lethargy, stupor, obtundation, or coma within a few hours or days.[36]

It is extremely important that physicians be alert to the fact that delirium may appear alone or with dementia and that they not attribute sudden changes, increases in confusion, or worsening cognitive disturbances solely to progression of dementia. Most acute brain syndromes, if diagnosed in time and appropriately treated, are reversible. An electroencephalogram (EEG), which shows an increasing frequency of slower activity during periods when the patient loses awareness,[23] may help in diagnosing delirium. The many other tests to rule out acute organic causes of mental impairment, which also should be considered, are discussed in the following sections.

Pseudodementia Versus Dementia

Aside from depression, a number of systematic disturbances produce mental changes which simulate dementia, but unlike chronic organic brain syndromes, these acute conditions are reversible partially or entirely if intervention is timely and appropriate. The term *pseudodementia* has been coined to describe such conditions and to encourage investigation into the source of all cognitive impairments. The physiological causes of pseudodementia are numerous, but a few should always be investigated.

Medication is an extremely common cause of dementialike symptoms, especially in older adults. The use of multiple medications or self-medication by the elderly results in a high occurrence of drug interactions and toxicity, either of which can cause deleterious mental changes. Physiological changes in the elderly lead to altered drug metabolism as well. For example, decreased protein synthesis slows the protein binding of drugs which, in turn, increases the active molecules available for protein attraction and absorption. Reduction in gastric acid production and gastrointestinal motility reduces the rate of absorption of acid-absorbed drugs. Diminished liver functioning and impaired glomerular filtration reduce drug detoxification, and an increase in body fat in proportion to body weight among elderly individuals increases the elimination time of fat-soluble compounds such as barbiturates or benzodiazepines. The half-life of diazepam, for example, one of the most commonly prescribed drugs in the United States, increases from 20 hours at 20 years of age to 90 hours at 80 years of age.[30] Portnoi[30] urges caution in prescribing drugs for the elderly. She notes that commonly used medications have adverse side-effects. Digitalis can produce central nervous system side-effects; reserpine and Aldomet can produce sedation and depression; diuretic treatment can cause mild dehydration leading to confusional states, and anti-Parkinsonian medication can produce paranoid delusions secondary to confusion. Table 15-3 lists some of the medications that may cause iatrogenic dementia.

Physicians should be alert to a number of considerations with respect to medication and dementia.

1. Even subtle mental changes accompanying medication regimens; drug-induced illness may go unnoticed in the elderly, since the symptoms frequently mimic stereotyped signs of old age such as forgetfulness, weakness, confusion, tremor, anorexia, and anxiety.[25]

TABLE 15-3 Medications That May Cause Reversible Dementia or Delirium

Psychoactives	Anticholinergics
Sedative–hypnotics	Atropine and related compounds
Minor tranquilizers	Antispasmodics
Major tranquilizers	
Tricyclic antidepressants	**Other**
Lithium carbonate	
	L-dopa
Antihypertensives	Narcotics
	Steroids
Methyldopa (especially combined	Digitalis
with haloperidol)	Quinidine
Clonidine (especially combined	Diuretics
with fluphenazine)	Oral hypoglycemics
Propranolol (or other beta blockers)	Anti-inflammatory agents
	Disulfiram
Anticonvulsants	Bromides
	Cimetidine
Phenytoin	
Barbiturates	

(Reproduced from Stoudemire A, Thompson TL: Recognizing and treating dementia: Geriatrics 36(10):115, 1981)

2. Drug prescriptions for the elderly should consist of decreased dosages of most medications. Levels can be increased gradually by titration until an effective dosage level is reached.
3. In most cases, the number of different drugs taken should be restricted, and drug consumption should be monitored periodically. The need for minor tranquilizers, sedative–hypnotic medication, and psychotropic drugs, which are frequently prescribed for older patients, should be evaluated; if no longer needed, the prescriptions should be discontinued.
4. Any investigation of cognitive impairment should include a detailed drug history.

Several *metabolic disorders* can lead to symptoms of senility. Liver and kidney disorders always should be thoroughly investigated. *Uremia* from renal failure is probably the most frequent metabolic basis for organic brain syndromes.[18] According to Gregory and Smeltzer,[18] when uremic episodes are of short duration, especially in young patients, the confusional state is likely to be completely reversible, but chronic uremia, especially in older persons, tends to damage cortical neurons irreversibly, and thus cause chronic dementia. Both hyper- and hypocalcemia may produce mental changes. *Hypercalcemia,* which can lead to lethargy and confusion in the elderly, may be caused by a number of factors including metastatic cancer of the lung or breast, multiple myeloma, Paget's disease, thiazide administration, and hyperparathyroidism.[27] Immobility can also potentiate any of these conditions. *Hypocalcemia,* on the other hand, mimics senile dementia and may result from hypoparathyroidism, malabsorption problems, or renal failure. *Hypoglycemia,* another metabolic disorder that may produce pseudosenility,[27] can result from a variety of metabolic disturbances, but most commonly diabetes. Hypoglycemia may be severe enough to produce acute brain syndromes with or without epileptic-type seizures.[18] Diabetic-type chronic brain syndromes are frequently accompanied by arteriosclerosis. *Hypernatremia,* a high concentration of serum sodium, may result from excessive sweating, administration of a hypertonic saline solution or a high protein diet, inadequate fluid intake, or a breakdown of the regulating center of the brain following a cerebral concussion. *Hyponatremia* (a hypo-osmolarity syndrome) also may occur as a consequence of an increase in antidiuretic hormone (ADH) secondary to hypothyroidism, stroke, congestive heart failure, or iatrogenic effects. Both of these disorders produce reversible dementia syndromes. Thyroid function and blood sugars tests should be performed routinely in all cases of organic brain syndrome of unknown origin.

Endocrine disorders, another source of reversible dementia, especially those involving the adrenal cortex, thyroid, parathyroid, anterior pituitary, and pancreatic islet cells may result in lethargy, confusion, and behavioral changes. For example, hypothyroidism causes a generalized impairment of cellular function, including that of the brain. Hypothyroidism has a subacute onset and may result in lethargy, depressed mood, pessimism, poor self-esteem, and a diffuse slowing of EEG waves. Congenital hypothyroidism (cretinism) leads to mental retardation but is partly reversible if diagnosed and treated promptly.[18] Untreated myxedema (hypothyroidism in older adults) has been known to progress to psychoses.

Malnutrition, which is present in more than 10% of all elderly,[27] can play a role in central nervous system dysfunction and thus can lead to changes in cognitive functioning. Deficiencies in the vitamin B complex—thiamine, niacin, and vitamin B12, make patients especially vulnerable to mental impairments similar to those in hypothyroidism; thiamine deficiency is an important component of Wernicke's and Korsakoff's syndromes. The classic symptoms of pellagra, which results from niacin deficiency, include dermatitis, diarrhea, delirium, dementia, and death. Vitamin B12 deficiency, which can lead to pernicious anemia, malabsorption syndromes, and encephalopathy, may involve inadequate supplies of other important nutrients necessary for adequate mental functioning and self-care activities.

Chemical, drug, or alcohol *intoxication* can lead to severe mental disorders. Certain gases such as carbon dioxide, carbon monoxide, carbon tetrachloride, oxygen at greater than two atmospheres of pressure, or conditions of hypoxia or anoxia, may cause diminished mental abilities. Metals, including mercury, manganese, aluminum, and lead, also are implicated in brain disorders. For example, Wilson's disease, a hepatolenticular degenerative disorder secondary to chronic copper intoxication, can lead to a progressive decrease in intellectual function. The onset of Wilson's disease usually occurs between the ages of 20 and 50 years. Alcohol or barbiturate intoxication, or their abrupt withdrawal after long-term use (*e.g.,* during hospitalization), can produce acute dementia within hours to days. Since patients may not volunteer an accurate drug or alcohol history, a correct diagnosis may be difficult. Physicians should consider that withdrawal from sedatives may be a diagnostic possibility whenever patients exhibit acute mental symptoms within a short period of time after admission to a hospital.

Other factors implicated in pseudodementia include cerebral or systemic infections (*e.g.,* neurosyphilis, meningitis, malaria, pneumonia, febrile conditions), head trauma, tumors, stroke, hydrocephalus, multiple sclerosis, Parkinson's disease, and cardiopulmonary conditions such as cardiovascular insufficiencies, congestive heart failure, emboli, emphysema, and the like. In addition to the many physiological factors previously discussed, environmental conditions may also play a role in causing acute brain syndromes. Such factors include sensory deprivation, social isolation, immobilization, relocation to unfamiliar environments, sleep deprivation, and other stressful events.[41] Table 15-4 summarizes some of the causative factors in pseudodementia.

Mental Status Examination (MSE)

A brief mental status examination should be performed by the primary care physician when cognitive impairments are evident or suspected. Mental status examinations have been found to be useful in establishing diffuse brain dysfunction and appear to correlate with diagnoses made by psychiatrists.[41] Some physicians neglect to examine patients with respect to orientation or memory for fear of embarrassing or insulting them by asking obvious questions. However, most patients are cooperative if the testing is explained to be a regular facet of the general health examination. The abbreviated MSE may help in detecting occult organic deficits or in confirming suspected dementia states. For example, demented patients are likely to give "near miss" answers or indicate that they do not know the answer to a question, whereas patients with affective disorders tend to give symbolic replies or show little cognitive disturbance.[41]

Although there are a number of mental status examinations cited in the literature, many test only memory and orientation functions. The FROMAJE test, designed by Libow,[27] is a short and useful status examination which, in addition to testing memory and orientation, assesses reasoning, judgment, emotional state, and general social functioning as well. The test is fashioned as a mnemonic device, each letter representing one aspect of mental functioning. This facilitates remembering and administering the test: F = function, R = reasoning, O = orientation, M = memory, A = arithmetic, J = judgment, and E = emotional state. Each category is individually scored; the overall rating determines whether an organic impairment is present, and whether it is minimal or severe. The FROMAJE evaluation is designed for an experienced clinician to take approximately 10 to 15 minutes to complete. The test, explained below in detail, is presented with permission of the publishers:[27]

F = function refers to an individual's mental ability to maintain himself adequately in the community and at home. In the case of a patient in a nursing home, the question is whether the patient has the mental ability to return home and maintain himself with respect to food, shelter, clothing, hygiene, and not behaving in socially unacceptable ways, including not wandering in the street, not failing to pay the rent, avoiding starvation, and so on. This rating refers only to mental strength and competence. An individual who has adequate capabilities but is physically incapable of maintaining himself at home (after a stroke, for example) would be rated as +1 for function.

To arrive at this rating properly, the interviewer must ask a relative, a friend, or a nurse about the patient's mental function in recent weeks or months

TABLE 15-4   Reversible Causes of Mental Impairment

Therapeutic Drug Intoxication
Depression
Metabolic
  Azotemia uremia or renal failure (dehydration, diuretics, obstruction, hypokalemia)
  Hyponatremia (diuretics, excess antidiuretic hormone, salt wasting, intravenous liquids)
  Hypernatremia (dehydration intravenous saline)
  Volume depletion (diuretics, bleeding, inadequate fluids)
  Acid-base disturbance
  Hypoglycemia (insulin, oral hypoglycemics, starvation)
  Hyperglycemia (diabetic ketoacidosis, or hyperosmolar coma)
  Hepatic failure
  Hypothyroidism
  Hyperthyroidism (especially apathetic)
  Hypercalcemia
  Cushing's syndrome
  Hypopituitarism
Infection, fever, or both
  Viral
  Bacterial
  Pneumonia
  Pyelonephritis
  Cholecystitis
  Diverticulitis
  Tuberculosis
  Endocarditis
Cardiovascular
  Acute myocardial infarct
  Congestive heart failure
  Arrhythmia
  Vascular occlusion
  Pulmonary embolus
Brain disorders
  Vascular insufficiency
    Transient ischemia
    Stroke
  Trauma
    Subdural hematoma
    Concussion/confusion
    Intracerebral hemorrhage

Epidural hematoma
Infection
  Acute meningitis (pyogenic, viral)
  Chronic meningitis (tuberculous, fungal)
  Neurosyphilis
  Subdural empyema
  Brain abscess
Tumors
  Metastatic to brain
  Primary in brain
Normal pressure hydrocephalus
Parkinson's disease
Pain
  Fecal impaction
  Urinary retention
  Fracture
  Surgical abdomen
Sensory deprivation states such as blindness or deafness
Hospitalization
  Anesthesia or surgery
  Environmental change and isolation
Alcohol toxic reactions
  Lifelong alcoholism
  Alcoholism new in old age
  Decreased tolerance with age producing increasing intoxication
  Acute hallucinosis
  Delirium tremens
Anemia
Tumor (systemic effects of nonmetastatic malignant neoplasm)
Chronic lung disease with hypoxia or hypercapnia
Deficiencies of nutrients such as vitamin B12, folic acid, or niacin
Accidental hypothermia
Chemical intoxications
  Heavy metals such as arsenic, lead, or mercury
  Consciousness alerting agents
  Carbon monoxide, carbon disulfide
Psychiatric
  Depression
  Chronic schizophrenia
  Repeated electroconvulsive therapy

(Adapted from Task Force of the National Institute on Aging: Senility reconsidered: Treatment possibilities for mental impairment in the elderly. JAMA 244(3):261–2, 1980)

and combine this information with his own impression. The test of function is scored as follows:

+1 = Mental function is adequate enough so that no at-home support is necessary.
+2 = Because of mental impairment, patient will need some at-home support at least part of the day or week (from family, friends, visiting nurse service).
+3 = Because of mental impairment, patient needs some 24-hour per day, 7-day per week, at-home support and supervision.

R = reasoning is tested by asking the person to explain the meaning of a proverb. If unsure whether or not the request is understood or if the proverb is familiar, ask another one. If educational or cultural background (non-English speaking) suggests that the person does not comprehend the question, use another proverb or saying that is appropriate to this patient's education and culture (through an interpreter). Assign a rating based on the use of an appropriate proverb and language. Sample proverbs are "The early bird catches the worm," or, "A stitch in time saves nine." The test of reasoning is scored as follows:

+1 = Well explained, with general connotation given.
+2 = Some semblance of meaning given, but some incompleteness or inability to generalize noted.
+3 = Completely unable to ascribe any meaning, or gives a totally incorrect explanation.

O = orientation. In responding to the items below, if the person does not spontaneously make a statement revealing orientation, choices are presented. Thus: Day of week? Is it Monday, Tuesday? Is it June, July, and so on.

1. Time—inquire about
   Day of week
   Month and date
   Year
2. Place—where are you now? (If necessary, present choices: Is this your apartment; your house or hotel; a nursing home or a hospital?)
3. Self
   Name
   Approximate year of birth or age

The test of orientation is rated as follows:

+1 = Generally accurate, with only minor errors in time, place, and self
+2 = Significant error in one area: Time, place, or self
+3 = Significant errors in two or three areas: Time, place, and self

1. Distant
   President of the United States during World War II who was in wheelchair? (Answer: FD Roosevelt)

United States president assassinated within the past 25 years: (Answer: JF Kennedy)

Where were you born?

2. Recent

What did you have for breakfast today?

Where were you yesterday?

Remember the number "8."

3. Immediate

What did I ask you about the presidents of the United States?

What number did I tell you to remember?

The test of memory is scored as follows:

+1 = Generally accurate, with only minor errors in distant, recent, and immediate memory

+2 = Significant error in one area: Distant, recent, or immediate memory

+3 = Significant error in two or three areas: Distant, recent, and immediate memory

A = arithmetic. Sample questions to test arithmetic:

1. Count from 1 to 10
2. Count backwards from 10 to 1
3. Subtract 7 from 100

The test of arithmetic is scored as follows:

+1 = Generally accurate with only minor errors

+2 = One significant error

+3 = Two or more significant errors

J = judgment. Sample questions to test judgment:

1. At night, if you need some help, how do you obtain it?
2. If having trouble with your neighbor, what do you do to improve the situation?
3. If you see smoke in a wastepaper basket, what action(s) do you take?

The test of judgment is scored as follows:

+1 = Generally sensible response

+2 = Demonstrates some poor judgment

+3 = Extremely poor judgment

E = emotional state. The patient's manner is observed during the interview. The patient is asked about crying, sadness, depression, optimism, and future plans. The patient's behavior is considered in relation to his situation; some sadness or depression is quite appropriate for a significant illness or loss. The test of emotional state is scored as follows:

+1 = Emotional state seems reasonable and appropriate for patient's situation

+2 = Extensive or inappropriate depression, or grandiosity, or anxiety

+3 = Extremely unreal or inappropriate ideas (delusional or hallucinatory behavior; extreme depression or suicidal ideas).

An overall score on the FROMAJE of:

7 or 8	= No significant abnormal behavior or mentation
9 or 10	= Minimal organic mental syndrome (dementia) or emotional illness
11 or 12	= Moderate organic mental syndrome (dementia) or emotional illness
13 or more	= Severe organic mental syndrome (dementia) or emotional illness

For example, if the following numerical values were recorded for each of the FROMAJE categories, the total score would be 10, indicating that the patient had minimal organic mental syndrome.

F = 2
R = 1
O = 2
M = 2
A = 1
J = 1
E = 1

An E (emotional) rating of 3 will produce a total score of +9, even if the patient scores normal (+1) on all of the remaining FROMAJE ratings. Thus the total of +9 or greater may be a false positive for senile dementia, but does allow this mental status evaluation to highlight emotional illness.

F = +1
R = +1
O = +1
M = +1
A = +1
J = +1
E = +3
———
+9

Numerical ratings serve mainly to assist less experienced interviewers. Experienced clinicians can use the FROMAJE format to arrive at a subjective overall rating of normal status or minimal, moderate or severe organic brain syndrome. Responses can be recorded for later use in re-evaluation comparisons or therapy management planning.

Conventional mental status tests, although used as simple, primary diagnostic tools in the evaluation of organic brain syndromes, have major limitations.

1. Few mental assessments are specifically designed for elderly persons. Older people tend to have less education, be in a lower socioeconomic group, and have poorer health than the younger people for whom the exams are designed, and therefore some of the items on the test may have little relevance to them.
2. Few tests take into account the cultural background of the patients being tested. Many proverbs, a frequent subject on mental status examinations, may not be readily understood by non-English speaking persons; in the FROMAJE test, Libow suggests that proverbs or sayings native to the culture of the person being tested be employed when English proverbs are not familiar.
3. Faulty examination ratings may also result from impaired functioning secondary to hostility, anxiety, depression, easy fatigability, lack of cooperation, inattention, and communication difficulties.
4. Aphasics cannot be evaluated with the FROMAJE examination, as performance rests upon receptive and expressive language facility. For the same reason, patients with sensory impairments, such as visual and hearing problems, should be evaluated beforehand to assess any problems that might interfere with accurate test results.
5. Acute mental syndromes frequently have fluctuating levels of awareness. Mental status examinations may need to be repeated over the course of several days or weeks to establish valid results.

The mental status examination is useful only as a general indicator of cognitive function. Psychologic and neurologic consultations are necessary for a detailed evaluation. The examination does not conceptualize the patient's mental performance in terms of overall functioning. The use of the FASQ, as discussed in Chapter 2, may help coordinate the findings on the mental status examination with a patient's ability to perform activities of daily living. Difficulty in performing tasks listed on the FASQ as involving cognitive or affective states (*e.g.,* grocery shopping, handling finances, conversing, concentrating, driving an automobile, and so on) may help the physician to associate mental limitations, as determined by the mental status examination, with functional limitations in everyday living skills, and focus treatment strategies on areas that are deficient. It should be noted that, although only certain activities are listed on the FASQ as dependent upon cognitive and affective skills, the performance of any activity is directly or indirectly related to these mental states.

Diagnostic Workup for Dementia

Complete evaluation of the patient with possible dementia requires a detailed neurologic history and physical examination. Special points to be covered in the history include questions regarding any prescription, over-the-counter, or illicit drug use. Alcohol-intake habits should also be reviewed. Physicians who are doubtful of a patient's replies may need to have a family member survey the home medicine cabinet; such an inventory may disclose that the patient is still taking drugs prescribed long ago, may be taking medications prescribed for other family members, or may have similar prescriptions from several physicians. If still in doubt, blood and urine samples may be analyzed for drug alcohol or high metallic content. The history should also examine recent losses in the patient's life and his present reaction to them, responses to past crises, current changes in employment or social roles, family interactions, and current emotional state.

Listed below are some common symptoms of organic brain syndrome.[8] Questioning in these areas during the history part of the examination may provide insight into a diagnosis of dementia.

1. Sudden onset ("functional" disorders may appear to have a sudden onset, but the patient has usually been having trouble for days to months)
2. Fluctuating symptoms (typical of multi-infarct dementia)
3. Older patient (younger patients also may develop organic brain syndrome)
4. Negative past history of psychiatric disorder
5. Onset or worsening at night ("sundowning")
6. Disorientation to time and place
7. Short-term memory disturbance
8. Illusions and visual hallucinations
9. Absence of obvious psychological precipitants

Dubovsky and Weissberg list symptoms that may present in more subtle cases of dementia.[8] In these instances, replies on the abbreviated MSE may be completely normal, especially if patients are able to compensate for mild disorders in alertness, attention, orientation, or memory. The physician should suspect possible chronic organic brain syndrome in patients who present with one or more of the following complaints:

1. Vague complaints from the patient or his family that he "isn't up to par"
2. Multiple somatic complaints
3. Difficulty concentrating
4. Forgetfulness
5. Subtle changes in personality, especially if accompanied by depression, apathy, or emotional lability
6. Errors in judgment at home or at work
7. Uncharacteristic irrational or impulsive behavior
8. Failure to grasp all facets of complex problems or situations
9. Suspiciousness
10. Fatigue
11. Social inappropriateness
12. Frequently getting lost
13. Incontinence
14. Chronic lateness in patients who are usually punctual
15. Insomnia

During the physical examination, sources of sensory impairment should be considered. Testing for abnormal reflexes should also be included in the examination. Although primitive reflexes are present in the normal elderly population, they are more prevalent in those with dementia. Reflexes to be checked include the Babinski, palmomental, grasp reflex, and glabella.

The neurological workup should also include a *CT scan,* helpful in identifying tumors, subdural hematomas, intracranial hemorrhage, cerebral infarction, and cerebral atrophy. Normal aging adults as well as demented patients may have atrophy, and a reversible dementia may be present even though cerebral atrophy has been documented; therefore, atrophy findings cannot establish a definite diagnosis of dementia. A *lumbar puncture* and examination of cerebral spinal fluid may be helpful but should not be performed if there are any signs suggesting increased intracranial pressure, such as papilledema, severe headache, or focal neurological findings.[36] The mental status examination previously discussed should be a part of all neurological assays.

Additional tests should be performed when dementia is suspected. Impaired spatial perception is almost always present in dementia. Constructional dyspraxia, the inability to perform a constructional task when motor and sensory pathways are intact, is frequently caused by diffuse brain disease or disease localized to either parietal lobe.[7,16] To test for constructional dyspraxia, the physician should first draw several figures on a paper and then ask the patient to copy them. Any figure can be drawn (square, Greek cross, three dimensional box), so long as the physician is aware of the way normal patients and patients with organic brain syndrome copy them. Rounding of the angles, closing in of the figure, rotation or fragmentation of the object and loss of three dimensionality are characteristic of patients with dyspraxia. Patients also should be asked to draw one or more figures on command (*e.g.,* without copying them). For example, a patient may be asked to draw a clock with the hands pointing to 5 o'clock. Patients also should be observed for the performance of simple motor tasks. As an example, physicians should ask patients to do rapidly alternating hand movements (see Chap. 4) and note whether the patient has any difficulty stopping and starting, or whether he has problems because of forgetting the activity sequence. Observation of dressing (buttoning a blouse) may also offer clues to the physician indicating the presence of dyspraxia. Routine laboratory examinations should include the following:[38]

1. Hematologic examination (blood cell counts, hematocrit reading, hemoglobin level, and sedimentation rate)
2. Urinalysis (albumin, glucose, and ketone levels, and microscopic examination)
3. Stool examination, including a test for occult blood
4. Evaluations of levels of serum urea or BUN and glucose; serum electrolytes (sodium, potassium, carbon dioxide, chloride, calcium, phosphorus); bilirubin; vitamin B12; and folic acid
5. Test for thyroid function
6. Serological test for syphilis

Chest X-rays, cerebral angiography, and electrocardiograms may also be used to supplement clinical findings. Although the tests are numerous and seemingly expensive, they may be invaluable in detecting a treatable form of dementia before it progresses to a state of chronic, irreversible mental impairment.

Management of Dementia

Although dementia often represents a chronic, progressively deteriorating disorder without cure, therapeutic intervention may help reduce the severity of its manifestation and improve the quality of life for both patient and family.

The first step in the management of the senile dementia patient is to rule out treatable causes of mental impairment. There are numerous drugs, metabolic disturbances, and environmental factors, as discussed in the section on pseudodementia, which can simulate chronic organic brain disease. Additionally, acute mental disorders may be superimposed on chronic organic brain syndrome; by alleviating the reversible causative factors, mental functioning may improve significantly.

Since drug toxicity is one of the major causes of dementia, and since elderly patients have an increased sensitivity to drugs, physicians should investigate the cognitively impaired patient's drug consumption thoroughly. It is important that the physician not take for granted that the patient has: (1) had a prescription filled, (2) understands or remembers how often to take the drug, (3) is on no medication other than that which the current physician is prescribing, (4) continues to take the drug, or (5) reports adverse reactions accurately.[25] Physicians should be specific with instructions for taking medication; for example, it is important to write down when, how often, and how to take the medication (e.g., three times a day after meals, with plenty of water), rather than to tell the elderly patient to take it as indicated on the package. Physicians should also try to restrict the number of medications prescribed in order to minimize drug interactions, and each prescription should reflect the lowest effective dosage. Since elderly patients show increased sensitivity to some tranquilizers, Valium and librium should be avoided during daytime hours, as should anticholinergics and antidepressant medication. Confusion is a common side-effect of antidepressants; sometimes the beneficial drug effects may be nullified by a patient's fear of memory loss or "going crazy."[12] Any medication that increases cognitive impairments or fails to achieve its desired effects should be discontinued.

Sudden changes in behavior, symptoms of delirium such as hallucinations or illusions, agitation, or memory loss should be investigated in conjunction with a thorough medical examination. Health-care providers should be alert for precipitating factors. Organic brain syndromes frequently appear following a psychological trauma, such as the loss of a loved one. A mourner may feel depressed, withdraw from social activities, and fail to eat adequately, leading to clinical malnourishment. Confusion and a reduced ability to perform self-care may result, secondary to the malnutrition. Dietary supplementation will usually return the patient to normal functioning. Physicians also should be cognizant of the fact that relocation, changed routines and staffing, and numerous tests or medical procedures during hospitalization may precipitate disturbed behaviors; these normally subside once the patient is returned to familiar settings. Similarly, patients admitted to the hospital with symptoms of acute brain syndrome should be re-evaluated before discharge plans are completed. Many hospitalized patients exhibiting acute mental disorders are sent directly to nursing homes or institutions by staff members unaware of the potential reversibility of such symptoms. Families should also be informed of the reversible nature of many acute conditions. It may help them to cope more easily with patients' tendencies to hallucinate, threaten suicide, react differently from normal, and so on, if they know the symptoms will abate in time.

For patients who have chronic organic brain syndrome, treatment is largely supportive. Zarit[41] pinpoints three main goals in treatment care plans: (1) Maintaining the impaired individual within the community; (2) providing information and support to the patient and family; and (3) focusing treatment plans on specific problem areas.

The role of the functional assessment in the management of senility and determination of patient's needs cannot be overemphasized. Mental status test results should be interpreted with respect to functional implications; for example, patients with impaired mathematical abilities will be likely to have difficulty paying bills, balancing checkbooks, and doing grocery shopping. Treatment strategies can then address these or similar issues. Many individuals with a substantial degree of impairment develop compensatory mechanisms, such as highly routinized activities, which decrease the need for spontaneous judgments and decisions. Such individuals may function remarkably well in a familiar environment. The validity of mental status test results, therefore, should be investigated by supplementing examination replies with information given by family members. Once the degree of dementia and specific areas of difficulty have been established, physicians should discuss prognosis, realistic expectations, and treatment plans with family members. Caregiver guides such as Mace and Rabin, *The 36-Hour Day,* should be strongly recommended to family members.[28]

Institutionalization is a frequent response to care plans for the demented patient; it is not, however, an inevitable nor necessary choice in all circumstances. Many patients living at home have impairments which are as significant as those of institutionalized dementia patients; on the other hand, institutional placement occurs more frequently when there is a breakdown in family support systems. Problems least tolerated by caregivers were determined in one study to be sleep disturbances, incontinence, and immobility.[41] However, in a study that evaluated caregivers' feelings of being burdened in relation to the degree of impairment or the patient's intellectual or self-care abilities, amount of behavioral or memory problems, presence of formal or informal assistance to the caregiver, and frequency of visits to the household by other people, only the latter variable was significantly associated with caregivers' feelings of being burdened.[41] Every treatment plan should therefore include an assessment of the patient's social network, which is especially important when evaluating the suitability of present living situations. Many programs are available that may increase social contacts for elderly or demented patients. Some communities have foster grandparents or volunteers available to look in on patients who live alone. In Sweden the postman checks on the health of all the older patients on his route;[17] a similar check by local postmen may be possible in some communities. There are also organizations such as Parents Without Partners, Widow to Widow, or Alcoholics Anonymous, which may be appropriate for some older patients. Support groups such as the Alzheimer's Disease and Related Disorders Association may help families engaged in the home care of chronically demented patients.

Patients should also be encouraged to participate in stimulating social interactions. It has been suggested that disorganized behavior, such as nocturnal wandering, is occasioned by the loss of environmental stimuli. The development of supportive, stimulating environments through the use of structured activities and encouraged social interactions has been found to improve a wide variety of behaviors in many nursing homes. In some communities, day care centers for the elderly are available to meet the need for socialization and to give caretakers a reprieve. Physicians familiar with available community resources or agencies can help families make the necessary contacts. Local agencies for the aged and handicapped may provide important information about the availability of homemakers, physical therapists, and mental health clinics.

Increasingly, respite care, a service designed to give caregivers time away from their impaired charges, is available. Many types of respite services exist, including in-home respite care (*i.e.*, respite-care providers coming into the home), community based respite care, and institutional respite. The latter two approaches require the caregiver to bring the impaired individual to the facility offering respite care. Institutional respite care, which is usually housed in a hospital or long-term care facility, is particularly helpful for persons with significant medical problems and for longer stays. Often families have difficulty separating from their caregiving roles and, as a consequence, do not elect to use respite, in spite of the intense caregiving burden they may be experiencing. Also the impaired person may resist receipt of this service. If appropriate, physicians should encourage both the patient and the caregiver to use this service to reduce the stress of one "36-hour day" of care giving.

Patients with dementia also are vulnerable to other physical ailments. Fecal impaction, incontinence, bedsores, and frequent falls may accentuate or initiate symptoms of dementia. Attention to diet and increased physical activity can help minimize these problems. Agencies such as Meals on Wheels can help to provide patients with at least one balanced meal daily. Neighbors or family members may also help in meal preparation or shopping. Exercise should be encouraged for demented patients—even simple exercises performed in a chair are beneficial. Studies have shown that patients who exercise have better short-term memories;[6] exercise also helps to maintain physical strength, lessen the frequency of falls, and reduce the incidence of nocturnal wandering. Incontinence problems may be minimized through the use of bedside commodes, catheterization, or diaper pads.

Dementia patients frequently exhibit a condition known as "sundowning," in which their symptoms worsen after early evening. For nighttime restlessness, thorazine or chloral hydrate may be prescribed; a glass of beer or wine may provide soporific effects for some patients. A healthier alternative is to encourage increased daytime activity. Since sensory impairments can also aggravate confusion, physicians should encourage patients to use eyeglasses, hearing aids, or other devices (large-print books and calendars, large-faced clocks and telephones, telephone amplifiers, and so on, that increase sensory awareness, when appropriate. A detailed listing of aids for patients with sensory impairments is provided in Chapter 13 and 14.

Management of dementia also involves attention to safety precautions. Access to firearms, gas ovens, and certain medications should be restricted. Precautions against wandering also should be planned. Scatter rugs and sharp furniture should be removed from the homes of patients who tend to trip or fall frequently.

Many simple strategies can be practiced by patients and their families to try to improve or maintain the functional status of the individual with dementia. A predictable and familiar environment seems to help.[31] Activities such as eating, exercising, and medication-taking should be scheduled at the same time each day. Devices such as containers that divide medication into daily portions may help impaired patients function more effectively. Visible calendars and clocks, lists of daily activities, and notes concerning basic safety measures may help aid orientation, reasoning, and memory. Several nursing homes have instituted a strategy called reality orientation, which involves staff members' helping to orient patients to person, time, and place through the use of calendars, newspapers, clocks, and the like. Whether such procedures actually help improve memory and orientation functions is still questionable, but at the very least such a strategy encourages interaction between patients and others involved in their care. When people who live alone have cognitive impairments sufficient to jeopardize safety in the performance of activities such as self-medication or bathing, a visiting nurse should be arranged if family supports are unavailable.

Cognitive retraining is a relatively new therapeutic intervention in which cognitive skills such as short-term memory, visual recognition, attention, organization of information, and comprehension are practiced. Unfortunately, a majority of the research on cognitive deficits and remediation has focused on impairments which occur in mental retardation and brain injury; the similarity between these groups and elderly individuals is not known. Studies have shown that at present there are no techniques or medications that restore or prevent further deterioration in chronic organic brain syndromes such as Alzheimer's disease, multi-infarct and Alzheimer's-type senile dementia. Nevertheless, many cognitive deficits assumed to be permanent may be changed in a positive way through training and practice, especially for patients with mild dementia or those with acute mental disorders superimposed on chronic dementia. Referrals to neurologists or psychologists should be considered to identify specific deficits and provide specialized cognitive remediation techniques. A battery of neuropsychological tests may be useful in directing this type of treatment intervention.

The primary care physician can also instruct the patient and family on many basic cognitive strategies. For example, patients can be taught to break down information into smaller pieces which are then mentally rehearsed, or they can be encouraged to pay more attention to items in the middle of a list when attempting recall. Mnemonic techniques are especially helpful in developing memory skills. Concentration on detail, which is important for activities such as use of medication, may be improved through practice exercises. For example, an individual can be presented with a shape and told to select the identical shape from a varied group of choices. Exercises can begin with simple shapes and progress to those in which the shapes have been rotated. Attention and visual scanning possibly can be improved by an exercise in which the individual is presented with a grid of letters and is then instructed to cross out a certain letter whenever it appears. Summarizing literature content after reading a brief passage may also help attention and memory recall. Awareness of time, which is useful in preventing confusion, apathy, and withdrawal can be improved through exercises in which the patient watches the second hand of a clock while counting aloud and then tries to identify a 10- or 20-second span without looking at the clock. Most of these exercises are outlined in *The Thinking Skills Workbook* by Tondat-Carter and colleagues[39] and can be used directly by patients and their families. The book also includes an examination which helps to identify the skills most in need of improvement.

The intent of these cognitive exercises is to help people function better, specifically to maintain or slow down the deterioration of skills. Because functioning is the goal, which exercises are to be used depends upon how well patients facilitate skills of high priority, such as telling time or keeping track of medication.

Counseling services can be helpful. Counseling may be provided either by the primary care physician or another team member, such as a psychologist, psychiatrist, social worker, or vocational counselor. When other people are involved in the provision of counseling services, the primary care physician should maintain contact and be aware of treatment strategies. Therapy sessions may be intended to help family members understand the nature of the disease process (*e.g.*, organic brain syndromes involve structural changes in the brain) and follow guidelines for alleviating some of the burden of caring. Physicians can be instrumental in helping to decide which activities the patient is still capable of pursuing (driving, cooking unassisted, living independently, and so on) and which should be curtailed. Although some of the affected person's responsibilities will have to be taken over, family members should be advised not to take away too much independence. Overprotectiveness on the part of the spouse or family will increase the patient's disabilities. Although demented persons may be unable to continue to do some activities, such as balancing a checkbook, they still may be able to function adequately in other realms, such as cooking or gardening. Counselors should explore activities a couple (or parent and child) enjoyed doing together in the past and see if they can still participate in the same or similar activities. Sometimes patients may be able to continue activities, but at a less optimal level; for example, they may take longer to dress or dress more casually than before. Whenever possible, family members should refrain from overtaking these tasks for the sake of efficiency or better appearance; instead, the demented person should be allowed to retain some control over his own personal care, unless it is endangering him in some way. Organizational strategies also can be suggested. For example, appointments or medication instructions can be written in a central place; keys can be assigned to a particular location. Routines can be set up for safety checks (for example, never leave the house without checking the stove burners, or always lock the wheelchair before standing up).

Behavioral techniques, having proved successful with many other clinical populations, are beginning to be used by clinicians treating people with organic mental disorders. A number of target behaviors that interfere with daily living are modifiable using these procedures. Hussian[20] describes a number of common, but difficult, behavior problems that have been treated successfully in this population. These behaviors include wandering, urinary incontinence, inappropriate sexual behaviors, and self-stimulation behavior. Treatment programs designed to change these behaviors have most often been implemented in long-term care facilities, although one can envision these programs being conducted in community settings, particularly to help prevent institutionalizations related to these disrupted behavior problems.

Health-care providers should realize that caring for a person with senile dementia or other cognitive impairments is a difficult task. For families of patients with Alzheimer's disease, financial burdens may increase substantially the trauma of the situation. Another common source of difficulty in caring for the demented parent is that care may be perceived as a reversal of parent–child roles, causing strong emotional responses. Sometimes the intact spouse may use the illness to seek revenge for long-standing marital problems or to change the family power structure. These issues require specific therapeutic interventions. Physicians should encourage family members to pursue outside interests, have periodic respites, and discuss problems as they arise. Counseling sessions may be needed occasionally just to bolster the confidence of caregivers in maintaining their roles or to reinforce their decision to institutionalize a loved one when home care is no longer possible. The affected patient should not be neglected in counseling efforts either. Patients frequently exhibit denial, withdrawal, depression, paranoia or dependency; they may need to discuss these feelings, fears of "going crazy," or the frustrating circumstances of their situation. In some cases patients will deny the need for counseling, indicating that they have no problems. In such instances, physicians should not force psychological treatment but should inform patients and families that services are always available if they are needed at some later date.

Summary

Since cognitive impairments can affect a person's ability to perform almost any activity, no functional assessment can be complete without an evaluation of a patient's cognitive abilities. Determination of a patient's mental status is important, not only in establishing a diagnosis, but also in developing timely and appropriate treatment plans.

In assessing mental status, it is important for the primary care physician to be able to differentiate between permanent and reversible cognitive impairments, as well as to distinguish between affective disorders and organic etiologies. As the population over the age of 65 continues to increase, physicians will be faced more and more with patients at risk for the development of senile dementia or other age-related mental symptoms. Depressive illness, metabolic disturbances, endocrine disorders, malnutrition, and chemical and drug intoxications can cause severe mental disorders, sometimes resulting in irreversible brain damage, obtundation, and death.

A differential diagnosis of dementia is made by obtaining a detailed neurological history, a thorough physical examination, specific laboratory test results to rule out reversible causes, CT scan, and sometimes lumbar puncture. A brief mental status examination which detects impairments in functioning, reasoning, orientation, judgment, memory, mathematical abilities, and emotional state, can help determine the presence or degree of cognitive impairments. Mental status examinations should always be evaluated in terms of resulting functional deficits.

Management of the demented patient requires the provision of counseling and informative services, activity guidelines, problem-solving oriented treatment plans, cognitive remedial strategies, and attention to the social and emotional consequences of caring for a mentally impaired person. Sensitive and informed physicians can enable a demented patient to remain in the community and function at his optimal level.

References

1. American Psychiatric Association: Diagnostic and Statistical Manual of Mental Disorders, 3rd ed. pp 111–112. Washington, American Psychiatric Association, 1980
2. Barnes RF, Raskind MA: DSM-III criteria and the clinical diagnosis of dementia: A nursing home study. J Gerontol 36(1):20, 1980
3. Bayne JRD: Management of confusion in elderly persons. Can Med Assoc J 118:139, 1978
4. Carter LT, Caruso JL, Languirand MA, Berard MA: The Thinking Skills Workbook: A Cognitive Skills Remediation Manual for Adults. Springfield, IL, Charles C Thomas, 1980
5. Cavenar JD, Sullivan JL: Depression: The great imitator—case report. Milit Med 144(11):752, 1979
6. Diesfeldt HFA, Diesfeldt-Groenendi JKH: Improving cognitive performance in psychogeriatric patients: The influence of physical exercise. Age Aging 6:58, 1977
7. Dubovsky SL, Weissberg MP: Clinical Psychiatry in Primary Care, pp 52–60. Baltimore, Williams & Wilkins, 1979
8. Freeman PM, Sack RL, Berger PA (eds): Psychiatry for the Primary Physician. Baltimore, Williams & Wilkins, 1979
9. Gans JS: Depression diagnosis in a rehabilitation hospital. Arch Phys Med Rehabil 62(8):386, 1981
10. Garcia CA, Reding MJ, Blass JP: Overdiagnosis of dementia. J Am Geriatr Soc 29(9):407, 1981
11. Gianutsos R: What is Cognitive Rehabilitation? J Rehabil 36–40, July–Aug 1980
12. Glassman M: Misdiagnosis of senile dementia: Denial of care to the elderly. Social Work 25(4):288, 1980
13. Glenner GG: Alzheimer's disease (senile dementia): A research update and critique with recommendations. J Am Geriatr Soc 30(1):59, 1982
14. Gold MS, Pottash ALC, Extein I, Sweeney DR: Diagnosis of Depression in the 1980s. JAMA 245(15):1562, 1981
15. Good MI: Pseudodementia and physical findings masking significant psychopathology. Am J Psychiatry 138(6):811, 1981

16. Granacher RP Jr: Basic Principles of Geriatric Psychopharmacology. J Ky Med Assoc 79(7):411, 1981
17. Greenblatt M, Becerra RM, Seratetinides EA: Social networks and mental health: An overview. Am J Psychiat 139(8):977, 1982
18. Gregory I, Smeltzer DJ: Psychiatry: Essentials of Clinical Practice. Boston, Little, Brown & Co, 1973
19. Heilbrunn G: Disorders of mental function. In Leitch CJ, Tinker RV (eds): Primary Care, Philadelphia, Chapter 28. FA Davis, 1978
20. Hussian RA: Geriatric Psychology: A Behavioral Perspective. New York, Van Nostrand Reinhold, 1981
21. Jacoby RJ: Depression in the Elderly. Br J Hosp Med 25(1):40, 1981
22. Jaffe JR: Functional psychiatric disorders. In Reichel W (ed): The Geriatric Patients. New York, HP Publishing, 1978
23. Karasu TB, Katzman R: Organic brain syndromes. In Bellak L, Karasu TB (eds): Geriatric Psychiatry: A Handbook for Psychiatrists and Primary Care Physicians. New York, Grune & Stratton, 1976
24. Kennie DC, Moore JT: Management of senile dementia. Am Fam Phys 22(6):105, 1980
25. Lamy PP, Vestal RE: Drug prescribing for the elderly. In Reichel W (ed): The Geriatric Patient. New York, HP Publishing, 1978
26. Lazar I, Karasu TB: Evaluation and management of depression in the elderly. Geriatrics, 35(12):47, 1980
27. Libow LS: Senile dementia and "pseudosenility": Clinical diagnosis. In Eisdorfer C, Friedel RD (eds): Cognitive and Emotional Disturbance in the Elderly, pp 78–79. Chicago, Year Book Medical Publishers, 1977
28. Mace MN, Rabin PV: The 36-Hour Day. Baltimore, Johns Hopkins University Press, 1981
29. McKinney AS: Appropriate investigation of stroke and dementia. Geriatrics 36(6):41, 1981
30. Portnoi VA: Diagnostic dilemma of the aged. Arch Intern Med 141(6):734, 1981
31. Rabin PV: Management of irreversible dementia. Psychosomatics 22(7):591, 1981
32. Reichel W: Organic brain syndromes. In Reichel W (ed): The Geriatric Patients. New York, HP Publishing, 1978
33. Sachar EJ: Evaluating depression in the medical patient. In Strain JJ, Grossman S (eds): Psychological Care of the Medically Ill: A Primer in Liaison Psychiatry, Chapter 6. New York, Appleton-Century-Crofts, 1975
34. Schneck ML, Reisberg B, Ferris SH: An overview of current concepts of Alzheimer's disease. Am J Psychiatry 139(2):165, 1982
35. Shraberg D: An overview of neuropsychiatric disturbances in the elderly. J Am Geriatr Soc 36(10):422, 1980
36. Stoudemire A, Thompson TL: Recognizing and treating dementia. Geriatrics 36(10):112, 1981
37. Strain JJ, Grossman S (eds): Psychological Care of the Medically Ill; A Primer in Liaison Psychiatry. New York, Appleton-Century-Crofts, 1975
38. Task Force of National Institute on Aging: Senility reconsidered: Treatment possibilities for mental impairment in the elderly. JAMA 244(3):259, 1980

39. Wilensky H: Diagnosis in old age. In Wolman BB (ed): Clinical Diagnosis of Mental Disorders: A Handbook. New York, Plenum Press, 1978

40. Yesavage JA, Westphal J, Push L: Senile dementia: Combined pharmacologic and psychological treatment, J Am Geriatr Soc 29(4):164, 1981

41. Zarit SH: Aging and Mental Disorders. New York, Free Press, 1980

CHAPTER 16
Mental Retardation

During the past two decades, there has been a large-scale relocation of mentally retarded people from institutional settings into the community. Also during this same time, persons at risk for institutionalization usually have remained in the community. This trend has significant implications for the community health care of mentally retarded persons. Whereas in the past, specialized care was most often given in institutional settings, currently the generic community health system is expected to function as an alternative system. Although numerous studies suggest that mentally retarded persons' quality of life seems to improve within the community,[58] we know very little about utilization patterns of these people once they are transferred to the primary care system. Garrard[18] suggests that subtle obstacles limit access to the generic health care system, which may include: (1) negative attitudes, (2) lack of training, (3) procedural uncertainties, (4) consent issues, (5) double standards in decision making, and (6) characteristics of the person.

This chapter is intended to inform the primary care practitioner of mentally retarded persons' health and psychosocial needs, so that obstacles to health care utilization in the community may be reduced, and to introduce the physician to some of the basic concepts in mental retardation, including definition, classification, and etiology. It will also provide material to sensitize the practitioner to the effects of mental retardation on the family unit and discuss the physician's role in the treatment and prevention of mental retardation.

Definition and Classification

Because of the functional perspective of this book, a definitional approach that includes an analysis of skills (adaptive behaviors) used by a person in his daily life is important. The American Association on Mental Deficiency's (AAMD)

370

definition requires an analysis of function as one element in the classification, as does the definition presented in P.L. 95–607, often referred to as the Developmental Disabilities (DD) definition. The elements of this definition include age (prior to 22), chronicity, 3 or more major life areas from a specified list in which substantial functional limitations are present, and the need for an extended array of long-term services from a multiplicity of service providers. This definition is a bold attempt to move away from categorical labels (*e.g.,* cerebral palsy, epilepsy, autism, mental retardation, and so on) and toward a functional perspective. Professionals using the DD definition do not label persons as developmentally disabled if they are functionally competent, living on their own, and not in need of services in spite of their IQ scores falling below 70. As Seltzer notes, "This definitional approach attempts to link planning, service provision, and eligibility determination to the level of competence a person displays in performing life sustaining and enhancing activities, not to a categorical label."[55]

Conceptual and operational definitions guiding the classification of mental retardation have been controversial throughout this century. The debate has focused on the importance that should be placed on such variables as IQ score, age, etiology, functional disabilities, and social and cultural circumstances.[58] The AAMD, a leading national, interdisciplinary organization of professionals concerned with mental retardation, offers the following definition:

Mental retardation refers to significantly subaverage general intellectual functioning existing concurrently with deficits in adaptive behavior and manifested during the developmental period.[20]

The three operational elements of this definition are (1) IQ score of 70 or below on standardized measures of intelligence; (2) functional limitations in personal care and instrumental (managing one's household) activities of daily living (*i.e.,* deficits in adaptive behavior); and (3) occurrence of the above two criteria prior to the age of 18.

A classification system is of critical importance for any scientific and clinical field; in mental retardation it serves many purposes. For example, it can be used to identify characteristics and problems of an individual, establish guidelines for evaluating the client's abilities and disabilities, evaluate needs in terms of help with daily living skills, plan education and vocational programs, determine eligibility requirements for programs, and identify treatment intervention needs. The building of knowledge from research rests upon definition and classification— that is, agreement as to who is or is not mentally retarded. In addition, understanding the incidence and prevalence of the condition, and encouraging relevant policy and financial allotments, depends upon definitional clarity and procedures used for case identification.

In spite of the research, planning, and policy and funding benefits of accepting a uniform system of classification, numerous classification systems have been developed by different disciplines to meet their own criteria and goals. In a 1983 review[55] of some of the most often used systems, such as the AAMD definition, *The Diagnostic and Statistical Manual of Mental Disorder (DSM-III)*, and *The International Classification of Diseases, 9th revision; Clinical Modification,* a trend is noted to adopt the AAMD definition as the standard and to adapt it to the particular nosology of each classification system.

Each system of classification has advantages and disadvantages, depending on its purpose and the type of discipline using it, and each reflects a different approach to categorization. For example, the *categorical approach* is based on the degree to which a phenomenon is present or absent. In mental retardation, the most commonly used criterion is intelligence. IQ scores provide inclusion/exclusion and level of retardation classes, so that two people who have the same IQ score actually can behave quite differently, and vice versa. An alternative is the *functional approach,* which classifies persons in terms of their behavior; that is, two persons with different IQ scores, but similar abilities and functional limitations, would be classified similarly. Most of the common classification schemes use one or both of these approaches. Factors such as age at onset, severity, prognosis, etiology, and degree of impairment are stressed to varying degrees by the different classification systems. The AAMD definition requires both a functional and a categorical approach.

Recently Zigler and colleagues argued that the definition and classification of mental retardation should be based on IQ score and etiology, and that diagnostic reliability and validity would be improved by eliminating adaptive behavior as a criterion.[79] They noted that because it is difficult to agree on the definition of adaptive behavior, measurement of adaptive behavior lacks validity. These authors asserted that, on the other hand, the organic versus the nonorganic etiological factors of retardation tend to be independent determinants of behavior and can be more easily measured than adaptive behavior because of known correlates of each of the etiological origins. A sample of organic, etiological correlates includes the high prevalence of other physical handicap (*e.g.,* epilepsy, cerebral palsy), higher mortality rate, IQs most often below 50, a wide distribution range of socioeconomic status lines, siblings usually of normal intelligence, and so on. Furthermore, Zigler and colleagues argue for the elimination of adaptive behavior and the inclusion of etiological factors and IQ, because it is their position" . . . that whatever mental retardation is, it is best conceptualized as a stable characteristic of a person rather than a creation of social agents who apply descriptive terms to children." These authors appear to dismiss the classification merit of using adaptive behavior measures that may vary because of social and environmental circumstances. By eliminating these measures of behavior, they are arguing for a categorical approach to classification—retardation is present or absent throughout one's lifetime. Their position represents one side of the controversy about the deleterious effects of using labels and IQ tests versus the benefits of using adaptive behavior as a criterion for classification.

Mercer and others argue that the social stigma of having a mental impairment can become a self-fulfilling handicap for persons with mild mental retardation or borderline normal intelligence.[45] Expected to be cognitively and behaviorally deficient, these people might functionally conform to these expectations. Moreover, when the label is based primarily on the results of an IQ score, it is disproportionately applied to minority and disadvantaged children. Also, professionals who would include adaptive behavior in the definition of mental retardation note that as each individual's behavioral demands vary situationally, it is possible for some people to be labeled retarded in some environments (*e.g.,* schools) and not in others (*e.g.,* ballparks, vocational settings). Those who are pro adaptive behavior tend to divide the population between those individuals whose significant physical, cognitive, and social deficits are stable characteristics and a sizeable number of other persons whose marginal problems rest upon who is employing which definition in what type of setting.[41] Those who agree with Zigler note the epidemiological problems in determining the incidence and prevalence of a condition that is chronic for some and variable for others.

Etiology

About 75% of persons with mental retardation have no known organic etiology and are often referred to in the literature as "familially retarded" or, as in the 1983 AAMD *Classification in Mental Retardation Manual,* as retarded due to psychosocial disadvantage."[20] Persons so classified present with no contributing organic etiology, have at least one parent and one or more sibling (if there are siblings) with subnormal intellectual functioning, and are usually from impoverished environments. An understanding of the etiology of familial retardation remains elusive, although many formulations utilize elements of the nature–nuture argument, contrasting polygenic explanations with sociocultural and environmental ones.[79]

On the other hand, mental retardation of biological origin has a sizeable number of known etiological agents. Grossman estimates that 9 out of 10 cases of mental retardation with a known organic etiology are prenatal in origin and present at birth or early in infancy.[20] Because of the overwhelming preponderance of prenatal etiologies, these problems will be stressed in the discussion that follows.

During the prenatal period problems can arise from chromosomal or fragile gene effects. *Chromosomal abnormalities* can occur in either the autosomal or the sex chromosomes. *Nondisjunction,* the most common cause of genetic aberrations leading to mental retardation, is a sorting error that occurs during cell division, more frequently during meiosis than mitosis. In Down's syndrome, nondisjunction of chromosome 21 occurs during the first meiotic division. During metaphase, when the chromosomes pair up, two of the number 21 chromosomes stick to each other and do not release during anaphase. As a result, at the end of meiosis one cell has 24 chromosomes and the other cell has 22, instead of each cell having 23 chromosomes. This error occurs much more frequently in the egg than in the sperm. The egg containing only 22 chromosomes cannot survive, whereas the egg with the extra chromosome can survive. If a sperm containing the normal 23 chromosomes then fertilizes this egg, the result is a child with 47 chromosomes (including three number 21 chromosomes). This phenomenon is also referred to as "trisomy 21." Down's syndrome children have characteristic physical stigmata and mild to moderate mental retardation. Other examples of trisomies include trisomy 13 (Patau's syndrome) and trisomy 18 (Edwards' syndrome). Physical stigmata, cardiac defects, microcephaly, and profound mental retardation are correlated with these disorders. Maternal age is the most significant factor currently recognized as being related to chromosomal nondisjunction.[8]

Another cause of chromosomal defect is *translocation.* During meiosis the chromosomes are close together for extended periods of time. They may touch, stick to each other for a while, and then separate. During separation a segment of one chromosome may attach itself to another chromosome. For example, in

Down's syndrome due to translocation a part of the number 21 chromosome might attach itself to the number 14 chromosome. If this occurs during meiosis, the cell will have the normal number of chromosomes but will contain both numbers 21 and 14/21 chromosomes. A child will result with 46 chromosomes, including two 21s and one 14/21. This partial trisomy will also cause Down's syndrome, although its occurrence is far less common than that caused by nondisjunction.

Another autosomal syndrome due to deletion is Cri-du-Chat syndrome. In this syndrome there is a deletion of part of the short arm of chromosome number 5. Affected children have characteristic physical stigmata, a variety of severe handicaps (including profound retardation), and are characterized by a high-pitched cry, likened to the mewing of a cat. Although Cri-du-Chat syndrome is the most frequent among the deletion syndromes, the estimated incidence is only between 1 in 50,000 and 1 in 100,000 live births.[68]

Sex chromosomal malformations can also occur and, in fact, are more frequent than autosomal chromosomal aberrations. In general, the physical and intellectual defects caused by sex chromosomal aberrations are less severe than those of autosomal chromosome syndromes.[4] The most frequent cause of sex chromosomal disorder is nondisjunction, as occurs in Turner's syndrome (X0 or 45X). Despite the absence of gonadal development, Turner's patients are phenotypic females. They have short stature, webbed necks, anomalies of ocular muscles, and sexual infantilism. Intelligence is usually normal, but there may be perceptual problems. Diagnosis is usually not made until puberty when amenorrhea, lack of sexual development, and short stature become evident. The incidence of 45X in newborns is approximately 1 per 8,000 female births.[24]

Two other common sex chromosomal abnormalities are XXY and XYY syndromes. The XXY disorder is known as Klinefelter's syndrome. The affected person is phenotypically male; however, because testosterone is inadequately produced, secondary sex characteristics fail to develop and the male is unable to form sperm. Klinefelter's males are normally tall and slender with breast development and small genitalia. Generally their IQs are in the normal or mildly retarded range. The XYY syndrome also affects males. These men are also tall, but have normal sexual development. XYY males frequently have lowered intelligence. This disorder also has been correlated with behavioral problems and aggressive behavior, as a relatively high incidence of XYY syndrome has been found among the prison population. Survey of consecutively born males indicates that Klinefelter's syndrome occurs in about 1 per 1000 births. Cytogenetic screenings of newborns have found the approximate incidence to be 1.1 per 1000 births.[68]

Mental retardation also can be caused by *single gene defects*. These can be autosomal recessive or dominant or sex-linked. *Autosomal recessive traits* normally involve degenerative nervous system disease caused by an enzyme deficiency. The enzyme deficit frequently causes a buildup of toxic materials resulting in mental retardation or early death. Recessive disorders only occur if two carriers mate; a carrier mating with a non-carrier will always produce normal children. Tay-Sachs disease, a lysosomal disorder, is an example of an autosomal recessive disorder caused by the absence of the enzyme hexosaminidase A, which normally catalyzes the degradation of Gm2-ganglioside. As a result, the ganglioside accumulates in the heart, liver, spleen and, most importantly, in the CNS, ANS, and retina. Affected infants appear quite normal at birth, but begin to manifest symptoms at 6 months. Then they show an abnormal sensitivity to sound (startle reaction) and progressive physical and mental deterioration, with motor incoordination, flaccidity, blindness, and increasing dementia. Eventually a vegetative state is reached, with death occurring usually between 2 and 3 years of age. Tay-Sachs disease is particularly prevalent among eastern European Jews. A screening blood test can detect Tay-Sachs carriers. Prepregnancy screening is recommended.

Finally, *X-linked disorders* involve defects in genes located on the X chromosome. Examples of X-linked disorders include muscular dystrophy, color blindness, baldness, and hemophilia. They are primarily manifested in males, but are passed on by carrier females. If a carrier female mates with an affected male, the resulting female child also can have the disorder. These disorders frequently involve biochemical abnormalities but, unlike autosomal recessive traits, usually do not involve mental retardation. Exceptions to this rule include disorders such as Lesch-Nyhan syndrome, a neuromuscular disease causing severe mental retardation and associated with self-mutilation; Menke's kinky hair syndrome, which is characterized by severe mental retardation and seizures; X-linked acquired aqueductal stenosis, which causes hydrocephalus and retardation; and Renpinning syndrome, which causes mental retardation without any other associated abnormalities.

Other prenatal causes of mental retardation include genetic mutation due to teratogens. A teratogen is any agent that can induce or increase the incidence of congenital malformations. Examples of teratogens include radiation, certain drugs, alcohol, cigarette smoke, environmental chemicals (e.g., industrial pollutants or food additives), and infectious agents.

Radiation

Radiation has long been known to cause genetic mutations. There is clear evidence that exposure to radiation increases the risk of cancer, particularly leukemia, especially before the child reaches age 10, if the mother has been exposed to radiation during pregnancy.[41] Radiation also may cause mental retardation. A high incidence of mental retardation and microcephaly has been reported in mothers exposed to massive doses of radiation from cancer treatment. In studies of survivors of Hiroshima and Nagasaki, a direct relationship was found between the distance the pregnant woman was from the focal point of the atomic bomb explosion and the resultant amount of damage her child suffered. Women who survived the explosion and were within ½ mile of it had miscarriages. Women who were about 1¼ miles had a high incidence of microcephalic children. Further away, the children were wellborn but were shown to have a high incidence of leukemia 20 years later.[4]

Since it remains uncertain how much radiation is harmful to an expectant mother, many physicians believe all elective diagnostic radiology should be confined to the preovulatory phase of the menstrual cycle, especially since many pregnancies are not detected until after the critical first month. Although the amount of harmful radiation is undetermined, there is evidence to show that immature cells are more sensitive to radiation damage. Thus, a child is most vulnerable during the first trimester of a pregnancy; however, he is still highly vulnerable through the entire embryonic period, and perhaps even into early childhood.[41]

Teratogenic Drugs

Although relatively few drugs have been positively implicated as teratogenic agents during the prenatal period, many drugs are suspected of having this potential. Most teratogenic effects are noted at birth, but occasionally problems appear only later in childhood. Such is the case with diethylstilbestrol (DES), an estrogen used primarily in the 1950s to prevent miscarriage. This drug now is correlated with an increased risk of vaginal and cervical cancer 20 years later in female offspring, as well as an increased risk of cancer in male offspring.

Drugs known to be teratogenic include thalidomide, Dilantin, anticancer drugs, sex hormones, antibiotics, alcohol, and tobacco.[4] Not all of these affect mental abilities. Thalidomide, for example, used predominantly in England in the 1950s to prevent miscarriages, resulted in shortened or absent limbs; Dilantin, an anticonvulsant, is known to cause unusual facial abnormalities, including a high incidence of cleft palate and lip.

In contrast, alkaloids, such as caffeine and nicotine, do not produce congenital malformations in human embryos, but may affect fetal growth. In heavy cigarette smokers (20 or more cigarettes a day), premature delivery is twice as frequent as in nonsmoking mothers, and birthweight is characteristically 1 pound less than that of a nonsmoker's baby. Nicotine also causes a reduction in the uterine blood flow, thereby compromising the oxygen supply to the fetus. This may cause impaired cell growth and mental deficits. In their literature review on the topic, Landesman-Dwyer and Emanual[37] report the results of three major studies that examine the long-term behavioral effects of maternal smoking. Overall, there appear to be decrements in intellectual and social performance among offspring of maternal smokers after controlling for social class, sibling order, and other intervening variables.

Alcohol is the most frequently abused drug. It breaks down in the body to form acetaldehyde, a highly toxic substance. Streissguth and colleagues, however, note that our understanding of the mechanisms by which alcohol works as a teratogen resulting in fetal alcohol syndrome (FAS) awaits further study.[65] Surprisingly, FAS has been described and studied as a major cause of mental retardation only recently.[33] FAS is associated with advanced stages of maternal alcoholism. Diagnostic criteria used by Landesman-Dwyer[36] include: (1) obvious growth retardation in height, weight, and head circumference; (2) damage to the central nervous system, as observed by marked impairment in intellectual and motor functioning; and (3) a characteristic phenotypic facial appearance. A milder form of the syndrome has been termed fetal alcohol effects. Little[38] notes that every study published on the topic shows some behavioral differences between children whose mothers were heavy drinkers and those who were light drinkers or abstainers. FAS may be a highly preventable form of mental retardation and other medical and behavioral problems. It seems reasonable to launch antialcohol policy and public information campaigns similar to those that have been effective against smoking.

Infections

A significant degree of mental retardation is produced by nonbacterial intracranial infections. Damage to the brain by viruses and other organisms may occur in either the prenatal or perinatal periods.[39] In some instances, the disease causes a failure in the development of intellectual functioning; at other times it causes loss of already acquired function. The principal causes of mental retardation due to infection include inflammation and destruction of the cortical cells of the brain. Unfortunately, while the placenta acts as a barrier to certain harmful substances, it is ineffective in preventing the passing of viruses from the mother to the fetus. Recent evidence suggests that the destructive effect on nervous tissue may be associated with fetal viral exposure before an antibody or inflammatory response can occur.[66] A group of viral infections, the TORCH infections, all cause similar malformations. Included in the group are toxoplasmosis, rubella, and infection with cytomegalovirus and herpesvirus.

The most commonly occurring and serious form of intrauterine infection is caused by cytomegalovirus (CMV). When urine is tested, CMV excretion is seen in 3% to 6% of pregnant women.[25] The nervous system of the fetus tends to be infected during the first and second trimesters. CMV causes an inflammation of brain tissue and results in meningoencephalitis. CMV infection may also affect other systems, resulting in low platelet counts, enlarged liver, and generalized skin rash. Neonatal seizures occur frequently in meningoencephalitis. In 95% of the CMV survivors, the presence of microcephaly and intracranial calcification is associated with mental retardation, deafness, seizures, and motor problems.[40]

Prior to 1969, when a vaccine was developed, rubella epidemics occurred every 8 years. Rubella is a fairly innocuous disease for adults, characterized by a rash and low-grade fever of several days' duration. If contracted during pregnancy, however, it can cause dire defects in the fetus. In the 1964 epidemic alone, 30,000 to 50,000 infants suffered handicaps, including mental retardation, heart disease, blindness, deafness, neurological defects, or death. Most affected children were born with multiple defects. The virus remains within the infant's body for up to 2 years after birth. The severity of the handicaps due to maternal rubella infection is correlated with the period of pregnancy during which the virus was contacted. If rubella infection occurs within a month *prior* to conception, there is a 42% risk of having an affected fetus; if contacted within the first trimester, 50% to 80% of infants have defects, and an additional 10% to 15% are spontaneously aborted. Later in pregnancy the incidence and severity of damage greatly lessens; infection after 26 weeks usually does not affect the infant.[4]

Toxoplasmosis is caused by a parasitic infection entering the mother's body through food (especially raw meat) or cat feces. Pregnant women should be warned therefore to cook their meat thoroughly and to try to avoid cleaning kitty litter boxes during pregnancy. Although the maternal infection is mild, the disease has devastating effects on the fetus, causing convulsions, blindness, hydrocephaly, microcephaly, feeding problems, and damage to the nervous system. Systemic manifestations are similar to those found with CMV, including skin rash, anemia, and liver damage. Mental retardation is present in 85% of children who survive prenatal toxoplasmosis.[59]

Syphilis, caused by a bacterial infection, was once a major cause of mental retardation; but with the advent of penicillin, the incidence of the disease diminished greatly. It has become an increasingly significant contributor recently, however, perhaps because of the changes in social trends and assumed increase in the number of sexual partners, which is associated with transmission of strains resistant to antibiotics.[39] In addition to mental retardation, cranial, ocular, olfactory, dental, skeletal, dermatological, and CNS abnormalities have been reported. The symptoms and manifestations of the disease vary, depending on the age of the individual. The symptoms of the child with congenital syphilis often include progressive mental degeneration, seizures, and bizarre behavior. Prenatal blood testing for syphilis is essential for early detection. Prompt treatment with antibiotics can cure the infection in the mother and prevent damage to the fetus, since little or no damage occurs before the 18th week of pregnancy.[41] Damage once done, however, is irreversible.

Maternal Nutrition

The relationship between maternal malnutrition and fetal abnormalities remains unclear. On the one hand, historical instances of mass starvation have not revealed any increased incidence of mental retardation in offspring of women who were pregnant during that time, although their offspring were small in size for gestational age. On the other hand, the fact that the fetus depends on the mother for its nutritional needs, including adequate supplies of carbohydrates, fats, proteins, vitamins, minerals, and water, can be seen by the failure of fetal development in children whose mothers lacked iodine during early pregnancy (endemic cretinism), and the mental retardation of infants born to mothers with PKU. Poor maternal nutrition also has been correlated with premature labor.

Postnatal Factors

Although postnatal organic insults resulting in mental retardation occur less frequently than prenatal insults, a number of such factors should be reviewed briefly. Postnatal infections can sometimes cause inflammation of the brain (*e.g.,* encephalitis and meningitis), leading to permanent mental and physical impairments. Lead encephalitis, once a common postnatal cause of mental retardation, is less problematic today.[20] The level of lead in the environment is believed to be increasing, however, and is seen as more toxic to children between birth and 6 years because of their high metabolic rate.[28] Even low levels of lead in children are associated with disorders in learning and behavior.[20]

Other postnatal factors that can cause mental retardation are head traumas, poisoning, brain tumors, and epilepsy. Direct injury to the head and brain, particularly because of the relative softness of the skull in early infancy, may result in retardation. There is increasing awareness of the possible connection between child abuse and neglect and head traumas. Postnatal nutrition may be another correlate of mental retardation; however, the effects of clinical malnutrition are difficult to tease out from social factors, particularly disadvantaged socioeconomic and hazardous environmental ones. Grossman[20] notes that it is best to view malnutrition and sociocultural factors as acting synergistically when suspecting these as etiologies for depressed physical and mental growth.

Diagnostic and Treatment Approaches

The physician is sometimes the first professional to suspect mental retardation in a neonate or young child, particularly in those cases with specific syndromes or significant neurological damage. The medical diagnostic workup for mental retardation is an important part of the total assessment of the child. A medical diagnostic workup for mental retardation should include a thorough history, physical examination, and assessment of psychosocial and cultural factors.

Although the bulk of this section focuses upon infants and children, it is important to consider the medical care system's involvement with mentally retarded persons throughout the life cycle. In fact, there seems to be a trend associated with improved methods of screening, prevention, and treatment that has reduced the incidence of mental retardation with a known organic etiology, but has increased prevalence of this disability as a function of improved medical technology and the resultant demographic bulge of older persons. In tandem with this trend, there is a rapidly developing literature on aging and mental retardation. Janicki and Wisniewski[32] have an excellent book on this topic, in which several chapters are devoted to the medical issues associated with aging and dementia in mental retardation.[76,77]

Taking a Developmental History

Medical information should include a history of pregnancy (including the month prenatal care began, maternal conditions such as syphilis, thyroid disease, exposure to radiation during the first trimester, prenatal rubella, maternal age, gestational age of the baby, prenatal exposure to chemicals, labor (duration and complications), and delivery (type of presentation, condition of the placenta and cord, use of instruments during delivery, prenatal convulsions or lethargy, Apgar scores, obvious abnormalities at birth, or need of neonatal resuscitation). The baby's birthweight and length, sibling order, survivorship of siblings, Rh incompatibility factors, and parent's consanguinity also should be determined. The presence of any hereditary disorders in the family, family history of retardation, speech delay, or other developmental problems should be investigated. Significant incidents in the child's life, such as accidents, infections, reactions to medications, convulsive seizures, cyanotic episodes, unusual crying spells, or behavioral disturbances, should be noted.

Developmental information should include delays in attaining motor and language milestones, for example, age of smiling, rolling over, sitting alone, walking, self-feeding, talking, and toileting. An example of the types of developmental delays associated with mental retardation appears in Table 16-1, which lists the developmental milestones timetable for normal and Down's syndrome children.

Developmental screening by pediatricians and family medicine practitioners using standardized instruments such as the Denver Developmental Screening Test may promote early identification of mental retardation. Children from birth to 2 years of age usually are first assessed by pediatricians or family physicians when obvious medical conditions or motor or sensory handicaps exist, or when significant delays of unknown etiology are suspected.

TABLE 16-1   Developmental Milestones

Milestones	Normal Child		Down's Syndrome Child	
	Average (Mo)	Range (Mo)	Average (Mo)	Range (Mo)
Smiling	1	½–3	2	1½–4
Rollover	5	2–10	8	4–22
Sit alone	7	5–9	10	6–28
Crawling	8	6–11	12	7–21
Standing	11	8–16	20	11–42
Walking	13	8–18	24	12–65
Talking, words	10	6–14	16	9–31
Talking, sentences	21	14–32	28	18–96

(Adapted from Canning CD, Pueschel SM: An overview of developmental expectations. In Pueschel SM (ed): *Down's Syndrome: Growing and Learning*. Kansas City, Andrews & McMeel, 1978)

Physicians should be especially alert to developmental delays in children with a history of high-risk factors, such as maternal illness, infections, use of teratogenic drugs or alcohol during pregnancy, prenatal exposure to environmental chemicals, familial history of retardation or developmental disorders, children with small head circumferences, and neonates with low birth weights. Kaminer and Jedrysek[34] report that a child weighing less than 1500 grams at birth has a greater than 10% chance of neurological or cognitive complications, as do babies over 2500 grams with postasphyxia seizures or meningitis. Children with neuromuscular, orthopedic, and cardiac disorders should also be considered at high risk.

It is important to realize that motor milestones usually are recalled more accurately than language ones; however, many children with mild to moderate and, even at times, severe mental retardation have normal motor milestones, unless concomitant degenerative processes are present. Similarly, many children with delayed motor milestones have IQs in the normal range. By 3 years of age, children should have speech intelligible to strangers. A lack of speech development, inattention to sound, and decreased visual alertness suggest the presence of a hearing or language disorder. A pattern of initial normal language development, but regression at 9 to 18 months of age, should alert the physician to the likelihood of either an organic or an emotional problem. A developmental language history should also include information about the educational level and literacy of both parents, ethnic background of parents, family interactional level, presence of economic or social deprivation, and educational achievement of the child, if of school age.

Physical Examination

Physical stigmata should be observed. Physicians should note the size of the child, including height and weight, cranial measurements (especially in relationship to the rest of the body), cranial malformations or irregularities suggesting craniostenosis, hydrocephaly, microcephaly, subdural effusion, size of thyroid gland, abnormal eye movements, corneal opacities and other optic abnormalities, inner epicanthial folds, low-set or malformed ears, flattened nasal bridge, protruding tongue, high arched palate, neck webbing, color and texture of skin (*e.g.*, cafe au lait spots, petechiae secondary to infection or neoplastic disease, ecchymoses secondary to trauma), single transverse palmar creases, digital abnormalities (*e.g.*, curved fifth finger, third toe longer than second toe), widely spaced nipples, undescended testicles, or hypertelorism. If one anomaly is present, others should be sought. For example, hepatosplenomegaly may be a symptom of galactosemia, and an enlarged spleen may correlate with Tay-Sachs disease. Dental aplasias are also common in mentally retarded youngsters.

Neurological examination should include testing of reflexes and cranial nerves. The physician should note any abnormalities in muscle tone, involuntary movement, impairment of fine movement, clumsiness, poor coordination, impaired two-point discrimination, or impaired rapid alternating movements. The patient's gait should be observed, with the physician looking for athetosis or chorea. The child may be asked to hop on one foot or crawl on hands and knees; in this way slight hemiparesis may be found which was not apparent on formal muscle testing. Handedness and manual dexterity should also be observed. Cerebellar integrity can be tested in young children by having the child manipulate small objects or play "pat-a-cake." The physician also should test the child's attention span and observe the child's play activity and reactions to a new environment. He should also look for signs of convulsions, hyperirritability, and hearing, speech or vision impairments. Because of the frequency of visual problems in mentally retarded persons, optic examinations always should include consideration of abnormalities in the fundus, retinal degeneration, or retroplastic disease.

Other Procedures

Prenatal tests include amniocentesis (to check for Down's syndrome, spina bifida), enzymatic tests (to test for Tay-Sachs), pH sampling of fetal blood (oxygenation and acidosis studies), fetal monitoring of vital signs. The most commonly administered neonatal test is the Apgar test, which can detect gross developmental disabilities, one of which may be mental retardation. The Apgar test checks pulse, respiration, activity (vigor and reflexes), appearance (skin color), and grimace at 1 minute and 5 minutes. Blood count, urinalysis, PKU testing (ferric chloride urine test or Guthrie blood test), and karyotype (if chromosomal abnormality is suspected) are also important neonatal tests.

Other tests may be administered: CT scans may be useful in limited conditions such as hydrocephalus, intracranial calcification secondary to toxoplasmosis, or tuberous sclerosis; x-rays of long bones of the hands and fingers can be performed to determine bone age; EEG cannot be used to distinguish normal from retarded subjects since mental retardation often involves diffuse cerebral dysfunction, but this test may be helpful in bringing to light a neuropathological condition associated with mental retardation, such as cerebral palsy, seizures, or hypsarrhythmia. Lumbar punctures may be valuable if a child is suspected of having a CNS infection, lead intoxication, or leukodystrophy.

Diagnostic Practices

The diagnosis of mental retardation is an arduous task. A minority of mentally retarded children are diagnosed at birth. More frequently, children are not brought to professional attention until they enter school. One reason for the long delay is that most mentally retarded children do not have significant abnormalities upon neurological examination. Also many neonates are normal in appearance and function at birth, but subsequently deteriorate over a period of months to years.

Although the physician may suspect mental deficiency, it may not be possible to specify its etiology. At present, over 200 identified causes and many instances of mental retardation of unknown etiology exist. Yet early identification of the etiological basis of retardation can be extremely important, because the condition in some instances can be reversed if caught early enough. Examples are hypothyroidism and some metabolic disorders; in other cases, such as phenylketonuria, although the primary cause of retardation cannot be eliminated, it can, with early treatment, be controlled through dietary means, thus preventing or minimizing intellectual deficits. Still other conditions, such as mental retardation secondary to hydrocephalus, are susceptible to surgical alleviation. Although for most mentally retarded children etiology is not that important, discovering the etiology is a part of the diagnostic process and can provide some prognostic parameters for health-care providers and families. In addition, as noted earlier in this chapter, Zigler and colleagues[79] argue that differentiation between organic and familial retardation is important for classification and epidemiological purposes.

Early etiological diagnosis is also important in preventing subsequent sibling retardation due to genetic or negligence factors. For example, if a child has been afflicted by neurofibromatosis, a hereditary disorder correlated with mental retardation, it is important to alert parents to the statistical probability of reoccurrence before a second pregnancy is planned. In disorders such as Down's syndrome or Tay-Sachs disease, particular age groups or ethnic backgrounds are known to have increased incidence rates, so potentially high-risk parents should be alerted and told of prenatal screening devices to help them decide whether or not to continue the pregnancy or to prevent future pregnancies. Lastly, early diagnostic approaches may be helpful in a variety of nonhereditary cases of mental retardation. Marshalling resources such as early intervention, counseling, and, in case of child abuse, social and legal services, may maximize developmental potential. In addition, an association between mental retardation and environmental chemicals is important public health information.

The diagnostic and assessment process in mental retardation is usually a multifaceted one, drawing on the strengths of many different disciplines. Since mental retardation may significantly affect cognitive, social, and emotional development, children subsequently may be at risk for general educational and vocational failures, behavioral problems, and limitations in coping skills. The number of areas involved makes interdisciplinary assessment an accepted practice in mental retardation. The core interdisciplinary team in a diagnostic clinic usually includes a family physician or pediatrician, educational or clinical psychologist, social worker, public health nurse, and vision, speech, and hearing consultants.

The following section provides an overview of the various disciplines and their functions in the interdisciplinary assessment process.

Role of Physician

The physician plays a strategic role in imparting medical information about mental retardation and treatment alternatives. A parent's ability to cope with the initial diagnosis of mental retardation may be largely related to the physician's attitudes and communication skills.[43] Many parents of retarded children also are strongly influenced by the physician's suggestions. For example, in one large-scale study it was found that 82% of families who had placed their retarded child in an institution had done so on the advice of a physician.[75] Physicians can initiate and coordinate referrals to other interdisciplinary members and community resources.

One problem in clarifying the physician's role in the care of mentally retarded children is that many of the needs and problems of patients and their families revolve around psychosocial crises rather than medical crises. With the shifting emphasis on deinstitutionalization and normalization, it is likely that physicians practicing without an interdisciplinary team will be called upon increasingly to offer advice and information about educational opportunities, behavioral problems, parenting skills, and available community resources, in addition to solving medical problems. Since many physicians function outside of the interdisciplinary team, a brief summary of their roles is presented.

The physician plays an important role in helping families accept the diagnosis, evaluate problems, formulate care plans, and prevent mental retardation in future pregnancies when possible. Effective interaction between the physician and family requires that the physician show consistent interest in the child and family, establish realistic goals for developmental changes in the child, provide a role model when talking to the retarded youngster, and be a source of advice to parents when needed.

Physicians should be able to direct the families to community resources and other health professionals (*e.g.*, day care services may be suggested to provide respite for the caregiver). Again, enlistment of other professionals is usually helpful. A visiting nurse or social worker may be able to suggest developmental objectives and techniques for parents to work more effectively with their children. The physician should exercise care in his use of referrals, lest the family feel tossed around from one agency to another without direction. The physician is an essential link and can act as case manager, providing aggressive follow-through after referrals to agencies, or following an interdisciplinary assessment with its attendant recommendations.

The *psychologist's* role is to assess the mental capacity and perceptual abilities of the child through the use of selective psychological tests. He also appraises behavioral and personality factors that may interfere with rehabilitation programs. In addition, the psychologist may help parents focus on ways to minimize behavioral problems, such as suggesting disciplinary techniques, stress-reduction maneuvers, or methods for averting common family disruptions.

The *social worker* obtains a complete history of the family, including structure, relationships, quality of interactions, and financial status. The worker helps parents to cope with the impact and realities of rearing a mentally retarded youngster and assesses the family's ability to comply with treatment recommendations. With older children, social workers may be involved in helping to overcome sporadic situational problems, providing therapy, or giving guidance to therapeutic groups. The social worker frequently is assigned primary responsibility for mobilizing community resources and helping to secure information about retardation for family members.

The *public health nurse* plays an important role in assessing family interactions and problems within the home. He or she also works to help the family deal with practical management issues. For example, the nurse may demonstrate proper feeding techniques for children with hypotonic neck control, or ways to help a retarded youngster learn to dress.

The *speech and hearing specialist* plays an important role in the program assessment by locating children who have been misjudged to be mentally retarded due to, or in addition to, deafness or hearing and language impairments. And since mental retardation is frequently accompanied by other physical handicaps, these specialists can identify mentally retarded youngsters who are also hearing or language impaired and assess ways to correct their problems or maximize their potential. Similarly, *vision specialists* try to identify any of the numerous visual handicaps that frequently accompany mental retardation—an especially common phenomenon when the cause of mental deficiency was anoxia at birth.

The comprehensive assessment results should incorporate information obtained from all of the above disciplines to provide an integrated picture of the child or adult. The goals of the diagnostic process should not only be to provide a diagnosis, but to develop short- and long-term care plans. The development of functional abilities should be encouraged along with the appropriate matching of services and skills. The use of the interdisciplinary approach does not diminish the physician's role; on the contrary, recent advances in the fields of genetics, enzymology, biochemistry, and obstetrics have further expanded the medical practitioner's role in interpreting medical facts and circumstances contributing to mental retardation.

Functional Assessment

Professionals in the field of mental retardation regularly use functional assessment procedures to determine who is or is not retarded, assess service needs, and monitor and evaluate the quality of the service plans. In fact, Halpern notes that management of mental retardation, probably more than any other disability, is dependent upon functional assessment procedures.[23] More specifically, he suggests that the best way to understand how functional assessment contributes to our knowledge and practice base is to examine the uses of functional assessment information.

Generally the two purposes of functional assessment are (1) diagnostic and service eligibility determination; and (2) cost and service planning, implementation monitoring, and evaluation. The two types of functional assessment procedures that usually parallel the above purposes, respectively, are: (1) IQ tests, and (2) adaptive behavior measures. That is, although most classification systems in mental retardation require both cognitive impairment and adaptive behavior deficits to be present for a diagnosis, in practice, IQs often are used by researchers and clinicians as the sole criterion for diagnosing and classifying mental retardation.[60] In contrast, even though IQ scores might provide broad program parameters, a program planner also needs to know the client's present skill level in order to design the short- and long-term goals of the service. Changes in adaptive behavior thus often become the outcome evaluation measures.

Another difference between the use of the two functional assessment procedures is that IQ tests attempt to measure learning potential, whereas adaptive behavior evaluation measures present performance. Because both types of functional assessments yield useful data for primary care practitioners, each will be reviewed. However, a greater emphasis is placed on adaptive behavior than on IQ, for the following reasons: (1) IQ testing usually is performed by psychologists and educators, often outside of the health-care system; (2) numerous good reviews of IQ testing and mental retardation exist,[55,79] whereas fewer are available on adaptive behavior; and (3) since IQ remains fairly constant, health-care planners and practitioners should find adaptive behavior more useful for assessing costs and program success.

Intelligence and IQ Testing

A number of intelligence tests have been developed which assess a person's knowledge, ability to learn, and predicted ability to cope with new situations. The most widely used tests are the Stanford–Binet and the Wechsler Intelligence Scales.

The Stanford–Binet assesses memory, information, verbal ability, and logical reasoning. At lower levels, it consists mainly of manipulative and pictorial items (testing object identification and eye–hand coordination); higher levels are increasingly verbal. At the adult level, this IQ test is highly abstract and verbal and includes vocabulary, sentence completion, and analogies. The Stanford–Binet is generally more sensitive than the Wechsler Test for very young children. It is also able to measure lower levels of intellectual functioning and is therefore important in assessing severely retarded school aged children. The Stanford–Binet has items arranged in discrete age-level test sections. The tasks are grouped in levels of difficulty corresponding to ½ year intervals between ages 2 and 5, 1 year intervals between ages 5 and 14, and 4 adult levels (average and superior adult I, II, and III).

There are three Wechsler scales currently being used—the Wechsler Preschool and Primary Scale of Intelligence (WPPSI), for ages 4 to 7 years, the Wechsler Intelligence Scale for Children-Revised (WISC-R), for ages 6.0 to 16 years and 11 months; and the Wechsler Adult Intelligence Scale-Revised (WAIS-R), for ages 16 to 70. Tasks on the Wechsler scales are grouped into subtests containing similar items, with items within each subtest arranged in order of increasing difficulty. The Wechsler intelligence tests have two domains of intelligence: *Verbal* scales, which measure long-term memory, immediate auditory memory, language comprehension, and mathematical reasoning, and *performance* scales, which test visual organization and sequencing, attention to detail, spatial relationships, eye–hand coordination, and visual memory.

Two factors that influence the predictive utility of these and other IQ tests are the age at which the child is tested and his degree of cognitive impairment. First, there is a great deal of controversy over the predictive value of psychological testing of young children, especially testing of infants up to 2 years of age. It is generally agreed that there is a positive correlation between the age of a child at the time of testing and the accuracy of the results. Tests such as the Gesell, Bayley Scale of Infant Development, and Cattell Infant Intelligence Scales have been designed to test children below the age of 2 years. However, the predictive value of these tests depends to a large extent upon the intelligence of the children tested; for infants testing in the average or near-normal range the predictive value is poor, while for children with more severe retardation there is a significantly greater correlation between infant test scores and future IQ and educational achievement. "Several studies agree that 1 child out of 4 or 5 judged definitely retarded even up to age 2 or 3 years will not be so judged later on."[50] Consistency of IQ test results tends to be greater when tested subjects are older at the time of the original tests, when the interval of time between testing is shorter, and when better standardized tests are used. Although in general lower IQs are more stable, 10 to 15 point changes during school years are frequent, and the IQs of some individuals do change dramatically over the course of several years.

An often cited reason for within-person variability of IQ tests is the associated influence which instrumental variables have on IQ tests. That is, IQ tests have been criticized on grounds of cultural and socioeconomic bias. Many test questions are based on white, Western, middle-class standards. On the average, nonwhite children score several points lower on IQ tests than their white peers. Mercer[45] and Mercer and Richardson[46], among others, have studied the disproportionately larger number of Mexican–Americans and blacks whose IQ scores have contributed to their being diagnosed as mentally retarded.

Furthermore, IQ scores may vary depending upon the child's own characteristics and his reaction to the testing situation. For example, behavior problems, distraction, family problems, preoccupation with something other than the test, uneasiness in a testing situation, or a desire to appear bright or dull are all factors that may affect test results. Institutionalized children with restricted experiences may present a further testing disadvantage. Children with vision, hearing, or speech impairments, or with motor coordination problems, may not perform to their capacity and may thus appear less intelligent than they really are.

Finally, IQ tests have been criticized because, although they can effectively predict educational achievement, they are not useful indicators of nonacademic intellectual capacity; for example, they may not indicate whether a child is capable of functioning in an adequate and responsible manner. Two children with the same IQ may have very different abilities; hence the need for adaptive behavior measures in the repertoire of functional assessment instruments. IQ tests alone are insufficient predictors of the diagnosis of mental retardation. Significant errors can be caused by problems in the construction of the tests, measurement standards, age of the testee, qualifications of the examiner, cultural and socioeconomic biases in test questions, and multisensory or physical impairments in the test takers.

Since 1959 the American Association of Mental Deficiency (AAMD) has included adaptive behavior deficits, in addition to subaverage intelligence, in their definition of mental retardation. Adaptive behavior refers to the degree to which an individual is able to meet the standards of personal independence and social responsibility expected of his age group and cultural group. Grossman states " . . . that adaptive behavior refers to what people do to take care of themselves and to relate to others in daily living rather than the abstract potential implied by intelligence."[20]

Adaptive behavior may also vary with environmental demands. For example, retardation is diagnosed more often in urban and industrialized areas where there are demands for individuals to tell time, read signs, and take public transportation.[2] Hence the behavioral expectations associated with social-role performance vary among cultures, geographic locations, and other sociocultural and environmental delimiters.

The domains used to assess adaptive behavior according to the AAMD Classification System are: (1) independent functioning; (2) physical functioning; (3) communication; (4) social functioning; (5) economic activity; (6) occupation; and (7) self-direction.

It is difficult to measure adaptive behavior. Numerous rating scales or interview techniques have been used for obtaining data but, in general, these are less reliable than standardized intelligence tests. A few of the most widely used scales are the AAMD Adaptive Behavior Scales (ABS), Minnesota Developmental Programming System, and Vineland Social Maturity Scale. The ABS enjoys wide popularity and is selected here as an example to illustrate this type of functional assessment tool.

The ABS is a functional assessment tool designed to be completed by anyone familiar with the person being assessed. Since it is based on information provided by an informant, the ratings are subject to errors because of the informant's problems of poor memory, unintentional or intentional distortion, and perception of the subject according to how he interacts with the informant, rather than the true score performance of the subject. The use of an informant methodology for data gathering on the ABS is not peculiar to this instrument and is, rather, the accepted approach. In fact, in the list of 19 scales of adaptive behavior found in Grossman,[20] only 1 scale is administered partly by testing and partly by observation, and one other as a test battery.

The ABS consists of 110 items in two parts. Part I includes domains considered to be important in independent daily living, while part II deals with inappropriate behaviors. Domains in part I include typical activities of daily living, as well as academic, vocational, and socialization domains. Part II domains run the gamut of maladaptive domains, such as violent and destructive behavior, socially aberrant behavior, self-abusive behavior, and the like. Reliability studies of the scale have shown that inter-rater reliability for part I is quite high, whereas it is only slightly better than 50% for part II.[56] After conducting reliability studies on the ABS, Isett and Spreat[30] concluded that part I had sufficient reliability, but that conclusions and research findings based on part II should be interpreted with great caution.

We have noted that adaptive behavior is a particularly useful functional assessment procedure for program planning, implementation, monitoring, and evaluation in mental retardation. The Individual Service Plan (known alternatively as Individual Educational Plan, Individual Habitation Plan, or Individual

Program Plan) enumerates the long- and short-term goals for a retarded person and delineates the services that will be required. It focuses not only on functional needs related to one's mental age, but also on consideration for the client's chronological age, including, for example, sex education courses for mentally retarded adolescents or retirement plans for elderly mentally retarded persons. The Individual Service Plan (ISP) also should be based on a developmental model, which perceives mentally retarded individuals as capable of continuing to develop new skills throughout their lifetimes.

In order for an ISP to be effective, there must be periodically updated information regarding a mentally retarded person's specific level of functioning. Change over time is observed by functional assessments and the ISP format and fits with the developmental model used in mental retardation. The quality of an ISP is measured by the amount of change. For useful change data to emerge, the discrete steps per skill being worked on should be listed, as well as the teaching method employed and who is providing the instruction. This level of detail promotes easily retrievable data for cost and program analysis.

The development of such a plan is usually an interdisciplinary effort and is formulated after the identification of functional needs by functional assessments using adaptive behavior measures and, often, behavioral assessments. The physician is expected to contribute to the functional diagnosis, as well as to clarify the relationships between the medical findings and the person's developmental status.

The use of the ISP format in conjunction with functional assessment procedures has contributed greatly to the success of the deinstitutionalization movement in mental retardation. Conceptually, community adjustment has moved beyond a focus on recidivism to an awareness of change in function associated with community placement. Moreover, since learning potential (IQ) varies among formerly institutionalized clients, it is important to focus not upon the absolute number of skills performed, but rather on the relative increase in skill performance over time. Hence, as Seltzer and Seltzer note, "A severely retarded person who increases his or her level of performance over time can be considered to be adapting more favorably than a mildly retarded person who makes no improvement. Although the mildly retarded person's absolute level of performance is higher, the extent of improvement displayed by the severely retarded person can be considered to be more adaptive."[56]

A final point about functional assessment comes from the work of Halpern,[22] who explored the relationship among improvement, handicap and disability, and functional assessment. He notes that impairment is usually measured with fixed norm comparison, disability with a conditional norm, and handicap with an evaluative norm. Both disability and handicap are subject to variability associated with environmental demands. Halpern suggests that a common error is assuming that limited intelligence is an impairment (with a fixed norm) and adaptive behavior a disability. He argues that the error emanates from grouping a mental impairment in the same class as a physical impairment. The difference, he states, is that measures of physical impairments describe characteristics of an object whereas measures of mental impairment describe the behaviors of a person. "Intelligence is not simply an attribute of a physical object; it cannot be defined or measured ostensively, that is by merely pointing to it at some location in our body."[22] He concludes that limitations in intelligence are better considered disabilities, as well as adaptive behavior. This solution would alter our functional assessment measurement of mental retardation and require consideration of both organic and environmental influences.

Family Considerations

Professionals could help parents more—and they would be more realistic— if they discarded their ideas about stages and progress. They could then begin to understand something about the devastating changes that life with a retarded son or daughter brings to parents and then they could begin to see that negative feelings—the shock, the guilt, and the bitterness—never disappear but stay on as part of the parents' emotional life.

This plea to professionals that they move beyond the stage theory approach to working with families strikes a blow to a sizeable body of professional literature.[35,48,62,78] In general, this literature suggests a flow of affective stages of assessment ranging from shock, denial, and grief to acceptance. Recently, a few investigators have begun to formulate alternative patterns of familial adjustment to having mentally retarded family members. Tymchuk,[69] for example, questions the axiomatic attitude in the literature that argues that having a mentally retarded offspring is traumatic, a position somewhat counter to that implied in the above statement. Wikler notes that adjustment is a cyclic phenomenon, punctuated by periods of crisis.[72] Her formulation is reviewed in more depth later in this section. In addition, Wikler and colleagues offer a perspective that may incorporate those of both Tymchuk and Searle.[74] They suggest that it is possible for parents to feel both chronic stress and sorrow and, at the same time, to gain emotional strength from the experience of parenting a handicapped child.

It is encouraging to see the literature on the family and mental retardation begin to reflect the complexities inherent in understanding the family system. In our society, this system is usually charged with the responsibility of providing for the economic and psychosocial growth and development of its members. Like the individual as he ages, the family moves through various age-related developments, moving from the birth of a child through older age and loss due to death. This section examines the impact of having a mentally retarded member on the family system as a whole and upon its individual members (parents, siblings, grandparents). The age of the mentally retarded family member is used as a guide to where the family system might be in relation to its life cycle. Of note is the bias in the literature toward parents and families who are most often white and middle-class. Impoverished families are generally overlooked in spite of the documented relationship between poverty and psychosocial retardation.[73]

Most babies who will eventually be diagnosed as mentally retarded are not recognized as such at birth, thus allowing their parents the opportunity to experience attachments before developmental disabilities are uncovered. However, in those instances in which a definite diagnosis is made near or at birth, it is important to examine parental reactions.

Intervention by professionals during the early stages should focus on encouraging parents to recognize the healthy and normal aspects of their baby's development during the first few months. Parents should receive information about normal infant behavior and care, and about what to expect from the retarded child. Severely retarded children may be more difficult to care for; they may have feeding and sleeping problems, cry excessively, be unresponsive, or have a hard time establishing routines. For example, children who are neurologically impaired may not be able to express their hunger urges or satisfaction with eating. Parents may need help in finding ways to gauge the effectiveness of their feeding efforts. The mother and father with an infant with uncontrolled hydrocephalus, for example, may need to learn how to limit vomiting, position the head, or administer tube feedings safely. It is equally important to discuss with parents ways to modify their schedules so that they can eat, sleep, relax, and care for other children. Parents should be informed that, for the most part, in the day-in and day-out care of the retarded baby there are more similarities than differences from the care of a non-retarded baby. Additionally, some problems, such as feeding difficulties, may not be a function of the mental retardation, but may be due to complicating factors such as low birth weight or prematurity and may eventually be outgrown.

Physicians should also be cognizant of the fact that, because of anxiety during the hospitalization and the physical and emotional fatigue caused by the shock of an abnormal birth, parents may be too distraught to remember what was told to them during the initial diagnostic period about how to handle the baby. Therefore, physicians should talk to the parents again before they leave the hospital with a newly diagnosed neonate. Parents may need to have some supportive assistance at home and should be told to call with questions once they have had some time to acclimate themselves to being at home with the child. Whenever possible, community resources should be mobilized; visiting nurses are frequently a good source of supportive care to parents of handicapped neonates. Contact with parents of other similar youngsters can be extremely helpful for both emotional support and practical advice.

The literature is replete with references to parental grieving associated with the loss of the fantasized normal infant.[16,48] Only recently have investigators begun to study the presumed consequences of these feelings on caregivers (usually mothers) and infant interactions. This study has been enhanced greatly by the introduction of attachment theory.[1,9,47] Blacher and Meyers[7] offer an excellent review of this theory as it applies to attachment formation between handicapped children and their parents. They note that in mental retardation, attachment behavior is most often studied in Down's syndrome infants. Blacher and Meyers summarize the Down's syndrome literature in this area and conclude that, . . . "Down's syndrome infants proceed through the same stages of attachment as do nonretarded infants, but at a slower pace and with less distress at separation." (p. 363). However, these authors do question the extent to which Down's syndrome children reach the highest level of attachment (phase 4) in which egocentrism gives way to reciprocity in primary relationships. The child is able to appreciate the caregiver's rights and ability to act for himself.

The introduction of attachment theory into observations of early infant–parent interactions may help professionals study the behavioral quality of the relationships. An understanding of these attachment patterns, together with parental reports of their affective status, may help reduce caregiver burnout, enhance family accord, and target early those families in need of additional services to prevent family dysfunction and placement of children out of the natural family home.

Since in the majority of cases mental retardation is not diagnosed at birth, by the time the parents reach a diagnostic clinic, they are usually aware that something is wrong with their child; however, they frequently focus on specific aspects of developmental problems. For example, they may suspect deafness as a cause for their child's language delay, or shyness as a cause of slow socialization skills. Behavioral problems, clumsiness, and immaturity are frequent complaints. Parents who focus on these isolated problems in their child's development are often shocked and griefstricken when a diagnosis of mental retardation is made.

Wikler suggests that among families of mentally retarded members crises similar to that which occurs at the time of diagnosis reoccur as a consequence of: (1) Discrepancies between expected and actual development; and (2) special events that happen when parenting a mentally retarded child. The latter range from the experience of the initial diagnosis through serious discussions about guardian help and care of the mentally retarded family member as parents and others in the system become elderly. The former class of experiences range from delays in the child's development of mental skills through to the twenty-first birthday when, symbolically, independence is achieved. Wikler asserts that by appreciating, anticipating, and perhaps predicting when family systems are most likely to experience vulnerability, the professional may help to lessen the deleterious impact of these events on the family.[72]

The entrance of the mentally handicapped child into the family has an obvious effect on siblings as well as parents. Initially parents may express their grief and disappointment by withdrawing from the parent role or becoming preoccupied with their grief. Siblings may be upset by the unexpected parental preoccupation with the newborn infant or with their continued sadness, irritability, or anger. They may especially resent the retarded child for taking up too much of their parents' time. This is especially true of the older sibling, who was previously the focus of attention. Now he or she may be called upon to do extra chores around the house while the parents attend to the baby or to actually help care for the retarded child. Older female siblings are especially at risk for being burdened with responsibilities for care of the handicapped youngster. Brothers and sisters may find it hard to comprehend the differences between the disciplinary methods and standards of behavior expected by the parents for themselves and their handicapped sibling, increasing sibling rivalry. They may also feel emotionally neglected, even by well-meaning parents, who are overwhelmed or overburdened with caring for the handicapped child. Family relationships and roles may be disturbed as young children are forced to take on adult responsibilities, or as the normal siblings develop skills and outgrow their older mentally retarded brother's or sister's achievements. Trevino delineates the following as the high-risk sibling combinations: (1) There are only two siblings, a normal and a handicapped child; (2) the normal sibling is close in age to, or younger than, the handicapped sibling, or is the oldest female child; (3) the normal child and the handicapped child are the same sex; or (4) the parents are unable to accept the handicap.[67]

As normal siblings reach adolescence, other problems may arise. They may become embarrassed about their retarded sibling when they bring their friends over. The normal siblings need to deal with their peers' reactions to the retarded youngster at an age when they are usually vulnerable themselves. Some children may refrain from bringing other children home because of their shame; others feel the need to warn their peers before they enter the house. Social contacts may become disturbed or curtailed. Normal siblings also may have pressures to be the achiever in the family and make up for the disappointments and frustrations caused by the retarded child. Sometimes normal siblings express guilt that they are not the affected child; other times they are glad that it is the sibling and not themselves who has the problem. Frequently, they worry about what will happen to their sibling when he grows up, especially if the parents have made the normal sibling promise to care for the retarded child in the event of a parent's death. Eventually, as sexuality awareness increases, they may begin to doubt their own capacity to bear normal children.

During annual checkup visits, physicians can query siblings about their attitudes toward their retarded brother or sister, responsibilities at home, and relationships with their parents. With older children the cause, if known, of the sibling's retardation should be explained, and the child should be given accurate and up-to-date information by the physician to help alleviate anxieties because of misinformation, fantasies, and fears. Uninformed children seem to be anxious. For example, sometimes they believe that mental retardation is catching, or they feel angry toward their mother, believing that it is her fault that the child she bore was retarded. As siblings reach puberty, their fears and questions regarding their own chances of producing a retarded youngster should be discussed at length. Throughout the years physicians should be available to discuss family issues or make appropriate referrals when family tensions are suspected or reported. Disturbances in siblings of retarded children may coincide with problems parents are experiencing, and the family system may need treatment. Berns points out that grandparents are also often part of the family system. Their planned involvement may aid the system; their ambivalence or resentment can foster a dysfunctional strife.[5]

Seltzer[57] notes that no research has studied the changing states of sibling relationships throughout the full life cycle in families with a retarded family member. She points out the growing need to explore the extent to which aging siblings continue their supportive relationship with their also-aging mentally retarded sibling.

In fact, issues related to the aging end of the family life cycle have recently come under closer study. Certainly a proportion of mentally retarded persons, usually those with nonorganic etiologies, have always lived into and past the sixth decade; however, the number of mentally retarded persons surviving to old age has increased substantially in recent years and is projected to continue to grow in the future. In old age, families tend to make the difference between staying in the community or entering an institution, all other variables being somewhat equal. Since the majority of retarded persons at any age do not live in public or private residential settings, we can infer that the number of aging mentally retarded persons who live with family members is considerable, although many of these persons are not currently in contact with the formal service systems. A related trend is that as family members age along with their retarded members, and parents die or become unable to care for their children, the formal service system is likely to become more involved.

The implication of these trends seems clear. There is a crucial need to develop a technology to support the natural advocates of elderly mentally retarded persons—the parents and other members of the informal support system—to become more competent, secure, and affectively connected to their aging mentally retarded members.

It is important for physicians to know that, when given a choice between information and counseling, family members usually choose information. Similarly, when given the choice between counseling and skill handling (parent training), the latter option tends to be chosen.[69,73] A sizeable body of knowledge has developed concerning the benefits of using behavioral parent training,[3,27,49] an intervention which has begun to be applied with families at different socioeconomic levels, over a wide range of etiological and presenting skill and behavioral problems, and at different developmental periods.[69]

In conclusion, families tend to be the natural advocates, trainers, and sources of support for persons with mental retardation. A common assumption related to the strain this role imposes is that the incidence of psychopathology, substance abuse, physical illness, and divorce must be higher among family members caring for a mentally retarded child. Wikler and colleagues[74] suggest otherwise. In their review of the literature, when social class is held constant, "the only repeatedly observed deleterious effects were . . . (1) increased risk of social isolation for the family; (2) increased stress experienced by the primary caregiver, usually the mother, and (3) an increased tendency for adolescent siblings who share the burden of care to develop problems." It seems then that, although having a mentally retarded family member dramatically changes a family system, the members of that system appear to cope over time with recurring crises and to maintain an adaptive level of functioning, perhaps growing emotionally in the process.

Summary

Mental retardation is a disorder that is particularly suited to the practice of functional assessment and primary care. There are opportunities for practitioners to intervene in each of the domains of impairment, disability and handicap. Given that 25% of persons with mental retardation have some organic etiology for their condition, traditional impairment status examinations are often warranted. Also on the impairment status level, practitioners committed to preventive interventions may be vigilant in managing such problems as fetal alcohol syndrome or PKU. On the disability level, practitioners challenged by interdisciplinary problem-solving may contribute their expertise of medicine and the behavioral correlates of health problems to the team's writing of an individualized service plan. For practitioners who are resolved to further the social, psychological, and health plight of citizens with disabilities, the field of mental retardation with its strong emphasis on community living, normalization, and developmental perspectives invites health-care practitioners to help retarded citizens gain or maintain access to a broad array of generic and specialized services.

In this chapter, the definition and diagnostic criteria used in classification of mental retardation are reviewed. Mental retardation is generally diagnosed before the age of 18, presenting with IQ scores of 70 or below and deficits in adaptive behavior. In three quarters of cases, there is no known organic etiology related to the disorder; we do, however, know of some 200 causes, most of which (90%) occur prenatally and present at birth or early in infancy.

Obtaining a developmental history and thorough physical and neurological examinations are important elements in the diagnosing and monitoring of the health care of persons with mental retardation. Often this occurs in the context of an interdisciplinary team. Other team members usually involved are social workers, psychologists, nurses, and speech and hearing specialists. The information gleaned from the above process is often used in tandem with functional assessment measures. Generally, functional assessments are conducted for diagnostic and eligibility purposes and to plan, monitor, implement, and evaluate service plans. Service plans typically require adaptive behavior information, whereas diagnostic and eligibility procedures may require both IQ and adaptive behavior scores.

The family plays a critical support and service role in mental retardation. The physician should be aware that living with a mentally retarded family member involves stresses throughout the life cycle. Nevertheless, family members learn to cope with and gain from the experience of living with and caring for a mentally retarded person. As the family system ages, all members are more likely to need health care for their physical and functional needs. The primary care physician is in the best position to be responsive to these needs, particularly if he is committed to coordinating services with other health care professionals.

References

1. Ainsworth MDS: The development of infant–mother attachment. In Caldwell BM, Ricutti HN (eds): Review of Child Development Research, Vol. 3. Chicago, University of Chicago Press, 1973
2. Albizu–Miranda C, Matlin N, Stanton H: The successful retardate. Hato Rey, PR: DUR Commonwealth of Puerto Rico, Mimeo, 1966
3. Baker B, Heifetz L, Murphy D: Behavioral training for parents of mentally retarded children: One-year followup. Am J Ment Defic 85:31–38, 1980
4. Batshaw ML, Perret UM: Children With Handicaps, p 43. Baltimore, Paul H Brookes, 1981
5. Berns JH: Grandparents of handicapped children. Soc Work, 25:238–239, 1980
6. Bicknell DJ: Living with a mentally handicapped member of the family. Postgrad Med 58(864):587, 1982
7. Blacher J, Meyers CE: A Review of attachment formation and disorders of handicapped children. Am J Ment Defic 87:359–371, 1983
8. Blackwell MW: Care of the Mentally Retarded. Boston, Little, Brown & Co., 1979
9. Bowlby J: Sadness and Depression: Attachment and Loss, Vol. 3. New York, Basic Books, 1980
10. Canning CD, Pueschell SM: An overview of developmental expectations. In Pueschel SM (ed): Down's Syndrome: Growing and Learning. Kansas City, Andrews & McMeel, 1978
11. Cohen P: Medical treatment of the mentally retarded. In Philips I (ed): Prevention and Treatment of Mental Retardation. New York, Basic Books, 1966
12. Crocker AC: Current strategies in prevention of mental retardation. Pediatr Annals 11(5):450, 1982
13. Diagnostic and Statistical Manual of Mental Disorders, 3rd ed: Washington, American Psychiatric Association, 1980

14. Dickerson MY, Social Work Practice with the Mentally Retarded. New York, Free Press, 1981
15. Eaton LF, Manolascino FJ: Psychiatric disorders in the mentally retarded: Types, problems and challenges. Am J Psychiatry 139(10):1297, 1982
16. Emde R, Brown C: Adaptation to the birth of a Down's syndrome infant: grieving and maternal attachment. American Academy of Child Psychiatry 17:299–323, 1978
17. French JH, Graziani LJ, Scheinberg LC: Treatment of metabolic and endocrine causes of mental retardation. In Poser C (ed): Mental Retardation: Diagnosis and Treatment. Harper & Row, New York, 1969
18. Garrard SD: Community Health Issues. In Matson JC, Mulick JA (eds): Handbook of Mental Retardation. Elmsford, NY Perganon Press, 1983
19. Gearheart BR, Litton FW: The Trainable Retard: A Foundation's Approach, 2nd ed. St. Louis, CV Mosby, 1979
20. Grossman H (ed): Classification in Mental Retardation, pp 11, 42, 149. Washington, DC, American Association on Mental Deficiency, 1983
21. Grossman H (ed): Manual of Terminology and Classification in Mental Retardation. American Association on Mental Deficiency, Washington, DC, 1977
22. Halpern AS: Functional assessment and mental retardation. In Halpern AS, Fuhrer MJ: Functional Assessment in Rehabilitation, Baltimore, Paul H. Brookes, 1984
23. Halpern AS: Mental retardation. In Stolov WC, Clowers MR (eds): Handbook of Severe Disability. Washington, US Dept. of Education, Rehab Services Administration, 1981
24. Hammerton JL, Canning N, Ray M, Smith S: Acytogenetic survey of 14,069 newborn infants. I, Incidence of chromosomal abnormalities. Clin Genet 8:223–243, 1975
25. Hanshaw JB, Dudgeon JA: Viral Disease of the Fetus and Newborn. Philadelphia, WB Saunders, 1973
26. Hart W: Psychiatric management of the mentally retarded child. In Poser C (ed): Mental Retardation: Diagnosis and Treatment. New York, Harper & Row, 1969
27. Heifetz L: Behavioral training for parents of retarded children: Alternative formats based on instructional manuals. Am J Ment Defic 82:194–203, 1977
28. Huber AM: Nutrition and mental retardation. In Matson JL, Mulick JA (eds): Handbook of Mental Retardation. Elmsford, NY, Pergamon Press, 1983
29. International Classification of Diseases, 9th rev: Clinical Modification. Ann Arbor, MI, Commission on Professional and Hospital Activities, 1978
30. Isett RD, Spreat SD: Test–retest and interrater reliability of the AAMD adaptive behavior scale. Am J Ment Defic 84:93–95 1979
31. Jakab I: Diagnosis and differential diagnosis of mental retardation. In Jakab I (ed): Mental Retardation. S. Karger, Basel, Switzerland, 1982
32. Janicki MP, Wisniewski HM: Aging and Developmental Disabilities. Baltimore, Paul H Brookes, 1985
33. Jones KL, Smith DW: Recognition of the fetal alcohol syndrome in early infancy. Lancet 2:999–1001, 1973
34. Kaminer R, Jedrysek E: Early identification of developmental disabilities. Pediatr Ann 11(5):427, 1982
35. Kennedy JF: Maternal reactions to the birth of a defective baby. Soc Casework 51:411, 1970
36. Landesman-Dwyer S: Maternal drinking and pregnancy outcome. Appl Res Ment Retard 3:241–263, 1982
37. Landesman-Dwyer S, Emanueal I: Smoking during pregnancy. Teratology 1:119–126, 1979

38. Little RE: Epidemiological and experimental studies in drinking and pregnancy: The state of the art. Neurobehav Toxicol Teratol 3:163–167, 1981
39. Lott IT: Perinatal factors in mental retardation. In Matson JL, Mulick JA: Handbook of Mental Retardation. Elmsford, NY, Pergamon Press, 1983
40. MacDonald H, Tobin J O'H: Congenital cytomegalovirus infection: A collaborative study on epidemiological, clinical, and laboratory findings. Dev Med Child Neurol 20:411–482, 1978
41. MacMillan DL: Mental Retardation in School and Society. Boston, Little, Brown & Co, 1977
42. Magrab PR: A primer for interpreting psychological test results. Pediatr Ann 11(5): 470, 1982
43. McDonald AC, Carlson KL, Palmer DJ, Slay T: Physician's diagnostic information to parents of handicapped neonates. In Ment Retard 20(1):12, 1982
44. Menolascino FJ: Challenges in Mental Retardation: Progressive Ideology and Services. New York, Human Sciences Press, 1977
45. Mercer JR: Labelling the Mentally Retarded: Clinical and Social System Perspectives on Mental Retardation. Berkeley, University of California, 1973
46. Mercer J, Richardson J: Mental Retardation As A Social Problem. In Hobbs N (ed), Issues on the Classification of Children. San Francisco, Jossey–Bass, 1975
47. Parkes CM, Stevenson–Hinde J: The Place of Attachment in Human Behavior. New York, Basic Books, 1982
48. Parks RM: Parental reactions to the birth of a handicapped child. Health Soc Work 2:51–66, 1977
49. Proctor EK: New directions for work with parents of retarded children. Soc Casework 57:259–264, 1976
50. Robinson NM, Robinson HB: The Mentally Retarded Child, 2nd ed. New York, McGraw–Hill, 1976
51. Roeher GA: Attitudes towards mental retardation: Implications for medical practice. Can Fam Phys 25:1337, 1979
52. Rubin AL, Rubin RL: The effects of physician counseling techniques on parent reactions to mental retardation diagnosis. Child Psychiatry Hum Dev 10(4):213, 1980
53. Schild S: The family of the retarded child. In Koch R, Dobson JC (eds): The Mentally Retarded Child and His Family: A Multidisciplinary Handbook. New York, Brunner/ Mazel, 1976
54. Schwartz CG: Strategies and tactics of mothers of mentally retarded children for dealing with the medical care system. In Berstein NR (ed): Diminished People: Problems and Care of the Mentally Retarded. Boston, Little, Brown & Co, 1970
55. Seltzer GB: Systems of classification. In Matson JL, Mulick JA: Handbook of Mental Retardation. Elmsford, NY, Pergamon Press, 1983
56. Seltzer GB, Seltzer MM: Functional assessment of persons with mental retardation. In Granger CV, Gresham GE (eds): Functional Assessment in Rehabilitative Medicine. Baltimore, William & Wilkin 1984
57. Seltzer MM: Informal supports for elderly mentally retarded persons. Am J Ment Defic 90, 3:259–265, 1985
58. Seltzer MM, Seltzer GB: Classification and social status. In Natson JL, Mulick JL (eds): Handbook of Mental Retardation. Elmsford, NY, Pergamon Press, 1983
59. Sever JL: Infectious agents and fetal disease. In Weisman HA, Kerr GR (eds): Fetal Growth and Development. New York, McGraw–Hill, 1970
60. Smith JD, Polloway EA: The dimension of adaptive behavior in mental retardation research: An analysis of recent practices. Am J Ment Defic 84:203–206, 1979

61. Sobol HL: My Brother Steven is Retarded. New York, MacMillan, 1977
62. Solnit A, Stark M: Mourning and the Birth of a Defective Child. Psychoanalytic Studies of the Child 16:523–536, 1961
63. Steele MW: Genetics of mental retardation. In Jakab I (ed): Mental Retardation. S. Karger, Basel, Switzerland, 1982
64. Stern A: Diagnosis, testing and assessment. In Gearheart BR, Litton FW: The Trainable Retarded: A Foundation's Approach, 2nd ed. St Louis, CV Mosby, 1979
65. Streissguth AP, Landesman–Dwyer S, Martin JC, Smith D: Teratogenic effects of alcohol in humans and laboratory animals. Science 209:353–361, 1980
66. Thompson JA, Glassow LA: Intrauterine viral infection and the cell mediated immune response. Neurology 30:212–215, 1980
67. Trevino F: Siblings of handicapped children: Identify those at risk. Soc Casework 60:1488–493, 1979
68. Trunca C: The chromosome syndromes. In Wortis J (ed): Mental Retardation and Developmental Disabilities: An Annual Review XI. New York, Brunner/Mazel, 1980
69. Tymchuk A: Interviews with parents of the mentally retarded. In Matson JL, Mulick JA (eds): Handbook of Mental Retardation. Elmsford, NY, Pergamon Press, 1983
70. US Dept. of Health, Education and Welfare: The Mentally Retarded Child at Home: A Manual for Parents. Office of Child Development, Pub No. 374–1959, 1971
71. Walker PW: Recognizing the mental health needs of developmentally disabled people. Soc Work 25:293–297, 1980
72. Wikler L: Chronic stress of families of mentally retarded children. Fam Relations 30:281–288, 1981
73. Wikler L, Keenan MP (eds): Developmental Disabilities: No Longer a Private Tragedy. Washington, NASW, 1983
74. Wikler L, Wasow M, Hatfield E: Seeking strengths in families of developmentally disabled children. Soc Work 28:313–315, 1983
75. Willer B, Goldberg B, Intagliata J, Kraus S: Current concepts in mental retardation. Fam Phys, 22(4):130, 1980
76. Wisniewski HM, Merz GS: Aging, Alzheimer's disease and developmental disabilities. In Janicki MP, Wisniewski HM (eds): Aging and Developmental Disabilities. Baltimore, Paul H Brookes, 1985
77. Wisniewski K, Hill AL: Clinical aspects of dementia in mental retardation and developmental disabilities. In Janicki MP, Wisniewski HM (eds): Aging and Developmental Disabilities. Baltimore, Paul H Brookes, 1985
78. Wolfensberger W: Counseling the parents of the retarded. In Baumeister AA (ed): Mental Retardation: Appraisal, Education and Rehabilitation. Chicago, Aldine, 1967
79. Zigler E, Balla D, Hodupp R: On the definition and classification of mental retardation. Am J Ment Defic 89:215–230, 1984

Index

Entries followed by "t" denote tables; entries followed by "f" denote figures.

DATE DUE

MAR 2 3 1994			
MAR 1 0 1994			

DEMCO 38-297